Training for Speed, Agility, and Quickness

Third Edition

Lee E. Brown
Vance A. Ferrigno

Editors

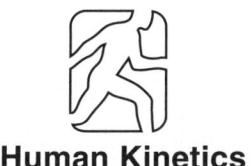

Human Kinetics

Library of Congress Cataloging-in-Publication Data

Training for speed, agility, and quickness / Lee E. Brown and Vance A. Ferrigno, editors. -- Third Edition.
  pages cm
  Includes bibliographical references.
  1. Physical education and training. 2. Speed. 3. Motor ability. 4. Coaching (Athletics) I. Brown, Lee E., 1956- II. Ferrigno, Vance, 1961-
  GV711.5.T72 2014
  613.7'11--dc23

2014013604

ISBN (print): 978-1-4504-6870-1

Copyright © 2015, 2005 by Lee E. Brown and Vance A. Ferrigno
Copyright © 2000 by Lee E. Brown, Vance A. Ferrigno, and Juan Carlos Santana

All rights reserved. Except for use in a review, the reproduction or utilization of this work in any form or by any electronic, mechanical, or other means, now known or hereafter invented, including xerography, photocopying, and recording, and in any information storage and retrieval system, is forbidden without the written permission of the publisher.

This publication is written and published to provide accurate and authoritative information relevant to the subject matter presented. It is published and sold with the understanding that the author and publisher are not engaged in rendering legal, medical, or other professional services by reason of their authorship or publication of this work. If medical or other expert assistance is required, the services of a competent professional person should be sought.

Notice: Permission to reproduce the following material is granted to instructors and agencies who have purchased *Training for Speed, Agility, and Quickness, Third Edition*: pp. 16 and 24. The reproduction of other parts of this book is expressly forbidden by the above copyright notice. Persons or agencies who have not purchased *Training for Speed, Agility, and Quickness, Third Edition* may not reproduce any material.

Acquisitions Editor: Justin Klug; **Developmental Editor:** Laura Pulliam; **Associate Managing Editor:** Anne E. Mrozek; **Copyeditor:** Patricia MacDonald; **Permissions Manager:** Martha Gullo; **Cover Designer:** Keith Blomberg; **Photograph (cover):** AP Photo/Michael Conroy; **Photographs (interior):** Doug Fink; **Visual Production Assistant:** Joyce Brumfield; **Photo Production Manager:** Jason Allen; **Art Manager:** Kelly Hendren; **Associate Art Manager:** Alan L. Wilborn; **Illustrations:** © Human Kinetics, unless otherwise noted; **Printer:** Sheridan Books

We thank California State University, Fullerton, for assistance in providing the location for the photo shoot for this book.

Human Kinetics books are available at special discounts for bulk purchase. Special editions or book excerpts can also be created to specification. For details, contact the Special Sales Manager at Human Kinetics.

Printed in the United States of America   10 9 8 7 6 5 4 3 2 1

The paper in this book is certified under a sustainable forestry program.

Human Kinetics
Website: www.HumanKinetics.com

United States: Human Kinetics
P.O. Box 5076, Champaign, IL 61825-5076
800-747-4457
e-mail: humank@hkusa.com

Canada: Human Kinetics
475 Devonshire Road Unit 100, Windsor, ON N8Y 2L5
800-465-7301 (in Canada only)
e-mail: info@hkcanada.com

Europe: Human Kinetics
107 Bradford Road, Stanningley
Leeds LS28 6AT, United Kingdom
+44 (0) 113 255 5665
e-mail: hk@hkeurope.com

Australia: Human Kinetics
57A Price Avenue, Lower Mitcham, South Australia 5062
08 8372 0999
e-mail: info@hkaustralia.com

New Zealand: Human Kinetics
P.O. Box 80, Torrens Park, South Australia 5062
0800 222 062
e-mail: info@hknewzealand.com

E6142

To Theresa. I owe you everything.

—Lee

For the love of a Savior who died to save me.

To Ann Marie, who loves and believes in me.

To Anthony and John: I couldn't be prouder to be your dad.

—Vance

Contents

Drill Finder.. vi
Accessing the Online Video xiii
Preface xv
Acknowledgments.. xvii

PART I   TRAINING ESSENTIALS

1   How the Training Works 2

2   Athlete Assessment 9

3   Incorporating Mental Skills Training 14

4   Speed Training 26

5   Agility Training 83

6   Quickness and Reaction-Time Training 175

PART II TRAINING PROGRAMS

7 Developing a Customized Program 254

8 Baseball and Softball 258

9 Football and Rugby 261

10 Basketball and Netball 265

11 Combat Sports 269

12 Track and Field 273

13 Soccer. 276

14 Lacrosse 279

15 Tennis and Badminton 282

16 Racquetball and Squash. 285

References. 287
About the Editors 291
About the Contributors 292

Drill Finder

Drill name	Drill #	Page #	Drill emphasis	Drill level*	VOD included?
CHAPTER 4 SPEED TRAINING					
Abbreviated B March	45	74	Maximal velocity	B	●
Abbreviated B Skip	46	75	Maximal velocity	I	●
Acceleration Heel Kicks	10	44	Acceleration	I	
Alternating Fast Leg	50	77	Maximal velocity	I	●
Ankling	11	45	Acceleration	I	
A Skip	16	50	Acceleration	I	●
Basic 40-Yard Model	18	51	Acceleration	I	
Bounding	22	53	Acceleration	B	●
Bound Into Acceleration	26	57	Acceleration	A	●
Broad Jump Into Acceleration	27	58	Acceleration	A	●
Bullet Belt	37	67	Partner-assisted acceleration drills	I	
Continuous Fast Leg	51	78	Maximal velocity	A	●
Continuous Wall Drill	4	39	Acceleration	B	●
Contrast Parachute Running	59	82	Maximal velocity	A	
Downhill Speed Runs	56	80	Maximal velocity	A	
Downhill to Flat Contrast Speed Runs	57	81	Maximal velocity	A	
Drive Wall Drill	2	38	Acceleration	B	●
Face and Chase	35	65	Partner-assisted acceleration drills	I	
Falling Starts	41	71	Start drills	B	
Forward A March	8	42	Acceleration	B	
Galloping	47	75	Maximal velocity	B	●
Gears	20	52	Acceleration	I	
Harness Pull	36	66	Partner-assisted acceleration drills	I	●
Heavy Sled Pull	30	61	Acceleration	A	
Hurdle Fast Legs	53	79	Maximal velocity	A	
Ins and Outs	19	52	Acceleration	I	
Light Sled Pull	29	60	Acceleration	I	
Medicine Ball Scoop Toss	44	73	Start drills	I	●
Medicine Ball Shovel Toss	43	72	Start drills	I	●

*Drill Level: B = beginner, I = intermediate, A = advanced

Drill name	Drill #	Page #	Drill emphasis	Drill level*	VOD included?
CHAPTER 4 SPEED TRAINING *(continued)*					
Mountain Climber Into Acceleration	28	59	Acceleration	A	▶
On-Command Wall Drill	5	39	Acceleration	I	▶
One, Two, Three, Five Step Wall Drill	3	38	Acceleration	B	▶
Parachute Running	58	81	Maximal velocity	A	
Partner-Assisted Tubing Acceleration	38	68	Partner-assisted acceleration drills	A	▶
Paw Drill (Cycling)	48	76	Maximal velocity	I	▶
Prancing	12	46	Acceleration	I	▶
Punch Wall Drill	1	37	Acceleration	B	▶
Quick Feet and High Knees	9	43	Acceleration	B	
Quick Feet Into Acceleration	24	55	Acceleration	I	▶
Resist from Behind	34	64	Partner-assisted acceleration drills	B	▶
Resist from Front	33	63	Partner-assisted acceleration drills	B	▶
Run-Through	52	78	Maximal velocity	I	
Sand Running	60	82	Maximal velocity	A	
Seated Arm Swings	6	40	Acceleration	B	
Single-Leg Fast Leg	49	77	Maximal velocity	I	▶
Single-Leg A Skip	17	51	Acceleration	A	▶
Single-Leg Bounds	23	54	Acceleration	A	▶
Skip for Max Height and Distance	13	47	Acceleration	I	▶
Split-Squat Jumps	54	79	Maximal velocity	I	
Stadium Stairs	32	62	Acceleration	A	
Standing Arm Swings	7	41	Acceleration	B	
Start From Parallel Two-Point Stance	40	70	Start drills	B	
Start From Staggered Two-Point Stance	39	69	Start drills	B	
Straight-Leg Bound Into Acceleration	25	56	Acceleration	A	▶
Straight-Leg Bounds	15	49	Acceleration	A	▶
Straight-Leg Shuffle	14	48	Acceleration	I	▶
10-Yard Burst	21	53	Acceleration	B	
30-Yard Flying Start	42	71	Start drills	B	
Uphill Acceleration Runs	31	62	Acceleration	A	
Uphill to Flat Contrast Speed Runs	55	80	Maximal velocity	A	
CHAPTER 5 AGILITY TRAINING					
Ali Shuffle	82	104	Line drills	B	
A Movement	116	129	Cone drills	A	
Backpedal–High Knees–Sprint	167	168	Backpedal drills	I	

Drill name	Drill #	Page #	Drill emphasis	Drill level*	VOD included?
CHAPTER 5 AGILITY TRAINING *(continued)*					
Backpedal–Shuffle–Sprint	109	123	Cone drills	I	
Backpedal–Sprint on Line	165	166	Backpedal drills	I	
Backpedal Weave	168	168	Backpedal drills	I	
Backward Cross-Step Bound	146	154	Agility ladder drills	A	▶
Backward Icky Shuffle	138	148	Agility ladder drills	A	▶
Backward Ladder Zigzag	140	150	Agility ladder drills	A	▶
Backward Roll Over Shoulder	172	172	Total-body agility	I	
Backward Run	164	166	Backpedal drills	B	
Backward Shuffle Bound	143	151	Agility ladder drills	A	▶
Backward Slalom Jump	136	147	Agility ladder drills	A	▶
Backward Twist Jump	137	147	Agility ladder drills	A	▶
Backward Zigzag	97	116	Cone drills	I	
Backward Zigzag Same In	142	151	Agility ladder drills	I	
Bag Jumps With 180-Degree Turn	163	165	Bag drills	I	▶
Bag Side Step	157	161	Bag drills	I	
Bag Side Step, Forward, and Back Combo	162	164	Bag drills	I	▶
Bag Side Step, High Knee Combo	158	161	Bag drills	I	
Bag Side Step With Double Step	159	162	Bag drills	I	▶
Bag Side Step With Sprint	161	164	Bag drills	I	
Bag Side Step With Two-Hand Touch	160	163	Bag drills	I	▶
Bag Weave	151	158	Bag drills	I	
Bag Zigzag	153	159	Bag drills	I	▶
Carioca	128	140	Agility ladder drills	B	
Change of Direction	150	157	Bag drills	I	
Combo Zigzag	98	116	Cone drills	I	
Comeback	76	100	Line drills	I	
Cone Spin	93	113	Cone drills	I	
Cone Zigzag	96	115	Cone drills	I	
Crossover Run	78	101	Line drills	B	
Crossover Skipping	77	100	Line drills	B	
Crossover Shuffle	147	154	Agility ladder drills	I	
Diamond Shuffle	108	123	Cone drills	I	
Double In–Out Shuffle	133	145	Agility ladder drills	I	
Double-Side Forward Jump	79	101	Line drills	B	
Double Step	127	139	Agility ladder drills	B	
E Movement	117	130	Cone drills	A	
Every Hole	126	138	Agility ladder drills	B	
F Movement	118	131	Cone drills	A	

Drill name	Drill #	Page #	Drill emphasis	Drill level*	VOD included?
CHAPTER 5 AGILITY TRAINING *(continued)*					
15-Yard Turn Drill	85	107	Cone drills	I	
15-Yard Z Drill	111	124	Cone drills	I	
55-Yard Line Sprint to Backpedal	69	94	Line drills	I	
Figure-Eight Cone Drill	122	134	Cone drills	I	
45-Degree Backpedal With Turn	73	97	Line drills	I	
40-Yard Line Backpedal to Sprint	67	93	Line drills	I	
40-Yard Line Backpedal Turn 180 Degrees and Sprint	68	93	Line drills	I	
40-Yard Line Shuffle	66	92	Line drills	I	
40-Yard Line Sprint	63	90	Line drills	B	
40-Yard Square Carioca	89	111	Cone drills	A	
40-Yard Square Multiskill	112	125	Cone drills	A	
40-Yard Square Shuffle	90	111	Cone drills	A	
Forward Cross-Step Bound	145	153	Agility ladder drills	A	▶
Forward Ladder Zigzag	139	149	Agility ladder drills	I	▶
Forward Roll-Backward Roll Combination	173	173	Total-body agility	I	
Forward Roll Over Shoulder	171	171	Total-body agility	I	
Forward Run With Lateral Shuffle	110	124	Cone drills	I	
Forward Shuffle Bound	144	152	Agility ladder drills	A	▶
Forward Zigzag Same In	141	150	Agility ladder drills	I	
H Movement	119	132	Cone drills	A	
Icky Shuffle	123	135	Agility ladder drills	I	
In–Out Shuffle	124	136	Agility ladder drills	I	
Ladder Quick Run With Sprint	149	156	Agility ladder drills	I	
Ladder Side Step	129	141	Agility ladder drills	B	
Ladder Side Step With Double Step	130	142	Agility ladder drills	B	
Lateral Shuffle	81	103	Line drills	B	
Lateral Weave	152	158	Bag drills	I	
M-Shuffle Drill	106	121	Cone drills	I	
Multidirectional Skipping	121	133	Cone drills	I	
90-Degree Backpedal With Turn	72	97	Line drills	I	
180-Degree Ladder Turn	125	137	Agility ladder drills	I	
180-Degree Line Turn	84	106	Line drills	I	
100-Yard Line Shuttle	70	95	Line drills	I	
Post—Corner	74	98	Line drills	I	
Post—Corner—Post	75	99	Line drills	I	
Pro Agility (20-Yard Shuttle)	61	88	Line drills	B	
Resisted Side High Knees	170	170	Mini-hurdle drills	A	
Scissors Step	83	105	Line drills	B	
Side High Knees	169	169	Mini-hurdle drills	I	
Side Left In	134	145	Agility ladder drills	I	
Side Right In	135	146	Agility ladder drills	I	
Side Shuffle–Angled Shuffle–Sprint	105	121	Cone drills	I	

Drill name	Drill #	Page #	Drill emphasis	Drill level*	VOD included?
CHAPTER 5 AGILITY TRAINING *(continued)*					
Single-Side Forward Hop	80	102	Line drills	I	
60-Yard Line Sprint	64	91	Line drills	I	
Slalom Jump	131	143	Agility ladder drills	I	
Snake Drill 1	113	126	Cone drills	I	
Snake Drill 2	114	127	Cone drills	I	
S-Pattern Run	101	118	Cone drills	I	
Sprint–Shuffle–Backpedal–Break	94	114	Cone drills	A	
Sprint–Shuffle–Sprint	104	120	Cone drills	I	
Sprint–Sprint–Backpedal	99	117	Cone drills	I	
Squirm	62	89	Line drills	I	
Star Drill	120	133	Cone drills	A	
Strides	155	160	Bag drills	I	▶
Strides With Double Step	156	160	Bag drills	I	▶
30-Yard Backpedal to Sprint	71	96	Line drills	I	
30-Yard T Drill	65	91	Line drills	B	
Triangle Drill	103	120	Cone drills	I	
20-Yard Rectangle	102	119	Cone drills	I	
20-Yard Square	86	108	Cone drills	I	
Twist Jump	132	144	Agility ladder drills	I	
V Drill	115	128	Cone drills	I	
W Backpedal Break	166	167	Backpedal drills	I	
Wheel	154	159	Bag drills	I	
W-Pattern Sprint to Quick Step Carioca	107	122	Cone drills	I	
X-Pattern Backpedal Sprint	91	112	Cone drills	A	
X-Pattern Multiskill	87	109	Cone drills	A	
X-Pattern Sprint to Backpedal	92	112	Cone drills	A	
Zigzag Crossover Shuffle	148	155	Agility ladder drills	I	
Z-Pattern Cuts	95	115	Cone drills	I	
Z-Pattern Diagonal Shuffle	100	117	Cone drills	I	
Z-Pattern Run	88	110	Cone drills	I	
CHAPTER 6 QUICKNESS AND REACTION-TIME TRAINING					
Ankle Jumps	196	201	Plyometrics	B	
Backpedal	260	252	Biomotor Reactive Drill	B	
Backpedal and Cut on Command	234	229	Directional change drills	I	
Backward Icky Shuffle With Reaction	256	248	Quick Feet Drills	A	
Backward Roll to Reaction	251	243	Whole-body reaction drills	A	
Ball Release	244	238	Hand-speed drills	B	
Barrel Roll to Reaction	250	243	Whole-body reaction drills	A	
Barrier Jumps	202	206	Plyometrics	A	
Barrier Jump With Cut and Sprint	203	207	Plyometrics	A	
The Bob	214	216	Reaction	I	
Bunny Jumps	210	213	Half agility ladder reaction drills	B	

Drill name	Drill #	Page #	Drill emphasis	Drill level*	VOD included?
CHAPTER 6 QUICKNESS AND REACTION-TIME TRAINING *(continued)*					
Card Snatching	245	239	Hand-speed drills	B	
Chubby Checker With Reaction	259	251	Quick Feet Drills	A	
Circle Reaction Drill	235	230	Directional change drills	A	
Color Dot Drill	228	225	Reaction	A	
Containing Opponent Drill	219	220	Reaction	I	▶
Crazy Ball Drill	242	236	Ground-base quickness drills	A	
Directional Foot Movement	229	226	Reaction	B	▶
Directional Hand Movement	230	226	Reaction	B	▶
Directional Mirror Drill	231	227	Reaction	B	
Dodge Ball	248	242	Whole-body reaction drills	I	
Explosive Reclined Pulls	194	200	Plyometrics	A	▶
Focus Mitt	247	241	Hand-speed drills	B	
Four-Box Plus Drill	226	224	Reaction	A	
Four-Point Pop-Up	238	232	Ground-base quickness drills	I	
Goalie Drill	179	187	Ball reaction drills	A	▶
Half Ladder Skill to Sport-Specific Skill	213	215	Half agility ladder reaction drills	A	
Hopscotch Drill	211	214	Half agility ladder reaction drills	B	
Hopscotch With Reaction	253	245	Whole-body reaction drills	A	
Hot Hands	243	237	Hand-speed drills	B	
Icky Shuffle With Reaction	255	247	Quick Feet Drills	A	
In–Out Shuffle With Reaction	257	249	Quick Feet Drills	A	
Jumping Jacks	208	211	Plyometrics	I	
Jump Rope With Multidirectional Jumps	207	210	Plyometrics	I	▶
Lateral Skaters	198	203	Plyometrics	I	▶
Lunge With Power-Up Jump	205	208	Plyometrics	A	
Lying-to-Stand Pop-Up	240	234	Ground-base quickness drills	I	
Medicine Ball Bull in a Ring	174	182	Ball reaction drills	I	
Medicine Ball Forward Scoop Toss, Bounce, and Catch	177	185	Ball reaction drills	I	▶
Medicine Ball Lateral Shuffle With Pass	175	183	Ball reaction drills	I	▶
Medicine Ball One-Arm Push-Off	190	196	Plyometrics	A	
Medicine Ball Release Push-Ups With Partner	186	193	Plyometrics	A	
Medicine Ball Squat, Push Toss, Bounce, and Catch	176	184	Ball reaction drills	I	
Medicine Ball Upper Body Shuffles	191	197	Plyometrics	A	
Medicine Ball Wall Chest Pass	185	193	Plyometrics	A	▶
Medicine Ball Wall Overhead Throw	189	195	Plyometrics	A	▶
Medicine Ball Wall Scoop Toss	188	194	Plyometrics	A	
Medicine Ball Wall Side Toss	187	194	Plyometrics	A	▶

Drill Finder

Drill name	Drill #	Page #	Drill emphasis	Drill level*	VOD included?
CHAPTER 6 QUICKNESS AND REACTION-TIME TRAINING *(continued)*					
Mirror Partner Sprints	218	220	Reaction	I	▶
Mirror Two-Box Drill	227	225	Reaction	A	
Mirror Two-Box Shuffle Drill	221	221	Reaction	I	
Mirror Two-Box Sprint Drill	220	221	Reaction	I	
The Parry	215	217	Reaction	I	
Partner Ball Drops	178	186	Ball reaction drills	I	
Partner Blind Tosses	180	188	Ball reaction drills	A	
Partner-Resisted Lateral Shuffle and Chase	217	219	Reaction	I	
Plyo Push-Ups	184	192	Plyometrics	A	
Push-Off Box Shuffle	206	209	Plyometrics	A	
Quick Feet	209	212	Half agility ladder reaction drills	I	
Rapid Fire	249	242	Whole-body reaction drills	A	
Rope Skipping	195	201	Plyometrics	I	
Ruler Drop	246	240	Hand-speed drills	B	
Scissor Jumps	197	202	Plyometrics	I	▶
Side Shuffle Reactive Drill	236	230	Directional change drills	A	
Single-Leg Hop	212	215	Half agility ladder reaction drills	B	
Sit-to-Stand Pop-Up	239	233	Ground-base quickness drills	I	
Slalom With Reaction	252	244	Whole-body reaction drills	A	
Snake With Reaction	258	250	Quick Feet Drills	A	
Speed Skips	204	208	Plyometrics	A	
Sprawl-to-Stand Pop-Up	241	235	Ground-base quickness drills	A	
Sprint and Backpedal on Command	232	228	Directional change drills	I	
Sprint and Cut on Command	233	229	Directional change drills	I	
Stability Ball Hops	182	190	Plyometrics	A	
Stability Ball Impact Lockouts	181	189	Plyometrics	A	
Standing Long Jump	201	205	Plyometrics	I	
T Drill With Ball Toss	254	246	Whole-body reaction drills	A	
Three-Point Fire Drill With Reaction	224	223	Reaction	A	
Three-Step Foot-Tap Drill With Sprint	223	222	Reaction	A	
Three-Step Foot-Tap Drill With Sprint to Ball Drop	225	223	Reaction	A	
Triangle Drill With Commands	222	222	Reaction	A	
Tuck Jumps	199	204	Plyometrics	I	▶
Upper Body Box Shuffles	193	199	Plyometrics	A	
Upper Body Shuffles	192	198	Plyometrics	A	
Vertical Jump	200	205	Plyometrics	I	
The Weave	216	218	Reaction	I	
Wheelbarrow Drill	183	191	Plyometrics	A	▶
X Drill	237	231	Directional change drills	A	▶

Accessing the Online Video

This book includes access to online video that includes 64 clips demonstrating some of the most dynamic exercises discussed in the book. In the drill finder and throughout the book, exercises marked with this play button icon indicate where the content is enhanced by online video clips: ▶

Take the following steps to access the video. If you need help at any point in the process, you can contact us by clicking on the Technical Support link under Customer Service on the right side of the screen.

1. Visit www.HumanKinetics.com/TrainingforSpeedAgilityandQuickness.
2. Click on the **View online video** link next to the book cover.
3. You will be directed to the screen shown in figure 1. Click the **Sign In** link on the left or top of the page. If you do not have an account with Human Kinetics, you will be prompted to create one.

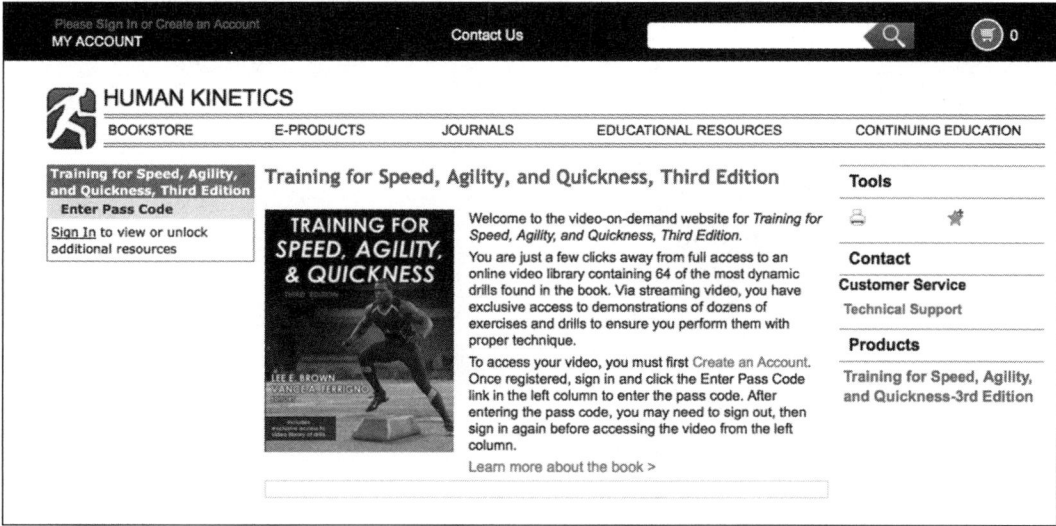

Figure 1

4. If the online video does not appear in the list on the left of the page, click the **Enter Pass Code** option in that list. Enter the pass code exactly as it is printed here, including all hyphens. Click the **Submit** button to unlock the online video. After you have entered this pass code the first time, you will never have to enter it again. For future visits, all you need to do is sign in to the book's website and follow the link that appears in the left menu.

Pass code for online video: **Brown-SKZQM-OLV**

5. Once you have signed into the site and entered the pass code, select **Online Video** from the list on the left side of the screen. You'll then see an Online Video page with information about the video, as shown in the screenshot in figure 2. You can go straight to the accompanying videos for each topic by clicking on the blue links at the bottom of the page.

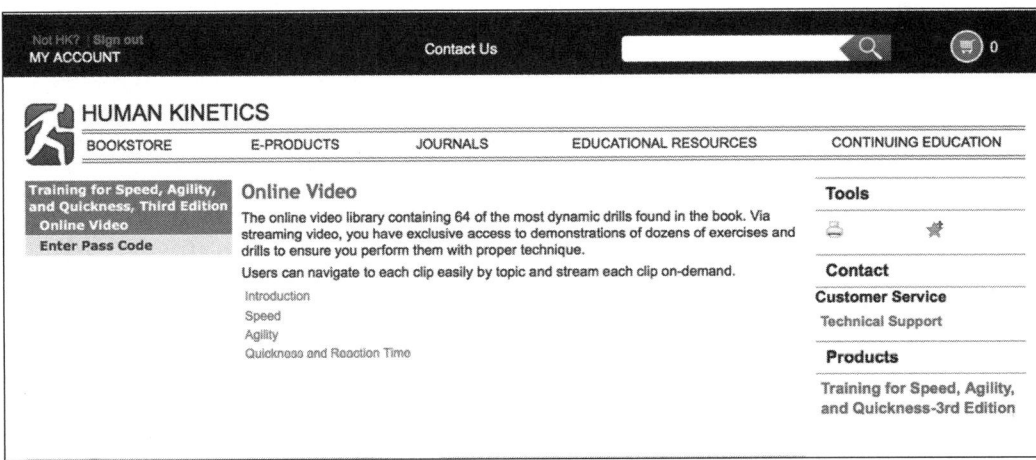

Figure 2

6. You are now able to view video for the topic you selected on the previous screen, as well as all others that accompany this product. Across the top of the page, you will see a set of buttons that correspond to the topics in the text that have accompanying video. Once you click on a topic, a player will appear. In the player, the clips for that topic will appear vertically along the right side. Just as in the print book, each topic contains two or more subcategories of drills; you can choose between these categories by clicking the tabs across the top of the player. Select the video you would like to watch and view it in the main player window. You can use the buttons at the bottom of the main player window to view the video full screen, to turn captioning on and off, and to pause, fast-forward, or reverse the clip. The video clips are arranged in this manner:

Speed Training
  Acceleration
  Partner-Assisted Acceleration
  Starts
  Maximal Velocity

Agility Training
  Agility Ladder
  Bag

Quickness and Reaction-Time Training
  Ball Reaction
  Plyometric
  Reaction
  Directional Change

Preface

Welcome to the third edition of *Training for Speed, Agility, and Quickness*! As editors, we hope you find it packed with new features that will enhance athletic performance while also increasing your ability to design sport-specific training programs for yourself or your athletes.

In this edition, you'll find that we have added new material on mental skills training as well as individual sport-specific training programs. We believe these new chapters will enhance your athletic performance as well as that of the athletes you train.

Additionally, this third edition uses an Internet platform for the drill videos. This enables you and your athletes to watch them in the field on any web-based device, thereby getting instant visual examples of proper execution. The drills that have accompanying video are noted in the Drill Finder and are also marked with this symbol in the text: ▶. Furthermore, the visual layout of the book has been enhanced with an increased number of drills in each chapter, including detailed instructions enriched by photos taken directly from the videos.

Here are the highlights of each chapter:

- Chapter 1, How the Training Works: This chapter discusses the important link between speed, agility, and quickness and sport-specific training. It provides the science behind training for explosiveness while discussing manipulation of the critical program design variables.

- Chapter 2, Athlete Assessment: Here we discuss the foundation of testing in order to properly design individualized training programs. We explain how to design an assessment strategy that uses the drills themselves as test tools to evaluate performance needs and gains.

- Chapter 3, Incorporating Mental Skills Training: In this chapter, we explain how to design, assess, and integrate mental skills in a training program. The chapter includes worksheets and activities that will enhance the sport psychology aspect of your athletes.

- Chapter 4, Speed Training: Speed is a complex skill made up of many component parts including acceleration, stride frequency, and stride length. This chapter breaks down each one and explains how to train them effectively to reach maximum performance. Also, proper sprinting technique is explicitly defined, including coaching cues.

- Chapter 5, Agility Training: Change of direction enhances athleticism. Therefore, this chapter provides for assessment strategies and training regimens to increase agility with supporting physiological rationales for performance.

- Chapter 6, Quickness and Reaction-Time Training: Quickness is often defined as the first step of speed. In this chapter, we explore how sport-specific quickness is achieved and improved. In addition, building reaction time drills into a program is explained as an integral aspect of any sport.

- Chapter 7, Developing a Customized Program: This chapter is a lead-in discussion of how to properly design and implement each aspect of a proper workout from warm-up to cool-down. There is also a special section on tweaking the workout for the best individualized results.
- Chapters 8 to 16, sport-specific training programs: These last chapters offer an overview of the specific demands of baseball, softball, football, rugby, basketball, netball, combat sports, track and field, soccer, lacrosse, tennis, badminton, racquetball, and squash. They provide a detailed eight-week strength, agility, and quickness training program complete with drills, sets, and reps.

Enjoy reading the book and watching the videos. We sincerely believe that following the programs and tenets laid out in this book will enhance any athlete's performance. Finally, remember there is only one speed . . . *fast*!

Acknowledgments

I thank my outstanding students at Cal State Fullerton for their willing assistance in filming the drills for this book.

—Lee

I thank Gary Gray and Dave Tiberio for their friendship, mentorship and patience in helping me to understand the GIFT of human movement.

—Vance

PART I

Training Essentials

Chapter 1

How the Training Works

Tori L. Beaudette and Lee E. Brown

Speed, agility, and quickness training has become a popular way to train athletes. With a continually increasing need to promote athletic ability, this type of training has proven to enhance the practical field abilities of participants in a wide variety of sports. Practiced in addition to conventional resistance training, it assists in the transfer of strength gained in the gym to performance in the arena of play. Nearly every sport requires fast movements of either the arms or legs, and speed, agility, and quickness training can improve skill in these areas. Hence, all athletes can benefit when speed, agility, and quickness training is integrated into their training programs.

Although this type of training has been around for a number of years, many athletes have not practiced it. This is primarily due to a lack of education regarding both its specific benefits and how to integrate it into a complete training program. In particular, speed, agility, and quickness training is intended to increase the ability to exert maximal force during high-speed movements. It manipulates and capitalizes on the stretch–shortening cycle (SSC) while bridging the gap between traditional resistance training and function-specific movements. Some benefits of speed, agility, and quickness training include increased muscular power in all multiplanar movements and enhanced brain-signal efficiency, kinesthetic spatial awareness, motor skills, and reaction time. The acquisition of greater balance and reaction time will let the athlete maintain proper body position during skill execution and react more proficiently to any change in the playing environment. Quick movements are useless if the athlete trips over his own feet.

Many athletes and coaches also do not realize that speed, agility, and quickness training can cover the complete spectrum of training intensity, from low to high. Each athlete comes into a training program at a different level, so the intensity must coincide with the athlete's ability. For example, at the lower-intensity end of the spectrum, the assorted biomotor skills illustrated throughout this book can be used to teach movement, warm-up, or the basics of conditioning. No significant preparation is needed to participate at this level of speed, agility, and quickness training. Higher-intensity drills require a significant level of preparation. A simple approach for safe participation and increased effectiveness is to start a concurrent strength-training program when beginning speed, agility, and quickness training.

Now we'll review how speed, agility, and quickness training works and how it can be implemented within workouts for complete conditioning.

Understanding the Muscles at Work

Understanding the basic physiology of muscular function is invaluable for understanding why this particular type of training is so effective.

Within your body, each skeletal muscle is made up of connective tissue, muscle tissue, nerves, and blood vessels and is controlled by signals sent from the brain. These components work together in a coordinated fashion to cause bones and therefore limbs to move in desired patterns. Muscle tissue is connected to tendons, which are noncontractile lengths of tissue that attach muscle to bone. Thus, tension developed within the muscle transfers to the tendon and then the bone.

On an even more intimate level, each muscle fiber contains hundreds or even thousands of thin longitudinal fibers. These fibers contain two opposing contractile and finger-like proteins (actin and myosin). The actin and myosin form attachments called crossbridges that pull against one another. Through a series of chemical reactions controlled via brain signals, these proteins work to repeatedly pull and release. This causes muscular contraction, resulting in force. The sum of this activity is what we measure as muscular strength. Training increases the muscle's ability to produce force and thus strength.

The stretch–shortening cycle is at the heart of speed, agility, and quickness training because these skills require explosive movements with changes in direction and velocity (Plisk 2000). The cycle involves a combination of eccentric (muscle-lengthening) and concentric (muscle-shortening) actions; it works like a rubber band that is stretched and then snaps back together. An eccentric muscle action is performed when an athlete lowers a weight, such as during the downward deceleration movement when landing from a jump or slowing to change direction. A concentric muscle action occurs during the upward phase, or the opposite movement in the exercises just described. When an eccentric action precedes a concentric action, the resulting force output of the concentric action is increased via more brain signals and the addition of the elastic force of the rubber band–like feature of muscle. This is the essence both of the SSC and speed, agility, and quickness training.

Examples of the SSC in sports occur in the swing of a baseball bat or a golf club, during which the intended motion is preceded by a windup or prestretch. However, if there is a pause between the preceding action and the follow-through, the increased force output will not occur during the concentric phase of the exercise. The SSC also takes place during everyday activities, such as walking and running, but it is greatly intensified during speed, agility, and quickness training.

Advantages derived from the SSC are both large and small at all levels of sporting competition. One example is the vertical jump. When the jumper precedes her jump by bending her knees and hips and then exploding upward, the resultant jump height will be greater than if she had stopped at the bottom of the knee bend for a few seconds. Another example can be seen in the baseball pitch. If the pitcher does not complete a windup, he is unable to generate as much force as would be possible by performing a prestretch motion, and thus the speed of the resulting pitch is slower.

SSC activities can be performed for the upper body as well as for the lower body and can be augmented by external devices, such as free weights, rubber tubing, and medicine balls. Devices such as these assist the athlete in performing both the concentric and eccentric portions of the exercise insofar as they require either acceleration or deceleration. However, speed, agility, and quickness training can be performed without assistive devices by simply using one's own body weight as resistance.

Integrating Speed, Agility, and Quickness Training

It is very important to remember that speed, agility, and quickness training should supplement traditional resistance training. In other words, it should be conducted in addition to and not instead of lifting weights. speed, agility, and quickness training at higher intensities should begin after a solid foundation of general conditioning has been established. This could mean six months to a year of foundational training for a beginner. The main point is to have enough of a strength base to adequately complete each speed, agility, and quickness exercise without undue strain. In addition, high-intensity speed, agility, and quickness training should normally be undertaken during the month or two just before the season and should last approximately 30 to 45 minutes per session, two days per week for beginners.

When writing an exercise program for any athlete, coaches need to take several parameters into consideration. First, consider years of training, level of fitness, and how often the athlete will be performing speed, agility, and quickness training. In addition to these considerations, there are seven critical training variables that require discussion. They are choice, order, frequency, intensity, volume, rest, and progression (CO-FIVR-P).

Choice

Choice of exercise for a training program should mimic the athlete's demands during competition. Exercises should be specific to the sport relative to direction of movement, velocity of movement, which muscles are utilized, and the metabolic demands of the sport. Every program must be designed with a specific goal in mind. For example, a training program for a sprint athlete may include short linear speed drills; however, a training program for a soccer player would incorporate more multidirectional drills and be performed for multiple repetitions and for longer durations.

Order

Order of exercise should follow three main patterns: Exercises should be executed from simple to complex, from low to high intensity, and from general to sport specific. This order should be used both within a single training session and over the course of an entire training program. Ordering the exercises in this manner allows an athlete to gradually prepare to perform the most complex, intense, and specific movements required during their peak event.

Frequency

Frequency of training refers to the number of training sessions completed in a given amount of time, usually per week. Frequency should be altered according to the ability levels of the athletes and where they are in their training program. For the novice athlete, begin by adding one or two basic speed, agility, and quickness training exercises to the current training schedule. In particular, it is important that athletes begin with the basic techniques of each exercise before advancing to more technical aspects. Furthermore, learning proper mechanics of basic exercises will allow them to progress to advanced exercises in a timelier manner. As an athlete becomes more advanced, his frequency of training will increase: from two to three or more times per week.

Intensity

Intensity applies to the quality of work performed during muscular activity and is measured in terms of power output (i.e., work performed per unit of time). Training intensity may also be defined by the ease or difficulty of a particular drill. Intensity of an exercise can be altered based on the velocity of movement, whether or not the movements are planned or unplanned, and the degree of angle for the movement. Intensity and volume are inversely related and therefore have significant influence on one another.

Volume

Volume is the quantity, or total number, of sets and repetitions completed in a training session. The inverse relationship between intensity and volume states that as intensity increases, volume decreases. Early in the program, volume is high while intensity is low. As the athlete nears competition, volume is progressively decreased as intensity increases. Measuring training volume (number of sets × number of repetitions) is vital for assessing training progression. Training volume within a given training session is based on the athlete's level of fitness. The proper combination of the number of sets and repetitions with variations in training intensity may also help augment training adaptations. These adaptations become evident through repeated testing sessions.

Rest

Rest is often the forgotten variable. It prevents overtraining and is critical for the success of a training program. The progression of a training program must include rest in order to maximize training adaptations that are specific to each sport. The harder a training session or activity, the longer an athlete will need to recover; therefore, rest should increase with increasing intensity.

Progression

Progression of the program should gradually increase as athletes reach their goals and should also be specific to the sport. Intensity should progress from low to moderate until movements are mastered, followed by a decrease in volume as the intensity increases. Progression from low to high intensity may depend on where the athlete is in the training year. The intensity level is generally lower for beginners to make sure they are able to perform the prescribed exercises correctly while also avoiding injury. Low intensity may consist of performing the exercises at 40 to 50 percent of maximal exertion, moderate intensity between 50 and 80 percent, and high intensity between 80 and 100 percent. Progression of volume is related to intensity; as intensity increases, volume decreases. Remember that as an athlete progresses, rest must be increased both within a training session and between sessions to allow for sufficient recovery. Coaches may employ different programs that allow for two or three days off per week. However, as the athlete nears competition, that number is likely to decrease.

Each critical training variable should be manipulated according to the athlete's level of training. Athletes can be divided into three major categories: novice, experienced, and advanced. The novice athlete is just beginning to exercise for sport. He might be an adolescent or even an adult who chooses to take up sport later in life. The potential for improvement is great. The experienced athlete has been training for one to five years and is involved in a regular program of exercise and sport. Although she is competing at a higher level, there is still great room for improvement. The advanced athlete competes at a national or international level, where events are decided by inches or hundredths of a second. Advanced athletes are near their genetic limits, and therefore their potential for improvement is small. The details of their programs must be precise. Training age (number of years training for a sport) is often more meaningful than chronological age in categorizing an athlete. By employing and manipulating the critical training variables, all athletes can be successful in their training program as they peak for their events.

Maximizing the critical variables of CO-FIVR-P in a training program can be accomplished through periodization, which involves the gradual alteration of primarily choice, frequency, intensity, volume, and rest throughout the year to achieve peak levels of fitness for the most important competitions (Plisk 2004). This planned variation is principally related to progression and organizes the annual training program into phases during which the athlete trains to meet goals particular to that phase. All the phases of a periodized program together constitute a macrocycle that might last a year. On its own, each phase constitutes a mesocycle, which may stretch over several weeks or months, depending on the goals set by the athlete and coach. The mesocycle may be further separated into even smaller sections called microcycles, which are generally periods of training around one week, depending on the type of event the athlete is preparing for. Microcycles are like puzzle pieces, with each being necessary to complete the overall goal of the training program.

In a linear periodized program, volume and intensity are manipulated throughout each phase to produce trends of decreasing volume and increasing intensity (Bradley-Popovich 2001; Graham 2002). The intensity of training sessions varies across a spectrum from easy to hard. Each of these training sessions has varying volumes and intensities. Without variation of the critical variables, athletes are at risk for overtraining and may not be prepared to peak at the time of competition.

Periodization should be used for athletes of all levels; however, implementation of the program will differ from one athlete to the next. It is important to assess and monitor the needs of each athlete individually to design an appropriate program. Table 1.1 is an example of a mesocycle within a linear

Table 1.1 Mesocycle Demonstrating Manipulation of FIVR for an Advanced Athlete

Week	Frequency	Distance	Intensity (%)	Sets	Reps	Volume*	Rest
1	2	10 yd	60	6	12	72	30 s
2	2	10 yd	75	5	10	50	30 s
3	3	20 yd	80	4	10	40	45 s
4	3	20 yd	70	5	10	50	45 s
5	2	10 yd	80	4	8	32	60 s
6	3	20 yd	85	3	8	24	60 s
7	4	30 yd	90	3	6	18	90 s
8	2	40 yd	80	3	8	24	90 s

*Multiply sets × reps to get volume.

periodized program for an advanced athlete. Trends of increasing intensity and decreasing volume are employed, as well as variation in frequency and rest. Exercise choice should be based on the needs of the athlete and progress from general to specific.

Preventing Injury and Staying Safe

An appropriate warm-up should precede every exercise session. Warm-up routines should begin with a low-intensity whole-body activity such as jogging. This will increase heart rate and blood flow to the muscles, thereby preparing the athlete for the higher-intensity workout to come. This general warm-up should be followed by a specific warm-up that consists of some of the session's exercises at a low intensity (Abad et al. 2011).

Male and female athletes have similar muscle structure, which allows them to follow the same training program. However, there are some differences between the genders. Male athletes have greater absolute strength and can therefore produce more power. This power contributes to the utilization of the SSC and enhances performance of speed, agility, and quickness drills. Decreased power production and increased risk of injury in female athletes is most often explained by neurological factors. When designing a program, however, gender is not a major factor. Rather, the focus should be on training age, the sport, and the athlete's ability.

Performance of female athletes can be affected by the female athlete triad. Low energy may be associated with eating disorders, menstrual disturbances, and low bone mineral density. Prevalence of the triad is common among females who participate in sports where lean body mass is critical (Nazem and Ackerman 2012). It is important to be aware of the seriousness of these disorders and to recognize their signs and symptoms.

An adolescent athlete should follow a periodized program similar to ones for adult males and females. A needs assessment is critical, as it will identify whether the adolescent athlete has mastered basic movement patterns. It is imperative to develop a strong foundation of motor skills before progressing through a training program to more intense and sport-specific exercises. A periodized program should be based on the needs and limitations of the athlete and not chronological age.

Injury prevention is a major part of any training program. It is vital that every athlete advance in a progressive and systematic manner when embarking on speed, agility, and quickness training. A properly conducted strength training program that emphasizes knee, hip, back, and ankle strength will reduce the possibility of injury when speed, agility, and quickness training is first introduced. Training should progress from simple to complex movements, from low to high intensity, and from general to sport-specific motor patterns. Moreover, factors such as frequency, intensity, volume, body structure, sport specificity, training age, and periodization phase should always be considered when designing speed, agility, and quickness training.

Here are a few more recommendations for athletes to help prevent injuries:

- Follow the proper progression of exercises, and wear proper clothing and shoes.
- Observe safety procedures while learning and mastering the speed, agility, and quickness drills in this book.
- Make certain all equipment is in proper working order before use.
- If exercising outdoors, make sure the area is free of any hazardous objects, such as rocks or trees.
- Be sure to understand each new exercise completely before attempting it for the first time.

When athletes first attempt a new exercise, they commonly experience muscle soreness. This soreness, called delayed-onset muscle soreness (DOMS), usually occurs 24 hours after the exercise bout, peaking between 48 and 72 hours (Dierking and Bemben 1998). The eccentric portion of the exercise is the primary cause of DOMS, and the prevailing explanation is micromuscle tears. The only way to reduce the development of DOMS is to adapt to the exercise stress. This requires repeating exercise bouts over several weeks, with sufficient rest between sessions. Since all speed, agility, and quickness training involves eccentric exercise utilizing the SSC, it is recommended that novice athletes perform no more than two exercise sessions per week separated by two or three days (Parsons and Jones 1998). Experienced and advanced athletes may exercise three or four days per week depending on their training phase.

In summary, speed, agility, and quickness training is high-intensity work that requires a foundation of strength. It may result in mild muscle soreness until the athlete adapts to the prescribed exercises. Regardless of gender and age, these exercises should be introduced slowly before progressing to drills of higher intensity and greater complexity. In the coming chapters, we describe the drills that make up speed, agility, and quickness training and show how to integrate them into a complete training plan.

Chapter 2

Athlete Assessment

Logan K. Schwartz and Vance A. Ferrigno

To determine whether a training program is truly moving an athlete toward the goal, testing and retesting of the athlete should be an integral part of the training process (Gambetta 1998). The initial testing is to determine a baseline of where the athlete is in terms of speed, agility, and quickness. It is difficult to know if an athlete is progressing if you don't know where he started. After this initial testing, subsequent tests should be done periodically to ensure the athlete is making gains.

In the previous editions of *Training for Speed, Agility, and Quickness*, this section on testing the athlete's functional strength was based on traditional models of assessment: basic strength, reactive resources, and strength deficit. In this third edition, we are taking a new approach to assessing the athlete based purely on baselining their speed, agility and quickness. It is a simple but effective approach that utilizes the very drills an athlete uses to train. There are more than 200 drills in this book, and each and every drill can be used as an assessment tool. Athleticism is based on symmetry and fluidity of movement. All top athletes can move in all directions with equal fluidity and grace. They make the transition from one skill to another look effortless.

Efficient movement is the foundation to athletic achievement. Simply put, the more efficiently a person moves, the better that person can perform. Efficient and effective movement is demonstrated through the qualities of speed, agility, and quickness. Human movement is complex, dynamic, individual, variable, and, at the highest level of performance, done on a subconscious level (Gray 2006b).

Assessing Your Athlete

One problem that many trainers and coaches confront is how to effectively and efficiently evaluate human movement. To authentically evaluate movement, we must understand one main principle of training: The "test is the exercise and the exercise is the test" (Gray 2004). The principle of specificity in training states that the body will adapt to the specific imposed stimulus. Therefore, if an athlete desires to improve in a specific skill, movement, or exercise, she must perform that exercise in training with multiple variations, or tweaks, to that drill. Because of the complexity of the human structure and human movement, specificity is paramount in training to reach the desired outcome. Another layer to this philosophy is that if the test is the exercise, then if the exercise is properly tweaked (complex variations), it will provide the best opportunity for an improved outcome (Gray 2006b).

The movement assessments presented in this book give coaches an example of one way to evaluate an athlete's ability to move foundationally. The drills can be tweaked however the coach deems necessary to fit his own personal situation and individual athletes (see table 2.1). In general, any drill presented in this book can be used to evaluate or test an athlete for whatever training parameter the coach deems requires improvement.

To choose proper drills, the coach must first evaluate the demands of the sport for that athlete and either develop or select drills that mimic those demands. Once the drill is selected, it can be used to monitor the athlete's functional progress with respect to her training program through subsequent retesting. In this way, the athlete's needs can be assessed and then rematched

Table 2.1 Drill Adjustments and Variables

Adjustment	Variables
Distance	Shorter Longer
Load	Weight vest Bungee cord Free weight Weighted sleds
Direction	Change dominant plane of motion of drill Reverse order of cuts Change angulations of drill
Speed	Half speed Three-quarter speed Full speed
Duration	Increase reps or sets Decrease reps or sets
Multiple tasks	Combine execution of drill with added task (e.g., catching and throwing a ball) React to whistle
Environment	Change surface on which drill is performed (e.g., grass to gym floor) Change level of the surface (e.g., uphill, downhill, side hill)
Angulation or plane changes	Change angles or planes on which drill is performed
Athlete feedback	Many athletes intuitively know what they are lacking; their feedback can be crucial in making the proper adjustments and progressions

or progressed to more complex drills (Brown et al. 2008). The goals of any training program should be based entirely on the needs of the athlete and the requirements of the specific sport.

Athletes move in a powerful yet effortless manner and are able to adapt to any demand necessary to accomplish the tasks of their sports. Movement quality needs to be assessed first so that an inefficient movement pattern is not placed under training loads, which can lead to increased movement inefficiency or worse, injury.

Once a drill has been selected for a given training quality, it can be timed to give the athlete his base-level time for that specific drill. During training, the same drill is repeated using one or more of the variables listed in table 2.1 or the complex variations for some of the drills in this book. This will create a new stimulus for adaptation, allowing the athlete to increase his performance for that given drill. Every four to six weeks the original drill can be retested, allowing the coach and the athlete to see his improvement on his base-level time.

The main goal of any movement assessment is to determine the successful abilities of the individual athlete. Once these are identified, the coach can go to work on improving those abilities to facilitate a more well-rounded athlete. There is no exact way to do each movement—each person will perform the movements differently because of her unique structure—but all efficient human movement has common characteristics. The coach should not get caught up in the finer details of assessing movement but rather should evaluate more globally, looking for efficient, smooth, graceful motion. This makes it easier to identify the specific tweaks the athlete needs to make to her drills in order to promote the desired outcome.

For example, athlete A may perform a certain drill in an uncoordinated way, stumbling out of cuts or unable to demonstrate gracefulness during the movement, while athlete B seems very comfortable coordinating the drill. However, athlete B has trouble decelerating and accelerating out of cuts. For athlete A, the proper tweak may be to slow down his speed during training, thus allowing him to learn the drill at a much slower pace. His speed can be progressively increased once his body adapts. Athlete B, however, may benefit from being loaded with a weight vest, bungee cord, or other device, allowing him to develop functional strength and power relative to the drill. This tweak will allow athlete B to progressively develop the ability to decelerate sooner and accelerate more explosively over the course of training.

Tweaks such as these are complex variations that allow specific adaptations to the drill. The complex variations in this book only scratch the surface of those possible to perform. Use your imagination, and remember that an athlete should always progress from easy to hard and from simple to complex (Gambetta 1998).

Ensuring Validity and Reliability

Test results are useful only if the test actually measures what it is supposed to measure. This is referred to as validity. For subsequent tests to be useful, they must be repeatable. This is referred to as reliability (Harman 2008). For testing to be valid and reliable, the tester must ensure that the environment stays as consistent as possible from test to test. Because these tests are measured in seconds not minutes, the test has to have enough sensitivity and reliability to provide the desired data. This means that flooring surfaces, shoes, turf conditions, and environmental conditions (e.g., heat, wind) all have to be controlled to ensure an accurate measure of whether the athlete is improving the biomotor quality or athletic movement being assessed. If the first test is performed on a dry field but eight weeks later is repeated on a dew-soaked field, the test will not be valid or reliable.

The procedures for reliable testing are as follows.

Testing Environment

First and foremost, the athlete's safety is the number one concern. Be sure the testing area is safe and doesn't have any holes, sprinkler heads, or anything else that could cause the athlete to trip, slip, or turn an ankle. Make sure the environmental conditions (e.g., temperature, humidity) are as similar as possible from test to test. For field sports, a hot, humid day will elicit different results than a cool, overcast day, especially on metabolic tests. This is less of an issue for court sports because indoor environments are more easily controlled than outdoor.

Athlete Fatigue Level

During training, athletes will develop a certain level of fatigue. Providing a day off between training and testing allows them to give their all and will contribute to validity and reliability. Also, ensure they have eaten and are properly hydrated. With prior communication regarding the test date, there is no reason the athletes shouldn't be rested, fed, and hydrated.

Recording Forms

Forms should be developed before testing so the tester can easily and efficiently record the required data without error. There is nothing worse than having an athlete put every ounce of effort into a performance test only to have the tester not record it properly.

Test Sequence

Explosive power-oriented tests or those with more complexity should be performed before more fatiguing tests such as drills for anaerobic endurance. Otherwise, power-oriented test results will be impaired and invalid.

Athlete Instructions

Instructions should be clear and easy to understand. Otherwise, the athlete will be focused on getting the test right and not on her maximal performance (Gambetta 1998). Also, standardize any verbal cues for motivation provided to the athlete from test to test (Brown et al. 2008).

Equipment

Keep test equipment to the bare minimum, and record exactly what is used. Also, each athlete should test in the same footwear they wear when competing.

Testing Protocol

Allow the same number of trials per test, using the same rest intervals between trials and between tests if performing a test battery.

Field or Court Measurements

When marking the test area (e.g., cones), use a measuring device to ensure you are using exact distances. Pacing off the area is inaccurate and renders the results invalid and unreliable.

Although most of the drills in this book can be used for testing, we recommend the following as starting points.

Speed Tests
10-yard burst (p. 53)
30-yard flying start (p. 71)

Agility Tests
30-yard T drill (p. 91)
F movement (p. 131)
Pro agility (p. 88)

Quickness Tests
Ankle jumps (p. 201)

Let's look at an example of an assessment using the 30-yard T drill. The tester should begin by explaining to the athlete exactly what will transpire during the testing slated for that day. After receiving instructions, the athlete begins a warm-up. Details of the warm-up must be recorded so the identical procedure can be used on the next testing session. The tester must also accurately record details of the environmental factors, equipment used, athlete's level of motivation, footwear, and other factors involved in the test.

The athlete performs three trials of the 30-yard T drill, with 2 to 3 minutes' rest between trials. All three times are recorded, as well as the exact rest time between trials. The fastest time becomes the athlete's base level for this drill. Coaches should always encourage their athletes during testing. With young athletes who are not competing on the national level, we discourage use of comparative norms. These norms will often deflate a person who is training hard but is not as athletically gifted as those from whom the norms were derived. As the athlete develops and is inspired to compete at a higher level, norms can be useful for setting goals.

Now that the test results for this drill are on record, the coach or athlete can tweak one of the parameters of the drill every time it is used in training. One week you can spread out the cones, adding distance between them; the next week, decrease the distance between the cones. One week use a bungee cord for resistance from the lateral side; the next week use the bungee for resistance in front or behind. Use a back shoulder turn to get around the cones one week and a straight turn the next week. Mix and match the variations to provide variety. Athletes retested eight weeks later will be faster. This encourages and motivates them for the next phase of training.

The goal of any training program is to create authentic results or adaptations that transfer directly to competition. Evaluation and testing of an athlete is paramount in determining if an athlete is progressing with her training program. Because of the amazingly complex nature of the human body performing athletic movements, the evaluation techniques and protocols must be carefully chosen in order to make sure the test is authentic to the athlete's goals. Initial baseline tests need to replicate drills being performed in the athlete's training program so the specificity of training adaptations are reflected in the testing. These same evaluation techniques can be manipulated using the variables listed in table 2.1 to train other athletic qualities relative to the same drill. This sets the athlete up for success whenever the drill is retested because of the principle of specificity of training.

Chapter 3

Incorporating Mental Skills Training

Traci A. Statler

Speed, agility, and quickness training, in conjunction with more traditional resistance and endurance training, has become a popular way to train athletes for a variety of sport-specific settings. This type of training, intended to increase athletes' ability to generate maximal force during the high-speed movements of their sports, is also a prime environment for training the mental skills needed for ideal sport performance. Because speed, agility, and quickness training occurs after a base foundation of strength has been established, this ensures that the athlete is already familiar with the traditional performance environment and expectations for success. This foundation—a more advanced understanding of and familiarity with the setting—sets the preliminary conditions for working toward improved mental skills in this training environment.

In reality, many athletes come to the training environment with some solid mental skills already in their repertoire, but often they have little understanding of how these skills evolved or even how to best utilize them for effective performance. This chapter introduces a model for integrating mental skills training into an athlete's program, thus providing a structure for understanding the interrelationships not only between the mental skills themselves but also between the mental skills and the physical, technical, and tactical skills being developed in the weight room and on the practice fields. Note, however, that these skills can only truly be effective if they are understood, practiced, and applied to the performance setting. Like the physical, technical, and tactical skills described throughout this book, the mental skills need to be taught, practiced, integrated into performance, and evaluated for effectiveness. Skills such as those in this chapter are most effective when their usage becomes seamlessly integrated into overall performance.

Designing a Mental Training Program

For a variety of reasons, the intentional structured integration of mental skills into existing physical skills training programs has been minimal. Whether this is because of a perceived lack of time to focus on this element, a belief that mental skills are personality characteristics rather than trainable components of performance, or a feeling of insufficient knowledge or training to teach these elements, the reality is that strength and conditioning and sport coaches are in an ideal environment to foster and develop these abilities in their athletes. Psychological and physical skills are taught, learned, and practiced in similar fashion and can be integrated simultaneously without much modification to existing training programs. Coaches and athletes already know that strength, speed, quickness, agility, and endurance can be developed if basic principles are followed. If the body is systematically and progressively overloaded over time, adaptation will occur and ability is improved. The same holds true for mental skills. Introduce these skills and practice them in a performance environment, and eventually they will become part of the athlete's automatic response patterns (Gould and Eklund 2007). As with the learning of anything new—whether mental, physical, technical, or tactical—the development of effective mental skills occurs in four distinct phases:

1. Assessment of current aptitude levels
2. Education in the new technique to be learned
3. Acquisition of the new skill and practice of it
4. Integration into automatic responses

Assessment

The first phase, *assessment*, starts with an evaluation of the performance environment, the goals of training, and the people with whom the training is being conducted. What are the specific mental skills needed for effective speed and agility training? If the coach needs to prioritize based on the specifics of the environment, what skills will she focus on and which ones will be eliminated? What are the central or core topics needed to optimize athlete performance? Additionally, at this stage the coach will want to examine the athlete's current ability level. What are his existing strengths and weaknesses? Once the coach has these answers, she can then determine which mental skills to focus on.

Some potential tools for assessing the athlete's existing strengths and weaknesses include a simple self-evaluation by the athlete or coach individually, or in conjunction with each other, or a psychometric mental skills test to identify what cognitive abilities the athlete excels at and which ones need improvement. To determine the athlete's starting point, a low-tech, no-cost exercise that can be conducted by the athlete or coach is a mental performance profile (Butler and Hardy 1992). This tool can be used to show discrepancies between current and ideal levels of proficiency in mental skills to show differences between a coach's and athlete's perceptions, or to compare where the athlete is today against where she wants to be.

Figure 3.1, the mental skills performance profile worksheet, is effective for generating awareness of an athlete's current psychological proficiencies and potential deficiencies. It brings awareness to how athletes feel about their current state of readiness for performance or competition. There are no right or wrong responses, and the profile focuses on what the athletes themselves feel

Figure 3.1 Mental Skills Performance Profile Worksheet

A performance profile is a tool often used to shed light on how performers are feeling about their preparation for performance. There are no right or wrong answers. Creating a performance profile for yourself may help improve your awareness of performance preparation and help direct your training focus.

1. What are the fundamental mental qualities of elite performance in your sport or position? In other words, what are the psychological qualities or characteristics of an elite athlete in your sport? List as many of these qualities as you can think of.

2. Taking into consideration your own personal performance style, go back and circle those *10* qualities you perceive as the most important for your effective performance.

3. Create your profile:

    a. Write each of the previously identified 10 characteristics in the outermost quadrant of the grid.

    b. Rate your current level of skill (on a scale from 1 to 10) for each of the 10 constructs.

    c. For each mental skill wedge, fill in your ranking from step b above, with 1 being at the center ring of the circle and 10 at the outermost ring.

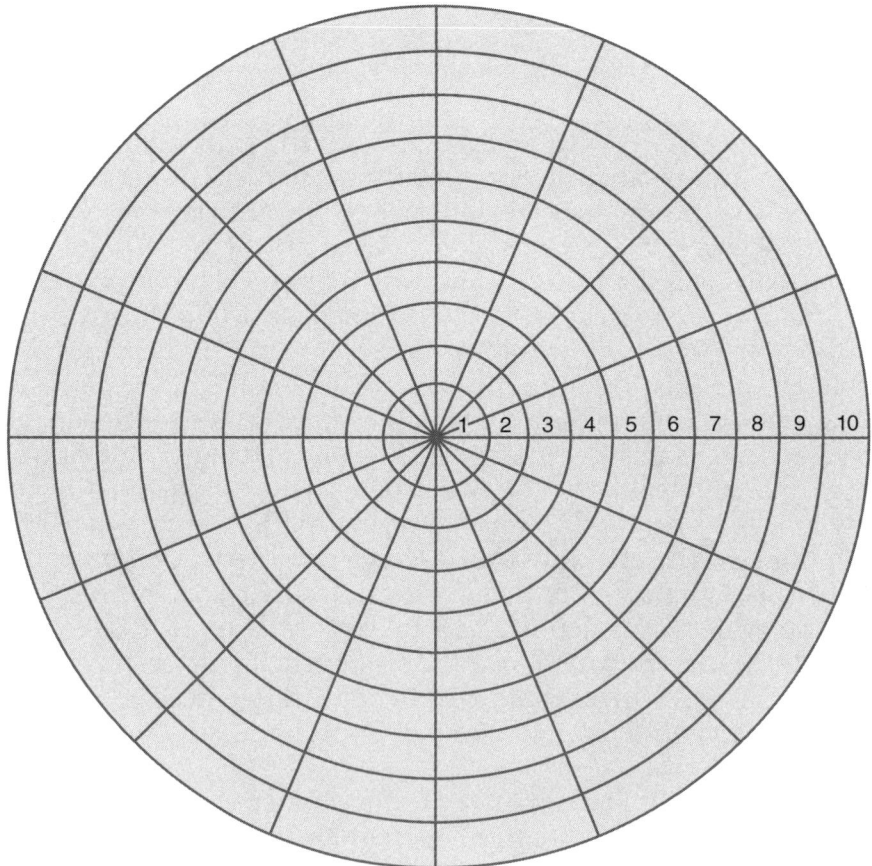

4. If you choose, ask your coach to add his/her rating of your proficiency with each of the skills identified, coloring in the wedges with a different color to see the differences.

From L. Brown and V. Ferrigno, 2015, *Training for speed, agility, and quickness*, 3rd ed. (Champaign, IL: Human Kinetics). Adapted from R.J. Butler and L. Hardy, 1992, "The performance profile: Theory and application," *The Sport Psychologist* 6(3): 253-264.

is important for effective performance. Also, a self-referenced evaluation often enhances adherence to an intervention program.

When completed, this profile provides a quick visual reference of the identified necessary mental skills, showing where the athlete has expertise (which can reinforce confidence and commitment) and where he should focus his energies for mental skills improvement.

Education

Once the coach has determined which of the athlete's skills to address, the next step, *education*, involves generating strategies for integrating these into existing training plans and actually teaching them to the athlete. The goal of this stage is to help the athlete recognize the importance of learning these mental skills and facilitate an applied understanding of how these skills can influence performance. Much of this chapter provides suggestions for how strength and conditioning coaches can do this.

Acquisition and Practice

The next phase, *acquisition and practice*, includes understanding the mental skills presented and then determining ways to individualize these to meet the athlete's performance goals. Many of the worksheets, questionnaires, and checklists in this chapter allow for individual assimilation of mental skills and provide tools for monitoring and evaluating progress in applying these skills.

Integration

The final stage, *integration*, is the end goal for a mental skills training program. This is where athletes find themselves making automatic adjustments and modifications to their performance, using their newly developed mental skills, to maximize their overall performance output.

Using the Cognitive Performance Pyramid

In reality, there are a number of potential mental skills that athletes might identify in the mental skills performance profile as being necessary for overall performance in their sport domains. However, for improved performance during speed, agility, and quickness training in and of itself, athletes and coaches should first focus on developing a few specific skills. These skills, the four Cs, form a hierarchical model of psychological skill development that will enhance any athlete's training program (see figure 3.2).

This model starts with *commitment* at its base. Commitment is the idea of dedicating yourself to a cause or making a promise to yourself. Embedded in this construct is the idea of motivation, for without motivation, a person is unlikely to commit to the action. The next level of the pyramid is *confidence*, or a belief in yourself and your ability to accomplish those tasks you set for yourself. Once an athlete forms a base of commitment and confidence, he needs to learn effective *concentration* skills. Attaining and maintaining appropriate focus during speed, agility, and quickness drills is imperative if the athlete is to get the most benefit from them. Last, in an effort to maintain consistency throughout the training cycle, the athlete will need to develop *composure*, or the ability to maintain

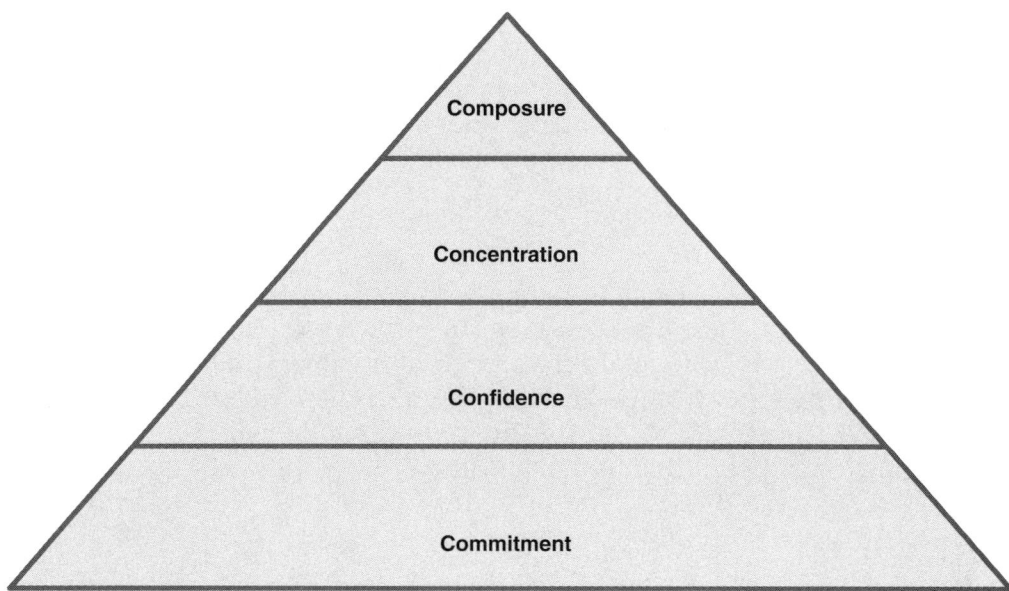

Figure 3.2 Cognitive performance pyramid.

self-control in performance. Once mastered, this progressional hierarchy of foundational psychological skills sets a base for further training in mental skills and can lead to the eventual development of mental toughness.

Commitment

Strength and conditioning coaches often wonder why some athletes seem highly committed to their training, are motivated each and every day they come to train, and constantly strive for success, while others seem to simply go through the motions, with little self-direction and minimal effort. The construct of commitment is challenging for coaches, predominantly because it is critically important for successful performance, and yet there is little the coach can do to mandate it. The athlete is solely in control of her own commitment levels. Others may help foster it, but ultimately, it is up to the athlete.

This construct of commitment goes hand in hand with motivation. Motivation is an inner condition that initiates, directs, and sustains one's behaviors. If an athlete is committed to his physical training program because he knows it will help improve his overall sport performance, he will likely show evidence of being motivated during training sessions. If he is lacking in commitment, low levels of motivation will result. An athlete who hates the feelings of fatigue that result from a hard speed workout may start slacking off during the drills, dropping intensity of motivation, or choose to avoid those training sessions altogether. This variable level of intensity can often be used as an outward indicator of an athlete's commitment level. Those who are highly committed to the training will choose to actively participate, make the most of every drill, and feel a sense of pride as a result of their participation in the activity.

Getting athletes to recognize that they—and only they—have control of their commitment levels is a needed first step for effective strength and conditioning training. Coaches can help athletes recognize this by initiating a conversation about why they are doing speed, agility, and quickness training in the first place. Asking them to identify what physical skills are needed to be effective in their sport will help them realize their own levels of commitment. Once they identify speed, agility, and quickness, coaches can explain how training plans will help get them there. This sets up athletes to think about their own commitment and motivation levels toward this training. The following Q&A exercise can be a good starting point. Coaches can ask the following:

1. How do you want to *feel* in regard to your ability to do your sport? What is your goal? What is the ideal?
2. What do you need to *do* to feel that way? What actions, behaviors, and beliefs will produce those outcomes?
3. *How* will you go about doing what you identified in the previous questions? What is your personal plan for generating the feeling you want to have?
4. What strategies will you use *when it gets challenging* to do what you set out to do? What is the plan for overcoming anticipated and unanticipated difficulties?

These questions force athletes to think about why they are doing the training, what they want to get from it, what they are willing to agree to in order to make it reality, and what they plan on doing when obstacles block their ability to be successful. When this is self-generated rather than imposed, it creates a sense of ownership over the training, and this ownership can enhance personal commitment.

Confidence

What we think influences what we feel, and what we feel in turn influences our behaviors. If we think confident thoughts, those thoughts generate feelings of excitement and determination. Feelings of excitement motivate us to take on challenges and push ourselves, thereby enhancing commitment to the goal. These are all necessary elements for successful physical training, but especially for speed, agility, and quickness because this type of training specificity often presents a new and challenging environment for the athlete. Lack of familiarity can generate feelings of apprehension and worry, which can in turn decrease an athlete's previously existing confidence levels.

Confidence is the belief that one's abilities in any given situation are greater than or equal to the imposed demands. It is the belief or trust that a person can successfully do what she set out to do. Confidence is critical for effective performance in any domain because of its vast range of influences. It can help regulate anxiety levels, facilitate effective focus, increase overall effort and commitment, motivate us to push ourselves past our perceived limits, and just generally helps us feel good.

Many athletes have their confidence shaken when introduced to new training methods. At the start of a new training cycle, the athlete may seem hesitant or resistant, choosing to revert back to methods that are more familiar to her. This is often a direct result of a perceived lack of ability in this new methodology. The athlete may not want to put herself in a situation where she will be shown her shortcomings or even where she could be perceived as less than skilled. Instead, she chooses to continue doing what she had been doing previously. This construct can be seen in a performer's volitions, or the choices she makes toward or away from certain activities. Confidence is a critical mediator upon a performer's choices. The spectrum of an athlete's volitions ranges from a stubborn "I won't do this" all the way up to an excited "I will commit to doing this" (Vernacchia, McGuire, and Cook 1996) (see figure 3.3). Confidence in oneself moves these volitions toward the positive end of this spectrum.

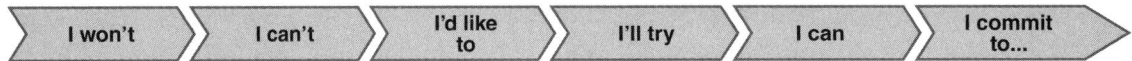

Figure 3.3 Spectrum of volition.

Moving athletes toward a willingness to try and eventually commit to new training modalities will come from improving their confidence in this new arena. Ways to generate confidence include creating situations where athletes can experience success, reinforcing successful efforts and progress as well as outcomes, and emphasizing how effective preparation and training will translate into greater likelihood of successful performance.

For coaches training a team or group, a great exercise for reinforcing training confidence is the activity on team training affirmations. Coaches training an individual can use other members of the training, coaching, and medical staffs as team members. To do this activity, list all team members' names along the left margin. Then make copies of this page and distribute them to each team member. Every team member writes one training strength he sees in each teammate listed. These can be strengths in mental, physical, technical, or tactical skills used in the training environment. Once all teammates have created affirmation statements, create a master list of all comments for the individual athletes, pulling all the relevant affirmations for each.

When athletes are introduced to new training modalities, it is all too easy for them to get hyperfocused and overly critical about those constructs they perform poorly. There are many new instructions and modifications to technique, all intended to improve an athlete's abilities in these new drills, yet as a result it sometimes becomes difficult to recognize what one does well. This affirmations activity can redirect the athlete's focus to what he is actually doing well, which is often a needed confidence boost during this time of unfamiliarity. This feeling of renewed confidence further challenges the athlete to continue striving for success even if he experiences temporary setbacks. This persistence is critical for the development of long-term performance gains such as speed, agility, and quickness.

Concentration

Concentration is the ability to maintain a clear and present focus on appropriate cues in a given situation and control responses to those cues for the execution of a particular skill. It is the athlete's ability to exert deliberate mental effort on what is most important in any given situation (Moran 2011). When performing new speed and agility training routines, many athletes need to improve their focusing and refocusing abilities—even if they have been taught these skills previously—because the nature of these drills can generate a number of distractions. Many of these activities occur outdoors, with multiple team members performing simultaneously, and require the athlete to follow specific instructions for safety and effectiveness—all characteristics that can strain an athlete's focus. Athletes in these environments will need to selectively attend to relevant information and ignore potential distractions while coordinating several simultaneous actions.

Distractions can be particularly detrimental for drills emphasizing speed of movement because speed and agility drills require more automatic processing of sensory feedback than other strength or endurance activities. This automated processing takes time and practice to generate. Controlled cognitive processing, which is generally seen in novice performers, creates slower movement patterns due to the level of instruction the performers are generating in their heads. Distractions at this stage of learning new skills, where athletes have yet to automate the movements, are particularly damaging because the athletes lose track of their cognitive instructions, inhibiting the completion of the activity. Once athletes attain automaticity in their technical skills, they tend to have extra mental capacity available to devote to other concurrent tasks, which can also increase distractibility if they are not trained to handle this appropriately (Moran 2011).

A focused mind requires deliberate mental effort and intentionality. In strength and conditioning training, particularly in the drills for speed and agility, a variety of factors can cause loss of appropriate focus. These include feeling anxious or uncertain about one's ability to perform the drill effectively, being fatigued from previous training or a cumulative fatigue from the events of the day, having inadequate motivation, or simply being distracted (thinking about other things). Additionally, a frequent cause of inappropriate focus in training drills is overanalysis of body mechanics while performing the drills. In essence, being overly focused on the kinesthetic can sometimes interfere with the appropriate focus on the overall movement activity.

A simple way of conceptualizing an athlete's concentration abilities uses terminology familiar to those in strength and conditioning environments. The ability to focus can be divided into three categories (USOC 2002):

1. *Strength of focus*: Is the athlete able to direct her attention to the proper point, keep it there, and shut out potential distractions?

2. *Flexibility of focus*: Is the athlete able to shift her focus quickly and accurately as needed during performance? Does she notice when focus is inappropriate and redirect it as necessary?

3. *Endurance of focus*: Is the athlete able to maintain her focus throughout the entire drill, even when she is fatigued or at the end of the training session?

A number of activities can help athletes better identify appropriate focus and manage their distractions in the performance environment, improving the strength, flexibility, and endurance of their focus. The first is simply a plan to increase recognition and awareness of the nature of the distractions and when they typically occur. During a designated training session, each athlete carries a three- by five-inch index card and a pencil. At any point during that training session, when an athlete recognizes distractions are present, she writes down what the distraction is—whether it is an external cue (e.g., other teammates, coaches watching drills, things in the environment) or an internal one (e.g., thinking about other things, distracting self-talk). At the end of that day's practice, the coach evaluates the types of distractions common to this group. If desired, this can be taken one step further by creating a team refocusing chart (USOC 2002) (see table 3.1) that adds coping responses and action plans for handling these distractions.

Table 3.1 Refocusing Chart

Distraction	Coping response to minimize negative impact	Self-talk cue
Negative comment by coach	Deep breath and positive affirmation	"I've got this. Stay focused!"
Self-doubt	Positive realistic affirmation	"This is a new skill. I'm getting it!"
Fatigue	Deep breath and motivational cue	"If it didn't make me tired, it wouldn't be making me better!"

Adapted, with permission, from U.S. Olympic Committee, 2002, *U.S. Olympic Committee coaches guide: Sport psychology training manual* (Colorado Springs, CO: USOC Coaching and Sport Sciences).

Another great activity for targeting appropriate focus can be integrated right into an athlete's existing training program: the "describe it" drill (USOC 2002). When the coach sees an athlete executing an speed, agility, and quickness drill correctly, he asks the athlete to stop and describe the feeling of the activity at that particular moment in her own words. The coach works with the athlete to develop targeted cue words that represent that feeling. These can be integrated into the athlete's self-talk to remind her of what she is trying to accomplish, and the coach can also use these reminders when communicating with the athlete the next time she does the drill. This activity also has the added benefit of enhancing confidence and commitment because it "catches" the athletes doing something right, which will often make them more excited to replicate the activity.

To generate endurance of focus, coaches can challenge their athletes to "lock in" their concentration for defined periods. Start small with a challenge to maintain appropriate focus throughout drills that can be completed in short spans of 30 seconds to 1 minute. At the end of each block, the coach takes a moment to evaluate how successfully the athletes were able to maintain focus. The activity is repeated with drills of slightly longer duration. Because this activity is done simultaneously with the existing training program, it adds only a few minutes of time (for the short debrief) to the overall daily training plan.

Recognizing, practicing, and repeatedly attaining the appropriate focus for any activity requires effort and intentionality. The ability to maintain concentration while immersed in a high-pressure environment is critical for optimal performance. Athletes cannot always eliminate distractions, but they can always control what they choose to focus on.

Composure

The final element of the cognitive performance pyramid is composure, or the ability to maintain self-control and manage emotion in any performance environment. Fatigue, inexperience, and frustration can all lead to a loss of composure during strength and conditioning training as well as in other performance environments. For athletes to perform effectively, they need to learn how to best manage their mental and physical energy levels. Athletes who deplete energy through worry, anger, frustration, or anxiety experience a greater likelihood of distraction and decreased self-confidence, and they have less energy for when they really need to perform.

Mental energy is generated, maintained, depleted, and refreshed via our emotions. Emotions are any strong feelings having both physical and psychological manifestations that energize behaviors. These energy-affecting emotions can have both beneficial and detrimental effects on human performance, often depending on how they are interpreted. Emotions can be beneficial to performance when they get us excited, cause us to feel motivated, elevate our self-confidence, and reinforce our commitment levels. However, emotion can be detrimental when there is either too much or too little (a performer being too "amped up" or too "flat") or when we lose control of our emotions and cease to function effectively in a performance environment (e.g., an athlete who cannot control his anger or frustration). Inappropriate energy levels can result in a lack of composure.

A strength and conditioning or sport coach is in an ideal position to help athletes develop their composure skills. The training environment provides a host of new and unfamiliar experiences that can produce anxiety. It also creates a multitude of opportunities to be evaluated for effectiveness, which can generate frustration and worry. By arming athletes with the mental tools to combat inappropriate thoughts, enhance confidence, and reinforce motivation and commitment, coaches are providing many of the skills necessary to allow athletes to maintain composure as well.

The goal of any composure-building exercise is to help the athlete think clearly under pressure and respond accordingly (TCUP + RA). Recognizing when inappropriate thoughts and feelings are draining energy and then doing something to regain appropriate focus is the first step. The energy awareness worksheet in figure 3.4 (USOC 2002) is an effective tool for helping athletes recognize what things drain or charge their mental and emotional batteries.

Every person has an ideal energy or activation level, so each athlete needs to determine what works best. With an awareness of his own activation level, the performer can take steps to elevate, decrease, or simply maintain his existing energy. Once an athlete realizes he is getting too "amped up" and needs to calm down, or recognizes he is too "flat" and needs to energize himself, the next step is coming up with a plan. The last two questions on the worksheet explore this idea. What has worked for the athlete in the past? What techniques is he already familiar with? The answers the athlete provides on those two questions are a good starting point for developing an action plan for handling composure issues.

If an athlete doesn't have a previously established technique for managing energy levels, there are a number of possible options. Following are several strategies athletes can try for both elevating and lowering energy levels for effective performance (USOC 2002).

- If an athlete is too energized and needs to calm down, following are a few tips that can help:
  - Slow down your breathing (take belly breaths).
  - Remove yourself from other people (take a personal time-out).
  - Remove yourself from chaotic surroundings.
  - Listen to calming music.
  - Choose a focal point and maintain focus on that spot.
  - Use calming self-talk.

Figure 3.4 Energy Awareness Worksheet

Think about how your mental and physical energy levels influence your ability to perform effectively in practice, training, and competition.

1. List three things that tend to **drain** your physical and emotional "batteries" for training, practice, or competition (things that make you feel drained, tired, or flat):

   a.

   b.

   c.

2. List three things that tend to **charge** your physical and emotional "batteries" for training, practice, or competition (things that make you feel fired up, energized, or psyched up):

   a.

   b.

   c.

3. Of the elements you have listed in the previous two questions, which do you have control over?

4. Which are totally out of your control?

5. What techniques would work for you when you need to charge your batteries (increase your energy levels for performance)?

6. What techniques would work for you when you need to intentionally drain your batteries (decrease your arousal level) to perform at your best?

From L. Brown and V. Ferrigno, 2015, *Training for speed, agility, and quickness*, 3rd ed. (Champaign, IL: Human Kinetics). Adapted, with permission, from U.S. Olympic Committee, 2002, *U.S. Olympic Committee coaches guide: Sport psychology training manual* (Colorado Springs, CO: USOC Coaching and Sport Sciences).

- If an athlete is too flat and needs to amp up, following are a few tips that can help:
  - Increase your breathing rate.
  - Get physically active.
  - Surround yourself with high-energy people.
  - Put yourself in high-energy environments.
  - Use energizing self-talk.

Finding and maintaining the appropriate energy level is essential, not only for maximum energy availability but also because of how it affects all the other concepts described in this chapter. For example, as energy levels increase past a desired level, the ability to focus appropriately decreases. Further, as anxiety, frustration, or anger increases, an athlete loses the ability to effectively process information. In essence, if an athlete's energy level moves outside of her ideal zone, it can lead to distraction and poor decision making. This is disastrous for speed, agility, and quickness training.

DEVELOPING MENTAL TOUGHNESS

People often talk about trying to improve their mental game because doing so will allow them to get into "the zone." This state of peak performance is absolutely a great thing to experience, but the reality is that the zone doesn't come along very often. Striving for this experience is an unrealistic goal, and expecting to reach it on any sort of regular basis is guaranteed to result in frequent disappointment. Furthermore, being in the zone is a passive experience—when you are there, you are somewhat like a spectator along for the ride. As soon as you recognize you are in the zone and then switch your focus to thinking about how great it is to be there, you are no longer in the zone. In reality, trying to get into the zone actually inhibits getting there.

Consistent effective performance in both training and competitive settings should not be motivated by an effort to get into the zone. Rather, it should be about developing consistent performance through effective motivation, commitment, focus, and composure. The characteristics of maintaining composure in challenging situations, keeping appropriate focus on a task, feeling confident, and being motivated to achieve success are foundational components for developing mental toughness. Mental toughness is the ability to consistently perform toward the upper range of your talent and skill regardless of competitive circumstances (Loehr 1986). It is about having the natural or developed psychological edge that enables you to generally cope better than your opponents with the many demands that sport places upon you, and to specifically be more consistent than your opponents in remaining determined, confident, and in control under pressure (Jones, Hanton, and Connaughton 2002). It is really about being able to think clearly under pressure and respond accordingly. A strength and conditioning coach, sport coach, or parent is in a prime position to introduce, influence, and reinforce a psychological skills training program for an athlete. Starting simply with the skills described in this chapter can create a solid foundation for improving performance in any domain, including training to enhance speed, agility, and quickness.

Chapter 4

Speed Training

Doug Lentz and Jay Dawes

The saying "speed kills" is used frequently in the sports world. For most sports such as football, soccer, basketball, field hockey, and tennis, the ability to start explosively from multiple positions is critical. Once an athlete initiates a sprint, he must be able to accelerate as quickly as possible for as long as 5 seconds. Beyond this point, and in many cases before it, an athlete may be required to slow down (or decelerate), change directions, and then reaccelerate to be effective. Consequently, learning how to start and accelerate in the most effective manner may mean the difference between victory and defeat.

To obtain maximal results from any speed program, athletes should incorporate drills that focus primarily on starting ability (or acceleration), maximal velocity, and speed endurance. This chapter includes guidelines and progressions that will enhance each of these attributes. In general, the drills range from basic to advanced. To enhance skill acquisition, athletes should learn and perfect the drills at slower speeds before going full speed.

Understanding the Main Components of Speed

Speed is generally thought of as simply moving fast. However, it can be broken down into several components. By gaining a better understanding of these components, coaches and athletes can determine which is most critical for their sport and focus on specific speed-development techniques that will provide the largest improvements in performance. In general, speed can be broken down into three main areas: (1) starting speed, or acceleration; (2) maximal velocity; and (3) speed endurance.

Acceleration

Acceleration can be defined as a change in the rate of velocity. Although in physics this change can be either positive (speed up) or negative (slow down), in the world of sports, acceleration typically refers to positive acceleration, whereas deceleration is commonly used to describe negative acceleration. For most sports, an athlete's ability to rapidly overcome inertia while in a stationary or near-stationary state to maximal or near-maximal speed is paramount to success. Several factors influence one's ability to accelerate. Improving any or all of them can enhance acceleration performance.

A considerable amount of research has been done on one of these factors, the starting technique of track athletes. According to Harland and Steele (1997), a sprinter leaves the starting blocks at a low angle relative to the ground (around 40 to 45 degrees from the horizontal plane). To minimize braking force, during the first two steps the body's center of mass should be well in front of the contacting foot (base of support). This allows the athlete to generate a large amount of force to overcome inertia and continue to accelerate down the track, particularly in the first 30 yards or meters.

In contrast to the track athlete, nontrack athletes do not have the benefit of using the blocks to accelerate. Rather, nontrack athletes must accelerate from a variety of stances, such as a stationary, rolling, or striding start. Typical field sport or court sport athletes initiate movement from an athletic stance, or ready position, whereby the ankles, knees, and hips are slightly flexed, with the feet either shoulder-width apart or in a staggered (split) stance. For these athletes, their weight should be shifted toward the forefoot while they remain balanced (e.g., not leaning too far forward, backward, or to the sides). Similar to a track start, athletes who initiate movement from this ready position must also project their center of mass forward so it is in front of their base of support.

Historically, athletes have been taught that it is counterproductive to sprint forward by first stepping back. This is commonly referred to as a false step. However, many professional athletes initiate movement from a stationary stance by utilizing this technique. In recent years, a mounting body of evidence has suggested that a quick back step, or rhythm step, may actually help optimize forward movement for some athletes. Recent studies suggest this technique may create greater impulse and more horizontal power, resulting in greater displacement compared with stepping forward first (Cronin et al. 2007; Cusick et al. 2014). This was found to be true in straight-ahead accelerations up to 10 meters (10 yards). Thus, teaching an athlete when and how to perform this technique may be beneficial for improving acceleration.

Maximal Velocity

Maximal velocity is the fastest velocity an athlete achieves in a speed bout. Many field sport athletes are able to attain maximal velocity at approximately 20 to 30 yards or meters. Track athletes are generally able to spend a greater time in the acceleration phase. These athletes typically reach maximal velocity between 40 and 50 yards or meters. This means they spend a greater amount of time in the acceleration phase than do field sport athletes.

When looking at the speed demands of athletes who participate in intermittent sports (most nontrack events), it becomes evident that these athletes are rarely able to reach their true maximal velocity (Duthie et al. 2006). This is due to the multiple changes of direction required over relatively short distances (5 to 15 yards or meters) to evade or elude a defender or to stop an attacker. For this reason, many coaches believe maximal velocity training is unimportant for these types of athletes. On the contrary, maximal speed training not only is a part of overall athletic development but also prepares these athletes for instances in which they are able to attain near-maximal velocity. However, it would likely be prudent to invest a significant amount of time learning how to start and accelerate more efficiently before spending a great deal of time learning and refining the mechanics that directly relate to maximal velocity.

Speed Endurance

The term *speed endurance* refers to an athlete's ability to repeatedly perform maximal or very near-maximal sprints at or near maximal speed. For track and field athletes competing in events over 40 yards or meters, it may not be the fastest athlete who wins the race but the athlete who slows down the least. For nontrack athletes, speed endurance may not necessarily be the ability to maintain speed during a single speed bout but instead the ability to maintain speed over multiple speed bouts. Outside of pure genetic potential, factors such as stride length, stride frequency, strength, power, mobility, flexibility, and proper technique all contribute to speed. Although not everyone can achieve world-class speed, most athletes can get faster via specialized training methods and techniques. This chapter includes guidelines for speed development, drills for maximal speed attainment, and information on other areas of significance that contribute to improved speed.

Stride Frequency and Stride Length

When seeking to improve speed, coaches try to influence two major components: stride length and stride frequency. Stride length is simply the distance covered with each subsequent foot strike, whereas stride frequency refers to an athlete's ability to repetitively cycle the legs quickly. Increasing stride length, stride frequency, or both will generally result in speed improvements.

Although these factors are interrelated, sometimes when athletes make a concerted effort to improve one they inadvertently hinder the other. For instance, in an effort to increase stride length, many athletes project the lead leg too far in front of the base of support. The end result is overstriding, with the athlete landing on the lead-leg heel. Consequently, this creates unwanted braking forces and a subsequent reduction in stride frequency, which inevitably results in a decrease in running speed. For this reason, it is critical when coaching to observe starts and acceleration to ensure the athletes maintain small shin angles (relative to the ground). This means the lower leg is always pointed in the intended direction of movement when in contact with the ground. Many of the elementary acceleration drills can help reinforce small, or positive, shin angles for the athletes.

Stride frequency, or the number of strides taken in a given amount of time or a specified distance, may be increased without sacrificing stride length if good form and technique are emphasized. Increasing stride frequency is important because the athlete can produce propulsive forces only when her feet are in contact with the ground. Therefore, the more often the feet touch the ground, the greater the athlete's potential to generate propulsive forces. However, during running the foot is in contact with the ground for just fractions of a second per stride. During this limited contact time, the athlete must generate a large amount of force to produce the power needed to generate explosive speed. For this reason, improving an athlete's overall strength and power, as well as her ability to produce force rapidly (rate of force development), is vital. In short, although a variety of methods can be used to improve strength and power, technique mastery allows the athlete to generate force rapidly via the optimal combination of stride length and frequency.

Recent research has explored the factors that differentiate acceleration ability in field sport athletes when compared with track athletes. It has been discovered that the amount of time the athlete's foot is in contact with the ground is a major step characteristic that distinguishes faster acceleration by field sport athletes and slower acceleration by the track sprinter. Contact time is a function of the force mechanics produced during the support phase of sprinting. Additionally, contact time and stride frequency were found to be the two most significant qualities for elite sprinters. It was deduced that for field sport acceleration, athletes who can accelerate faster will have lower contact times and may also have a higher step frequency.

Strength and Power

Researchers have also concluded that one's ability to produce force within a short time appears to be a key component in field sports. In fact, the majority of the current literature related to speed training reveals that faster field sport athletes tend to be more powerful and have greater strength in relation to their overall body mass. For this reason, it is suggested that strength and conditioning programs include explosive power movements (e.g., Olympic weightlifting, plyometrics, ballistic weight training) to help improve stride distance as well as high-speed movements (e.g., overspeed training, or assisted speed training) to improve stride frequency.

Mobility and Flexibility

Mobility generally refers to the amount and fluidity of movement around a joint, whereas flexibility refers to the extensibility of the muscle tissues. It is essential that athletes have the appropriate amount of mobility and flexibility to move the limbs through the required ranges of motion at the necessary speeds to produce efficient movement. For example, if an athlete has poor flexibility in the hamstrings, it may hinder the lift he is able to achieve on the lead leg, which would potentially restrict the athlete's hip mobility. This restriction may impede the athlete from getting his foot in the optimal position for the subsequent foot strike, causing reduced force production when the foot hits the ground. Poor flexibility and mobility not only may have a negative impact on performance but also may increase injury risk.

Proper Technique

Although the importance of strength and power for producing speed cannot be overstated, proper body positioning and proper sprinting technique should never be compromised when attempting to develop these attributes. Both coaches and athletes should be ever vigilant to emphasize proper sprint mechanics at all times when implementing speed and acceleration training programs. Proper mechanics allow the athlete to maximize the forces generated by the muscles at foot strike and reduce energy leaks as the forces are transferred from the ground up through the legs, trunk, and upper extremities. If poor technique is used, then greater biomechanical stresses are placed on the joints and the surrounding musculature, resulting in inefficient movement patterns and increased risk of injury. Good technique significantly improves neuromuscular efficiency and an athlete's ability to maximize her genetic potential. It also allows for smoother and more coordinated movements that contribute to faster running speeds.

There are three main elements to concentrate on with regard to proper sprinting mechanics: posture, arm action, and leg action (PAL) (Gambetta 2001).

Posture Posture refers to the alignment of the body. An athlete's posture changes depending on which phase of the sprinting cycle he is in. During acceleration, there is more of a pronounced lean. With track sprinters, body lean is around 40 to 45 degrees from the horizontal plane. This aids in overcoming inertia. As the athlete approaches his maximal running speed, posture should become more erect (around 80 degrees). Regardless of the phase of sprinting, one should be able to draw a straight line from the ankle of the supporting leg through the knee, hip, torso, and head when the athlete's leg is fully extended just before the foot loses contact with the ground.

The head should be in line with the torso and the torso in line with the legs (at full extension) at all times. Do not allow the head to sway or jerk in any direction. Making explosive starts and achieving maximal speed require extending the hip, knee, and ankle to maintain a relaxed neutral position with the jaw relaxed and loose. In regard to body lean, as previously mentioned, one should be able to draw a straight line, when looking from the side, through the center of the body at full leg extension during each stride. The body should have a pronounced forward lean during initial acceleration, progressing to a taller, more erect posture at maximal velocity. Athletes should concentrate on complete extension of the hip and knee joints as the foot pushes the body forward (training cue: "Think about pushing the ground away from you"). Younger athletes, who are not as physically developed, will have a tendency to become upright more quickly than older, stronger, and more powerful athletes.

Arm Action Arm action refers to the range of motion and velocity with which athletes use their arms. The movement of the arms counteracts the rotational forces generated by the legs. Because these leg forces are substantial, vigorous and coordinated arm movements are necessary to keep the body in proper alignment. This is important in all phases of sprinting, but it is crucial during the start and initial acceleration phase.

Aggressive arm action is a must. Each arm should move as a whole, with the elbow bent at 90 degrees. The hands remain relaxed, coming up to about chin level in front of the body and passing the buttocks in the back. Arm action must always be directly forward and backward, never side to side. Arm swing should originate from the shoulder without excessive flexion and extension of the elbows, which is a common mistake for many young athletes. During the downward motion of the arm, a slight straightening of the elbow will correspond with the longer leverage of the driving leg on the contralateral side of the body. The elbows should always remain close to the body. The hands may be kept open or slightly closed, but always relaxed. The athlete should keep the thumb side of the hand pointed forward and up at all times during the movement; the wrist should not move.

Leg Action Leg action refers to the relationship of the hips and legs relative to the torso and the ground. Making explosive starts and achieving maximal speed require extending the hip, knee, and ankle in a coordinated fashion to produce the greatest force possible against the ground. Also, in order to keep the stride frequency high and the stride length optimal, proper recovery mechanics—that is, what the leg does while it is not on the ground—are important.

The foot should remain in a dorsiflexed (toes up) position throughout the running cycle, except when the foot strikes the ground. In the acceleration phase, athletes should try to recover their heels quickly, with limited backside mechanics. In sprinting, backside mechanics refer to movements occurring behind the center of mass. Keeping heel recovery low (and noncyclical in nature) during starting and initial acceleration is very important. As the foot strikes the ground, weight should be on the ball of the foot (never on the heel), directly under the athlete. As the foot leaves the ground, it follows a path straight up toward the buttocks. Simultaneously, the knee rises up and the thigh is almost parallel to the ground. The foot then drops down below the knee. At this point, the knee is at an angle of approximately 90 degrees. The leg aggressively straightens down and underneath the body to the ground contact point. This process is repeated over and over with each leg. The greater the running speed, the higher the heel should kick up. Failure to achieve a high rear-heel kick will reduce stride frequency. Athletes should avoid placing the foot in front of the body when making contact with the ground. Foot placement in front of the body yields increased braking forces and significantly slower running speeds.

During acceleration, athletes should focus on trying to push into the ground with forceful steps. As the athlete transitions into more of a maximal velocity gait, he should practice running as lightly and quietly as possible with correct foot-to-ground contact. As he approaches top speed, the head is held high, the torso becomes more upright, the shoulders and head are relaxed, the driving leg is fully extended to the ground, and the heel of the recovery foot comes close to the buttocks.

Developing Speed Potential

Although there is no magic formula for developing or increasing maximal running speed, there are some specific guidelines that anyone can follow when training for speed improvement. Simply put, running brief and intense sprints with plenty of rest between repetitions is critical. Sound programs emphasize technique, starts, acceleration, plyometrics, speed endurance, and recovery. Following are guidelines for sound speed training programs:

Perform speed training at the beginning of the training session

The body's nervous system is responsible for muscular contraction speed and coordination. When trying to boost performance, it is critical that athletes perform high-quality work during each and every speed training session. Athletes who are training for increased sport speed must develop intense neuromuscular movements. When an athlete is in a fatigued state, it is more difficult to train with maximal effort as well as control the high level of muscular forces produced during sprint work. Consequently, the body is unable to maintain the appropriate body angles and positions necessary to transfer and generate the powerful forces produced at foot strike. Additionally, if the upper or lower extremities are fatigued, stride frequency may be compromised. Therefore, both the ability to learn and the ability to develop these movements are hindered, and it may even lead to injury as other muscle groups compensate to adjust to the stress being placed on the body. It is also a poor idea to conduct a speed training session if the athlete is significantly tired, sore, or fatigued from a previous training session. A tired, sore, or overtrained athlete cannot maximize speed potential.

Perfect practice makes perfect

Proper sprinting technique is mastered through the execution of numerous training drills and repetitions over a long time. Thus, it is critical when performing these drills that both the coach and athlete demand strict form and technique on every repetition. Otherwise, poor motor patterns are developed that lead to bad habits that inevitably will need to be broken to maximize sprint technique. Developing an athlete's optimal speed potential requires many months, and even years, of hard work emphasizing thousands of repetitions using purposeful training drills, such as the ones found in this text.

Changes in performance are usually much greater and more rapid during the initial stages of motor skill acquisition. As practice continues, the amount of improvement realized becomes smaller. This is known as the law of diminishing returns. As a person gets closer to recognizing her potential, the gains she experiences are much more marginal. A long-held motor skill acquisition theory embraces a three-stage process of motor learning that incorporates a cognitive stage, an associative stage, and an autonomous stage. During the cognitive stage of skill development, the greatest challenge for the athlete is to understand what is to be performed. The biggest challenge for the coach is conveying to the athlete what is to be done. Performance gains are normally quite large, especially during the initial part of this stage.

The athlete moves into the associative stage as he learns a movement strategy and performs the skill. The athlete then begins to modify how the movement is performed based on the coach's feedback. At this stage the coach should focus on asking athletes to evaluate their performance rather than simply telling them what they need to do. Asking athletes to provide feedback about how a movement felt, where certain body parts may have been when executing the task, and what they should focus on during the running task is important during this stage. This helps athletes improve their internal feedback mechanisms, reduces reliance on the coach, and moves them closer to the autonomous stage of learning (Jeffreys 2009).

The third and final stage of motor skill acquisition, the autonomous phase, appears after extensive training with hours and hours of practice. This stage can be characterized by motor movements being performed automatically and devoid of any real stress. It is during this stage that the athletes can train in a truly relaxed state. In essence, this is similar to cruise control when driving. The athlete does not have to make a conscious effort to move or execute a task in a specific manner—it just comes automatically.

Ensure all sets and repetitions within a speed workout are accompanied by adequate rest

Any sprint drill that lasts 6 to 8 seconds, at a maximal or near-maximal effort, will have placed significant stress on the short-term anaerobic energy system (ATP–CP) and the central nervous system (CNS). A one to four (1:4) work-to-rest ratio is recommended as a good estimate; however, slightly larger ratios may produce even better results if optimizing speed is the priority. The ATP–CP energy system relies heavily on stored adenosine triphosphate (ATP) and creatine phosphate (CP) to sustain exercise intensity during short, explosive bouts of training. In general the human body stores approximately three ounces of ATP and about five to six times this amount of CP. During intense bouts of exercise, stored ATP and CP are used relatively quickly because they are the preferred source of energy during these activities. To allow this energy system to fully recover would take up to 5 minutes between repetitions.

Exercise recovery refers to the bodily systems' return to a preexercise state after a bout of exercise. An athlete's ability to perform maximally on repeated exercise bouts is influenced by the activity and the subsequent recovery periods. In repeated exercise bouts, if the recovery period is less than a few minutes long, as is the case in many team sports, the ATP–CP stores may be only partially restored before the onset of additional exercise demands. This in turn will result in compromised performance on successive bouts.

The length of the recovery interval between high-intensity bouts of exercise will also affect recovery. Unfortunately, in sports requiring intermittent bursts of all-out effort, the recovery periods may last only a few seconds; therefore, performance on subsequent bouts may suffer.

Figure 4.1 shows the results of a 20-meter repeat sprint ability test. In this test the athlete was required to run 20 meters with only 10 seconds of rest between intervals. The test was terminated after the athlete ran 10 sprints. Although this is a common test to determine speed endurance for athletes in intermittent sports, there is a sharp drop-off in speed with each successive repetition. In contrast, figure 4.2 displays the same test with a 30-second rest between bouts. Notice as the rest intervals increase, the drop in speed is less dramatic. Thus, to train speed, a greater rest period would be needed to ensure that athletes are able to perform each sprint at closer to their best effort.

The same is true of speed training—a 30-second rest interval after 6 seconds of high-intensity speed work may appear sufficient; however, 45 to 60 seconds of rest would likely lead to even better results. Performing shorter rest intervals may promote the development of speed endurance. This attribute would be beneficial for athletes who are involved in mixed sports, such as basketball and soccer, which rely heavily on both the aerobic and anaerobic energy systems. This method of training should be used sparingly with younger athletes and be employed only after technique mastery has occurred. Furthermore, if the rest intervals do not allow athletes to maintain good form and technique, the training session should be either stopped or the amount of time between repetitions (rest) should be increased to allow greater recovery and better maintenance of technique.

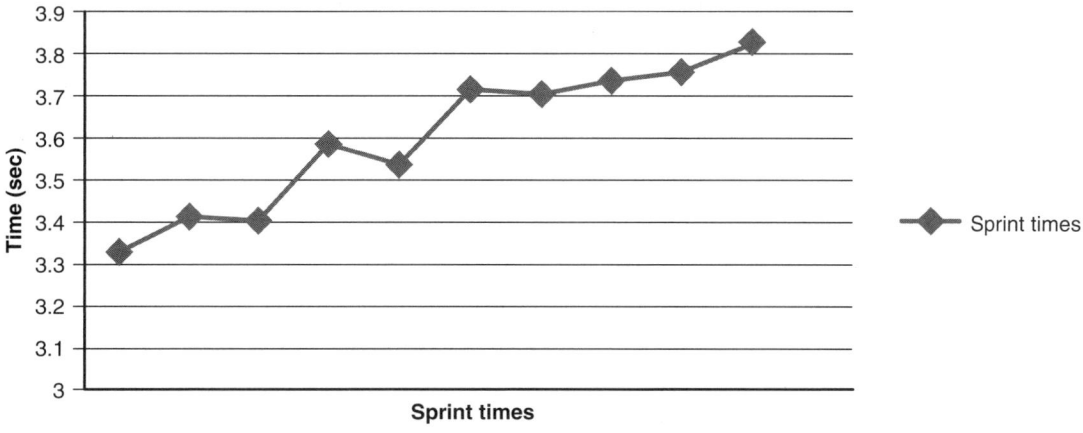

Figure 4.1 Repeat sprint ability times with 10-second rest.

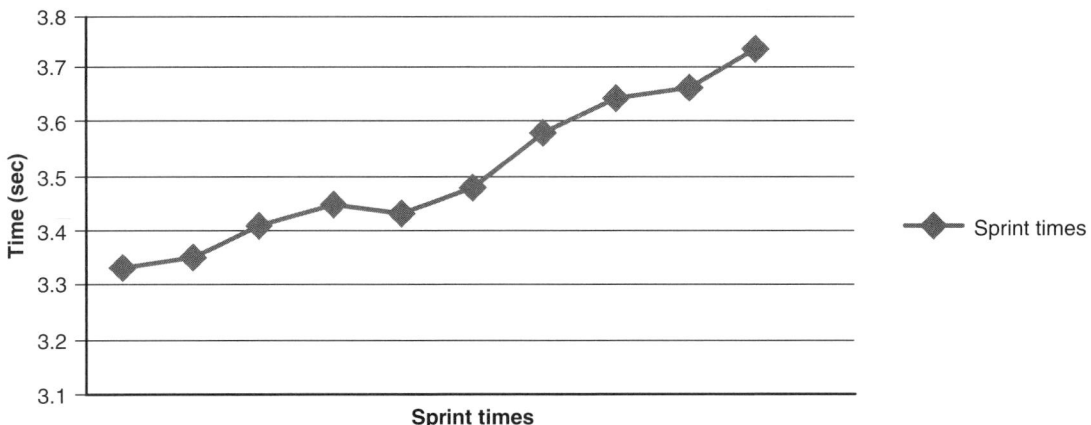

Figure 4.2 Repeat sprint ability times with 30-second rest.

Vary the intensity of the speed sessions between light, medium, and heavy days

Back-to-back days of hard sprint training would not be beneficial for speed enhancement because it may inhibit recovery. Coaches may want to distinguish their speed workouts by the intensity or speed, the duration (which is normally measured by time or distance), and the degree of total fatigue that is created by each drill and the total workout.

For example, a light workout might be characterized as having short to medium durations and low to medium stress or fatigue. A light day most normally follows a heavy day of sprint training within the total training program. A medium day might be characterized by medium to high intensity, short to long durations, and medium to high stress. For example, a coach who is planning a day of drills with high intensity would also incorporate longer rest intervals so as not to fatigue the athlete prematurely. A heavy day could be characterized by high intensity, medium to long durations, and high stress or fatigue levels. These are the most difficult of the speed workouts, and it is advised that they not be performed too close to a competition. Also, heavy speed training days should never be performed more than one day per week.

Track the total distance run by the athlete during each speed workout

As was previously mentioned, an overtrained or overly fatigued athlete will be unable to optimally reap the benefits of her speed workouts. Preplanning speed training workouts is every bit as important as preplanning the conditioning and strength or power component of a total workout plan. Failure to adequately plan for the speed training segment will most likely lead to injuries or subpar performances. Tracking the total distance of each speed session minimizes the chances of having less than desirable results.

To fully achieve maximal speed, the athlete must learn to run in a relaxed manner while at the same time producing maximal effort

This is much easier said than done, especially with junior and senior high school athletes. Overexertion will produce extraneous body movements, which will detract from the power required to go fast. Tight muscles do not move as quickly as those that are more relaxed. Relaxed athletes will sprint faster than similarly matched unrelaxed athletes. This is because they are better able to utilize the stored elastic energy created when the muscles are rapidly stretched during the sprinting motion. For example, when the arms are swung back, the muscles of the shoulders experience a rapid stretch. This stretch builds up potential energy within the shoulders and helps the athlete explosively swing the arms forward during the sprinting action. If these muscles are tightened through muscular contraction, not as much elastic energy will be stored as when there is less tension within the muscles.

Athletes must learn how to turn muscle contractions on and off extremely quickly; this is one critical aspect of sprinting. The ability to rapidly contract a relaxed muscle can enhance the speed and force of the muscular contraction. As with any learning process, for relaxation to become second nature, the skills must be rehearsed over and over during training.

Train acceleration, maximal velocity, and speed endurance separately

Whether an athlete should engage in more acceleration or speed training can be determined by taking split times to separate acceleration from maximal speed. For example, figure 4.3 shows a sample of the split times for four different athletes over 10 meters (acceleration speed) and 30 meters. In this example, both Joe and Devin had the best acceleration times as well as the fastest overall times. Between Steven and Mitch, you will see that Steven had a better acceleration time (10-meter distance) than Mitch; however, Mitch had a better 30-meter time. This chart helps clarify two points: (1) Each of these speed attributes is different, and (2) to improve each they should be trained differently. This information may also help guide a coach's training decisions. For instance, it appears that Mitch may benefit from more acceleration training, whereas Steven may benefit from more maximal velocity training.

All sports require some level of speed endurance; however, there is a significant difference between the speed endurance needs of a volleyball player versus a soccer player. All speed endurance programs should be designed with the respective sport's primary energy system in mind. Although the aerobic energy system may not be the predominant system called on during a particular sport, a well-conditioned aerobic system will aid in overall speed endurance maintenance. This is not to be confused with the need for a high $\dot{V}O_2$ max. Any attempt to maximize one's pure aerobic capacity will most likely result in overall speed decrements. Thus, altering the rest periods between certain speed drills or utilizing drills such as the 150- and 300-yard shuttle would be more suited to athletes in more strength and power sports. It should be noted that

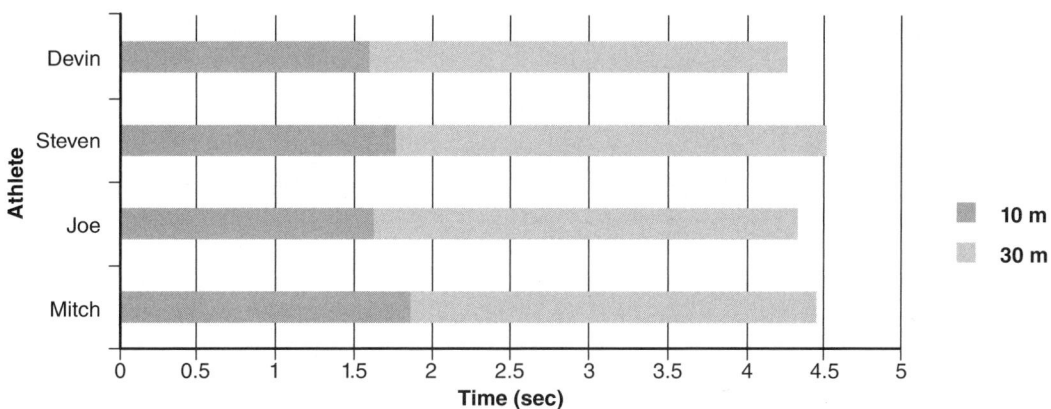

Figure 4.3 Split times for a 30 m sprint.

the recovery intervals selected to enhance speed endurance should always have the athlete's sport-specific needs in mind.

Speed endurance can be developed by running longer intervals, 165 to 440 yards (150 to 400 m), or by decreasing the rest between short intervals between 20 and 65 yards (18 and 50 m). The latter is a good choice for many sport-specific applications in which the sport is characterized by quick accelerations over relatively short distances.

Precede all speed workouts with a dynamic warm-up and flexibility routine, which will prepare the athlete for maximal efforts

According to Jeffreys (2009), performing a dynamic warm-up routine before speed training offers numerous benefits. A dynamic warm-up facilitates faster muscle contraction and relaxation of the agonist (working or contracting) and antagonist (opposing) muscle groups, improved blood flow and oxygen delivery to the active muscles, and decreased viscosity within the bodily tissues. This allows greater rates of strength, power, and force development to be displayed. Additionally, it may help improve quickness because it could potentially reduce total movement time via faster reaction times.

The warm-up is an essential component of any speed training session and should not be skipped. Many of the foundational movement patterns required to maximize speed should be addressed during this component of the workout. This portion of the speed training session should reinforce the motor skills that will be exhibited in the main speed session and should receive the same amount of attention. Basic progressions during the dynamic warm-up routine should transition from simple general mobility and flexibility drills to more specific and complex drills. Initially, drills should be performed at slower movement speeds and progress to faster speeds as the athlete's body temperature, respiration rate, and perspiration rate increase.

As athletes become more proficient at speed training drills, many of the drills that were once part of the speed session can be used as part of the dynamic warm-up. In many cases, if this portion of the warm-up is performed as just described, it may be difficult for athletes to differentiate between when the warm-up has been completed and the actual speed training session has begun. Accordingly, as the fundamental and remedial speed drills (which were originally introduced and utilized in the dynamic warm-up) are mastered, they may be replaced by slightly more advanced drills in the warm-up (e.g., begin with marches, then progress to skips, then progress to actual sprinting movements within the warm-up).

Speed Training Drills

The drills in this section focus primarily on the appropriate technique for starting from a stationary position, the technique for accelerating while in motion, and the foundations of top-speed mechanics. Mastering these techniques will significantly enhance an athlete's opportunity for success and provide the basic skills needed to reach his speed potential.

ACCELERATION DRILLS

Punch Wall Drill

1

Purpose
To reinforce proper body positioning and alignment, especially during acceleration. This drill is the first in the wall drill series.

Procedure
- Stand on the balls of both feet and lean against a wall at about a 45- to 60-degree angle, with the arms supporting the body.
- Keeping the body tall and tight, raise one thigh approximately parallel to the floor, with the ankle locked in a dorsiflexed position, on the command "Punch" (see figure).
- The recovery lower leg should maintain an angle that is parallel to the stance leg.

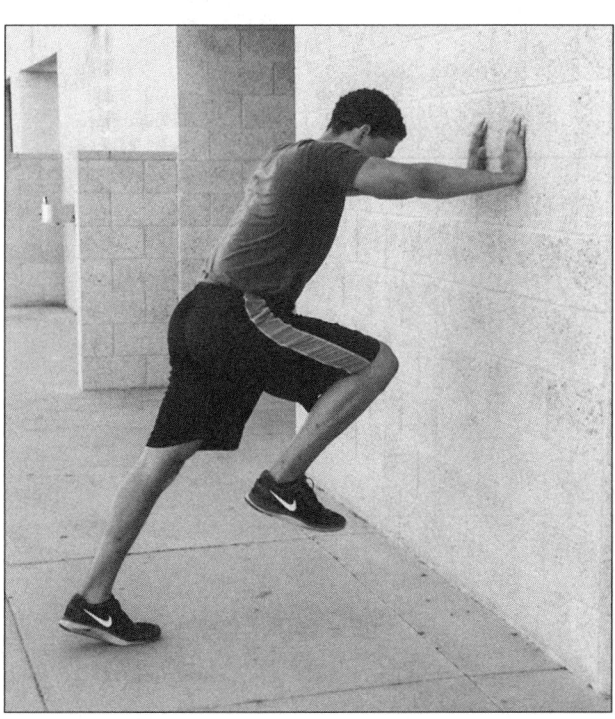

2
Drive Wall Drill

Purpose

To reinforce acceleration mechanics. This teaches the athlete to drive the ball of the foot back into the ground in a piston-like fashion. This drill should be mastered before moving on to the one, two, three, five step wall drill.

Procedure

- Stand on the balls of both feet and lean against a wall at about a 45- to 60-degree angle, with the arms supporting the body.
- Keeping the body tall and tight, raise one thigh approximately parallel to the floor, with the ankle locked in a dorsiflexed position.
- On the command "Drive," the recovery leg should drive down and back into the ground. Remain on the balls of the feet at all times.

3

One, Two, Three, Five Step Wall Drill

Purpose

To reinforce proper posture and leg action of acceleration mechanics. This drill should be mastered before moving on to the continuous wall drill.

Procedure

- Stand on the balls of both feet and lean against a wall at about a 45- to 60-degree angle, with the arms supporting the body.
- Keeping the body tall and tight, raise one thigh approximately parallel to the floor, with the ankle locked in a dorsiflexed position.
- Drive the leg down and back into the ground the number of times (one, two, three, five) called out by the coach.

4

Continuous Wall Drill

Purpose
To mimic a short acceleration sprint and ensure proper mechanics throughout the acceleration phase. This drill should be performed after the previous wall drills have been mastered.

Procedure
- Perform the wall drill in a continuous manner for 4 to 6 seconds.
- Ensure proper body position is maintained (do not round back or shoulders).
- Continue to drive the foot back and downward, and the opposite knee toward the chest throughout the drill rather than simply picking up the feet.
- Maintain a toe up knee up position.

5

On-Command Wall Drill

Purpose
This is an advanced progression in the wall drill series. The coach watches for proper mechanics while the athlete reacts and responds appropriately to the coach's commands.

Procedure
- This drill is performed in the same manner as the one, two, three, five step wall drill; however, the coach calls out a number (1, 2, 3, 5) at random.
- Respond by producing the appropriate movement pattern to the step count.

6

Seated Arm Swings

Purpose

To train the correct position of the arms as the hands pass the lowest point of the swing by avoiding contact with the ground.

Procedure

- Sit on the floor with legs straight out in front and arms at the sides at a 90-degree angle (see figure *a*).
- Swing the arms so that the hands come up to about shoulder level in front of the body and pass the gluteus in the back (see figure *b*). The hands are relaxed.
- Each arm should move as one unit, with the elbow bent at about 90 degrees. The arm action should be forward and back without crossing the midline of the body.
- Be careful not to bounce off the floor as the drill becomes more vigorous.

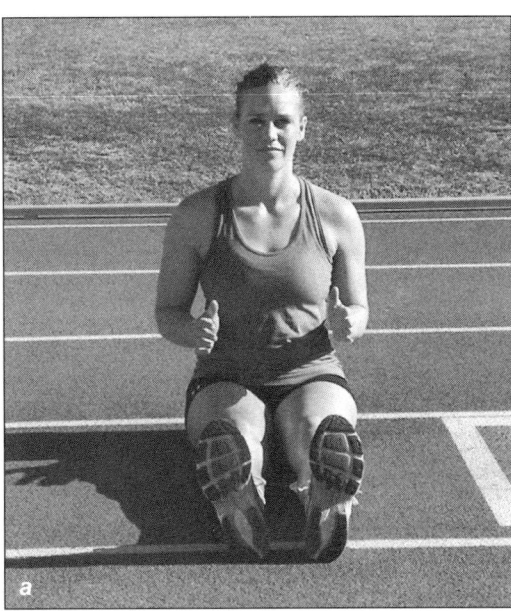 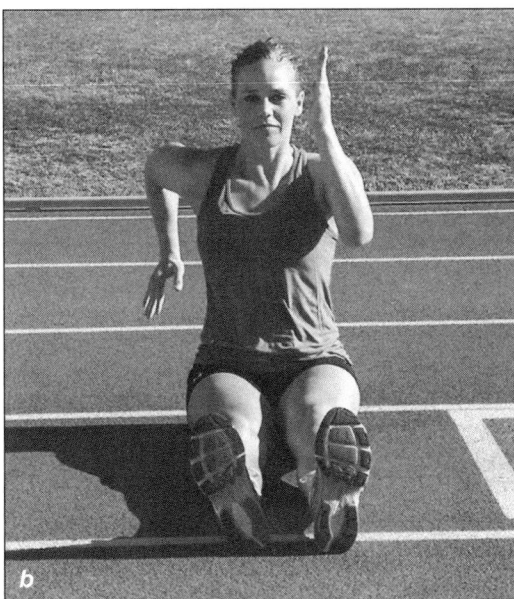

Standing Arm Swings

Purpose

To improve running mechanics and speed by providing teaching cues for upper body movement while in a stationary position.

Procedure

- Stand with the feet together and arms at sides at a 90-degree angle (see figure *a*).
- Swing the arms in a sprinting motion so that the hands come up to about shoulder level in front of the body and pass the gluteus in the back (see figure *b*). The hands are relaxed.
- Each arm should move as one unit, with the elbow bent at about 90 degrees.
- The arm action should be forward and back without crossing the midline of the body.

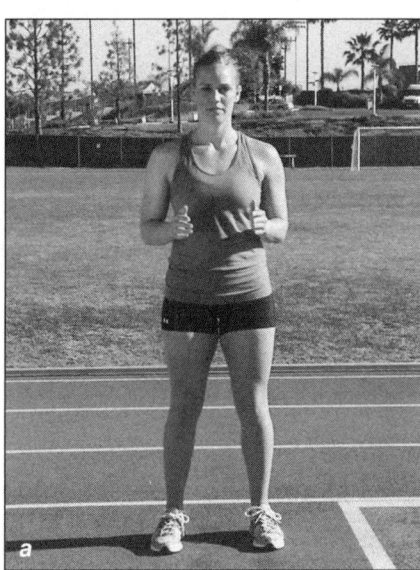 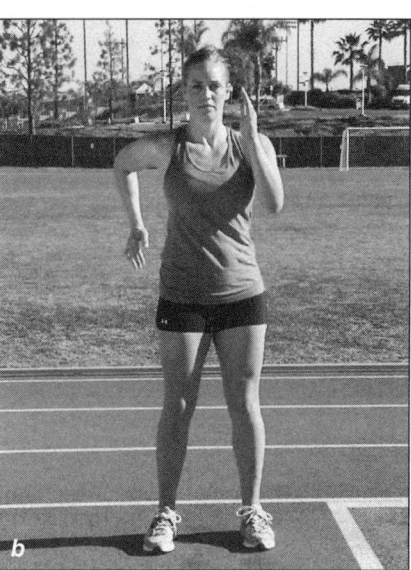

8

Forward A March

Purpose

The A march is a prerequisite to the A skip. The A march reinforces proper acceleration mechanics and foot speed. This drill should be mastered before moving on to more advanced drills.

Procedure

- March using perfect posture and arm action.
- Bring the knee on the recovery leg high, and keep it fully flexed while keeping the ankle close to the gluteus and dorsiflexed (see figure *a-b*).
- When the recovery knee is at the highest point, the opposite ground foot should emphasize plantar flexion.

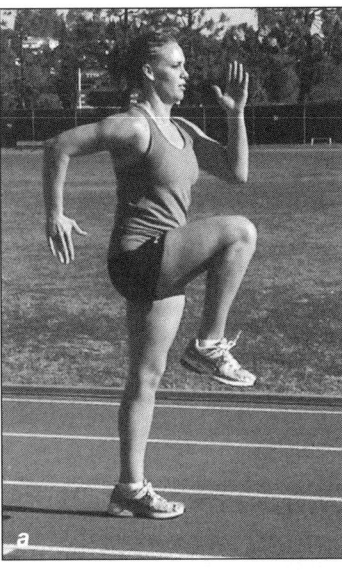 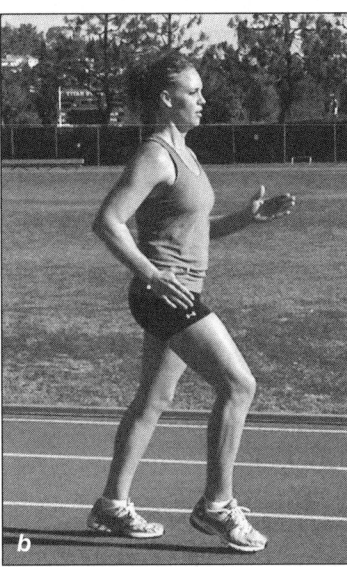 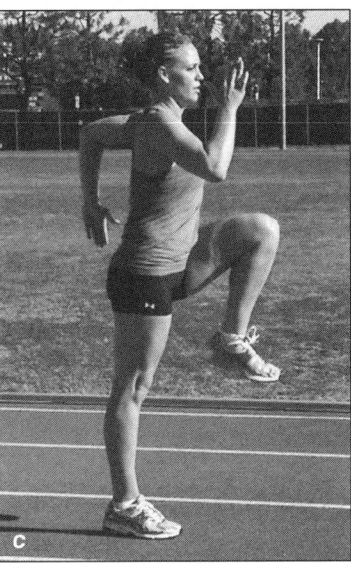

Quick Feet and High Knees

Purpose

To work on stride frequency while maintaining proper sprinting (acceleration) mechanics.

Procedure

- This drill is performed in the same manner as the A march; however, there is a greater emphasis on stride frequency within a relatively short distance.
- Thighs should *not* exceed parallel to ground height.
- Focus on striking the ground forcefully with the balls of the feet while spending as little time in contact with the ground as possible (see figure *a-b*).
- To emphasize the speed of movement required, visualize the feet landing on hot coals.

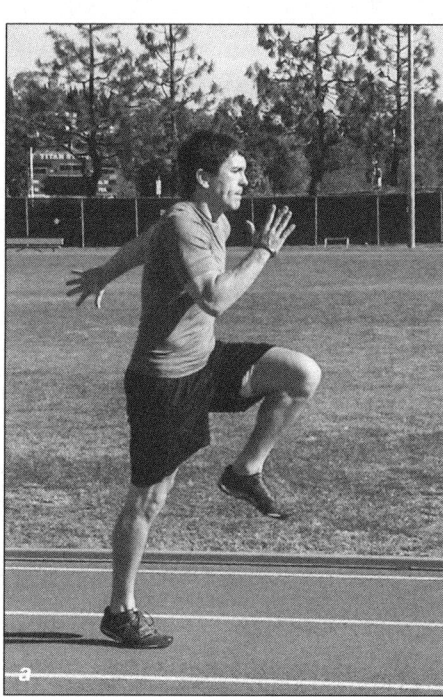
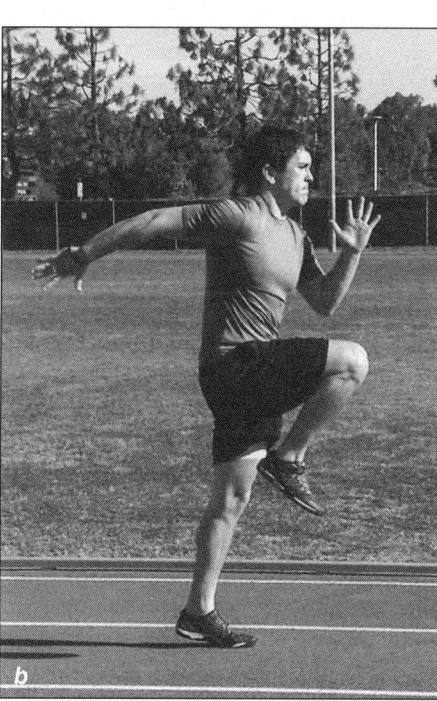

10
Acceleration Heel Kicks

Purpose

To increase foot speed while minimizing backside mechanics.

Procedure

- From a jog, pull the heel of the lower leg up to bounce off the gluteus (see figure *a-c*).
- As the leg bends, the knee should come forward and up.
- During acceleration, especially the first six to eight steps, you want to minimize backside mechanics, which refer to movements occurring behind the center of mass.

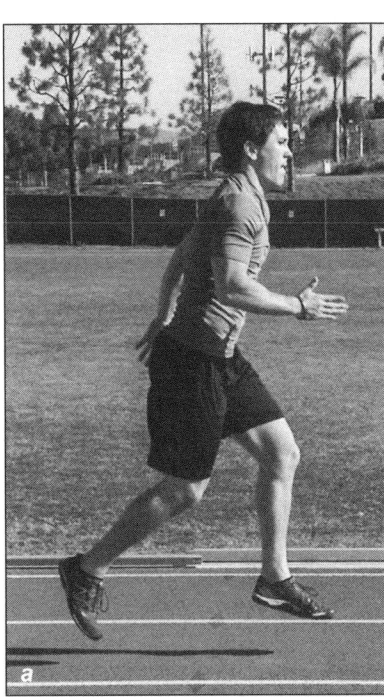 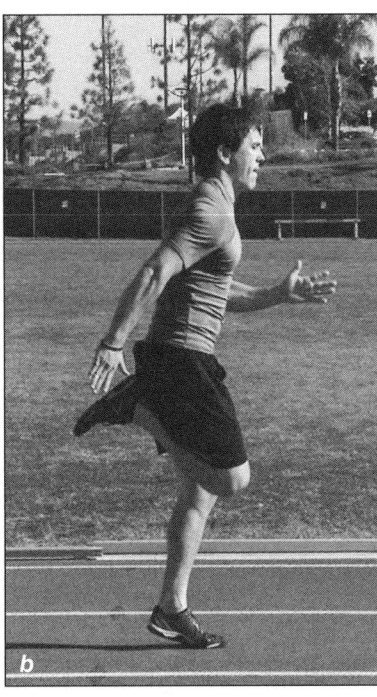 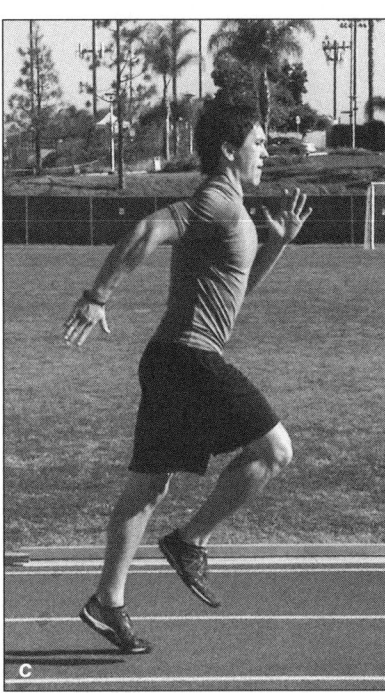

Ankling

Purpose

To increase foot speed and elastic ankle strength.

Procedure

- Jog with very short steps, landing and pushing off the balls of the foot (see figure *a-c*).
- Minimize ground contact and maximize foot contact.
- Emphasize the plantar flexion phase of ground contact and low foot recovery.
- Keep quiet but fast feet.

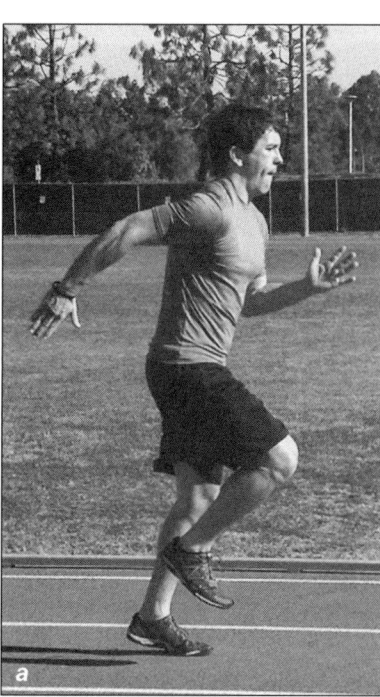
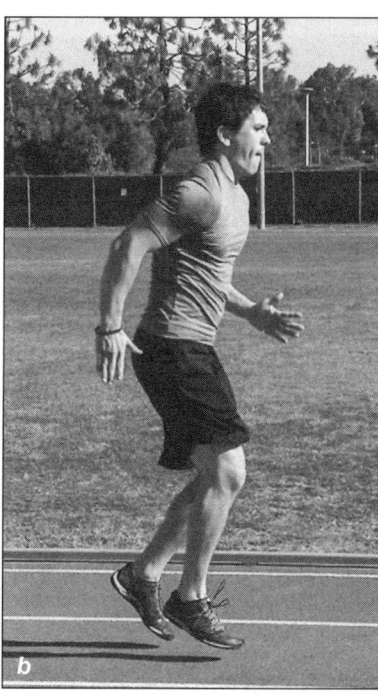
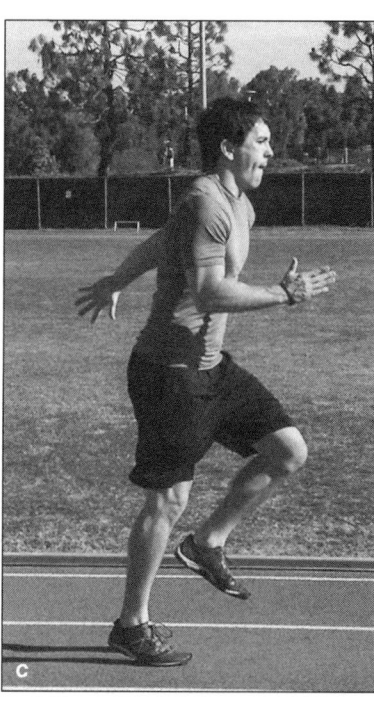

12 Prancing

Purpose

To introduce an elementary progression for bounding.

Procedure

- Begin in a standing position with a slight knee bend and the hips in a forward tilt position.
- During takeoff, push the hips forward and upward, with the knee of one leg recovering forward (see figure *a* and *b*).
- After landing, repeat the takeoff with the opposite knee recovering forward (see figure *c*).
- Both feet should land simultaneously, and both ankles remain in a dorsiflexed, or locked, position.

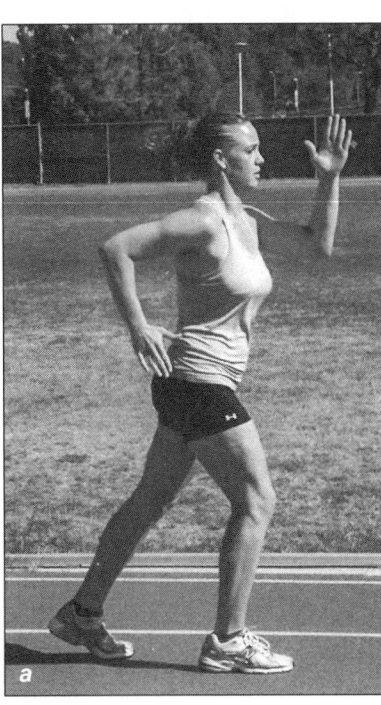 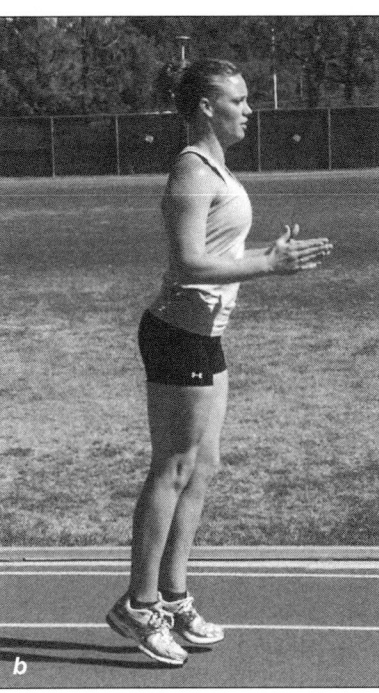 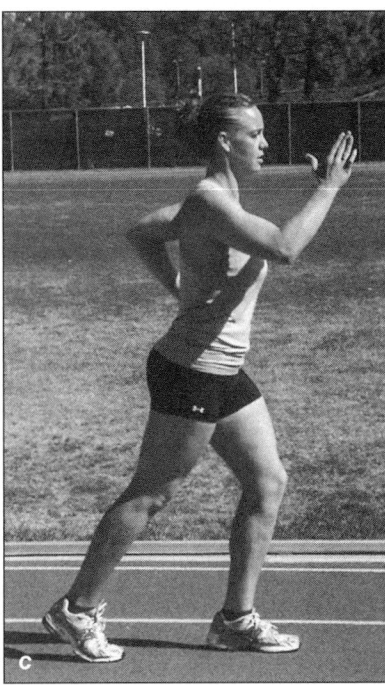

13

Skip for Max Height and Distance

Purpose

To increase hip extension and flexion strength, improve ankle-muscle stiffness, and enhance hip and leg power and stride length.

Procedure

- Skip, driving the free knee upward as aggressively as possible (see figure *a-c*).
- Use an aggressive arm action.
- Try to skip as high and as far as possible on each jump.

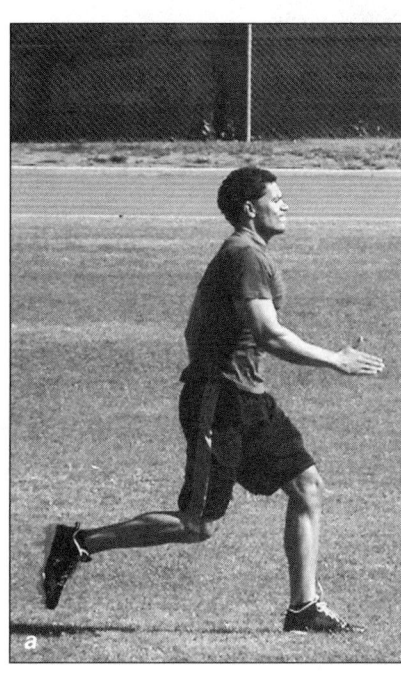
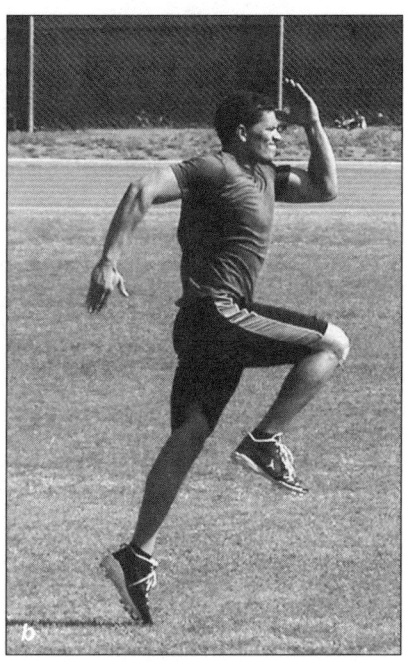
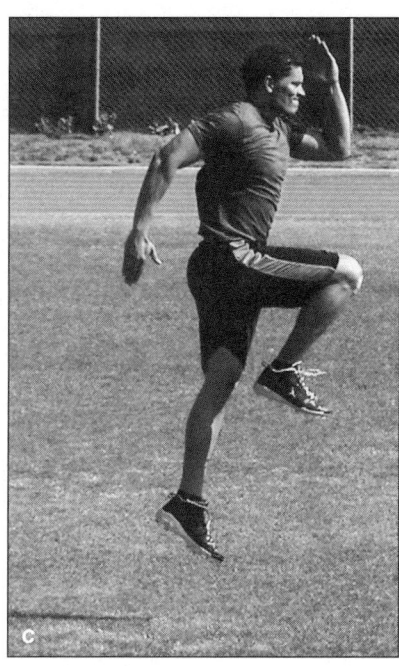

14

Straight-Leg Shuffle

Purpose
To increase hip strength and elastic ankle strength.

Procedure
- Run while keeping the legs straight and the foot dorsiflexed (see figure *a-c*).
- Emphasize fast ground contacts with the ball of the foot and pulling through with the hips.

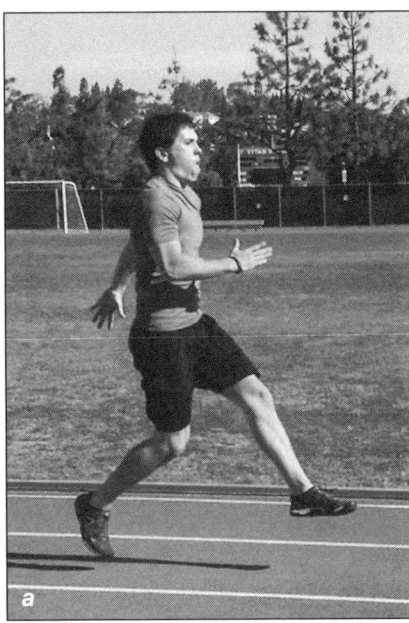
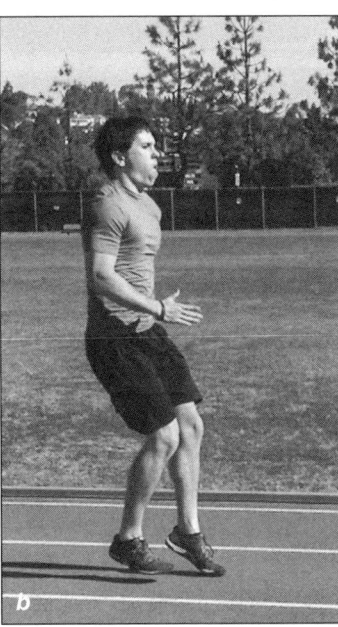
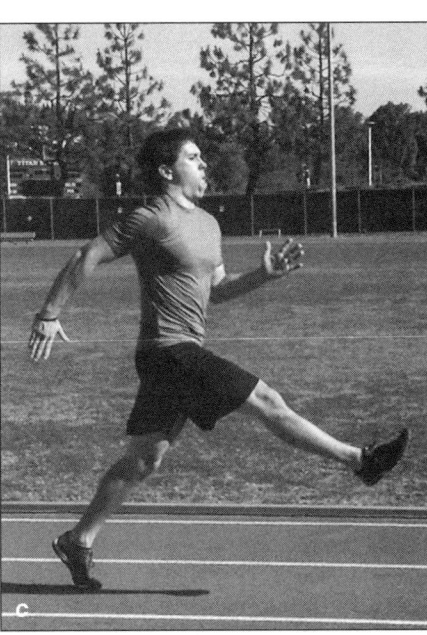

Straight-Leg Bounds

Purpose

To increase hip strength, elastic ankle strength, and stride length.

Procedure

- Run explosively while keeping the legs straight and the foot dorsiflexed (see figure *a-c*).
- Emphasize fast ground contacts with the ball of the foot, and spring forward while keeping a tall posture and without leaning back.

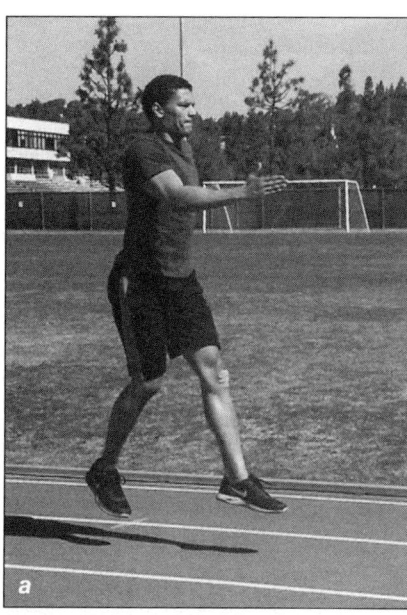 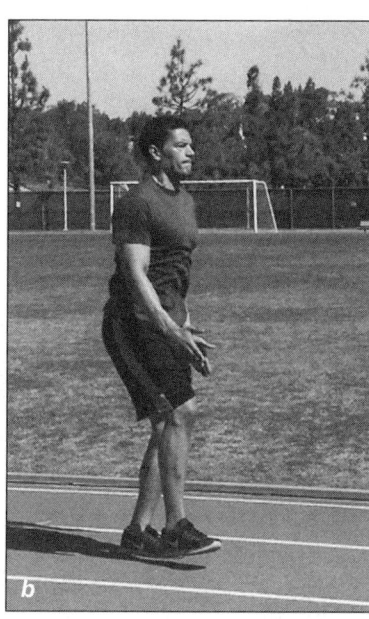 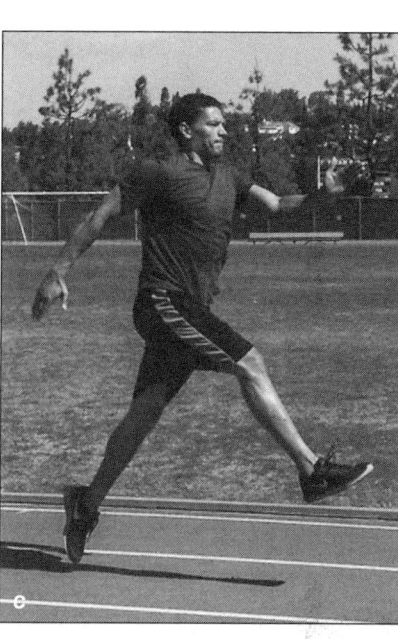

16

A Skip

Purpose

To increase hip extension, flexion strength, and ankle-muscle stiffness.

Procedure

- Skip using perfect posture and arm action. Bring the knee on the recovery leg high and keep it fully flexed while keeping the ankle close to the gluteus and dorsiflexed (see figure *a-c*).
- While in the air, emphasize the high recovery posture used in the A march.
- Keep the upper body in an upright and steady position at all times; the foot strike should be quiet but explosive, emphasizing muscle stiffness at the ankle.
- Be careful not to slam the foot onto the ground.

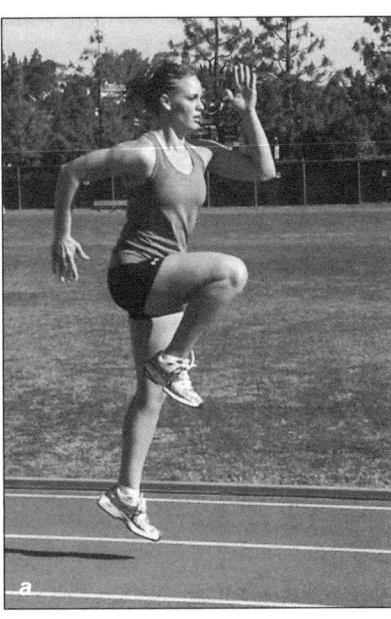 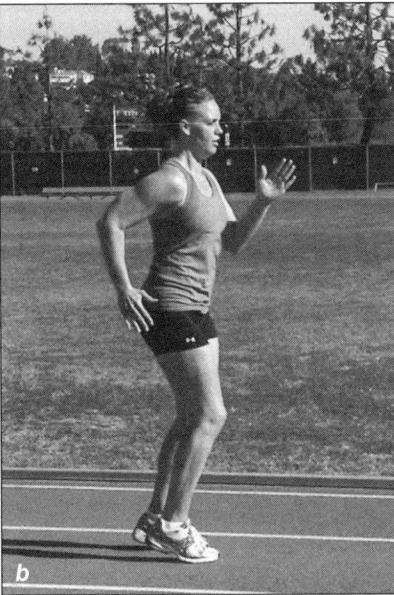 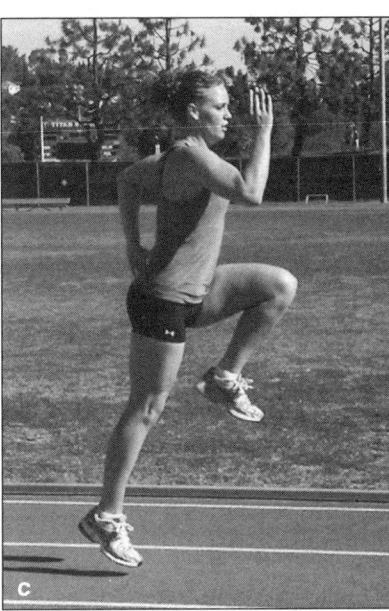

17

Single-Leg A Skip

Purpose

To increase hip extension, flexion strength, and ankle-muscle stiffness. This is a progressive variation of the A skip.

Procedure

- Skip with the same mechanics as for the A skip, except skip with the right leg only, making sure to drive the right foot into the ground; keep the left leg straight.
- The trail leg should remain slightly behind the body and be used as support during each skip.
- Stay on the ball of the foot at foot contact.
- Be sure to fully extend the hips, knees, and ankles.
- Maintain a good arm swing throughout.
- Repeat on the other leg.

18

Basic 40-Yard Model

Purpose

To teach starting, acceleration, and maximum-speed integration; enhance 40-yard (36.6-meter) test performance.

Procedure

- For 40-yard sprint times greater than 4.7 seconds, follow this sequence:
  - Visualize the start.
  - Inhale, assume the starting position, hold your breath, and begin.
  - Split your arms, drive the back leg, focus on hard leg drives for about 10 yards (9 meters). Exhale and inhale, drive tall in an upright posture.
  - At about 20 yards (18 meters), exhale and inhale again, and finish tall.
- For 40-yard sprint times less than 4.7 seconds, follow this sequence:
  - Visualize the start.
  - Inhale, assume the starting position, hold your breath, and begin.
  - Split your arms, drive the back leg, focus on hard leg drives for about 15 yards (14 meters). Exhale and inhale, drive tall in an upright posture, and finish tall.

19

Ins and Outs

Purpose

To improve transition acceleration and enhance ability to change speeds.

Procedure

- Space five cones 15 yards (14 m) apart (see figure).
- Start at cone 1 and accelerate to submaximal speed by the time you reach cone 2.
- At cone 3, try to go faster than you have ever attempted to go (try to break your maximal speed record).
- At cone 4, reduce intensity but try to maintain stride frequency.

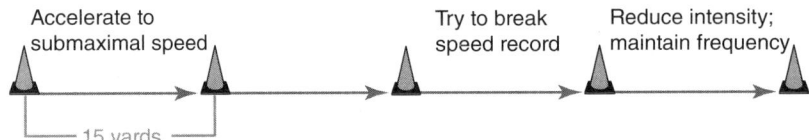

20

Gears

Purpose

To improve transition acceleration and enhance ability to change speeds.

Procedure

- Space five cones 20 yards (18 m) apart (see figure).
- Vary running intensity between cones, which will teach you to accelerate and shift (transition) between various speeds (or gears). For example, run in second gear (half speed) between cones 1 and 2, third gear (three-quarter speed) between cones 2 and 3, first gear (one-quarter speed) between cones 3 and 4, and fourth gear (full speed) between cones 4 and 5.
- You can change the order of the gears to any order you wish. You can also use fewer cones for specific transition work or more cones for conditioning work.

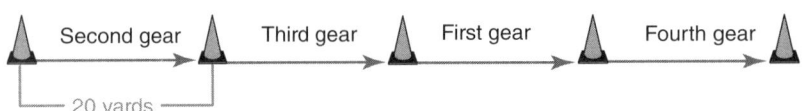

21

10-Yard Burst

Purpose

To test and improve acceleration mechanics and first-step explosive power.

Procedure

- Assume a two point stance.
- Accelerate as hard as possible for 10 yards.

22

Bounding

Purpose

To increase hip extension and flexion strength, improve ankle-muscle stiffness, and enhance leg power and stride length.

Procedure

- Run, driving the free knee so that the thigh reaches a parallel position with the ground; jump a little on each step (see figure *a-c*).
- This should look like a bouncy run with longer than normal strides.
- Be careful not to reach forward at ground contact.

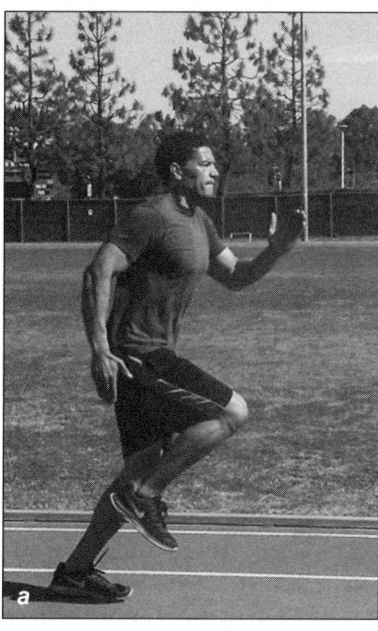
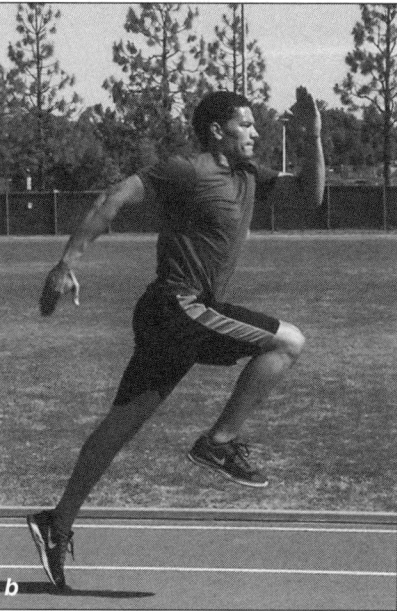
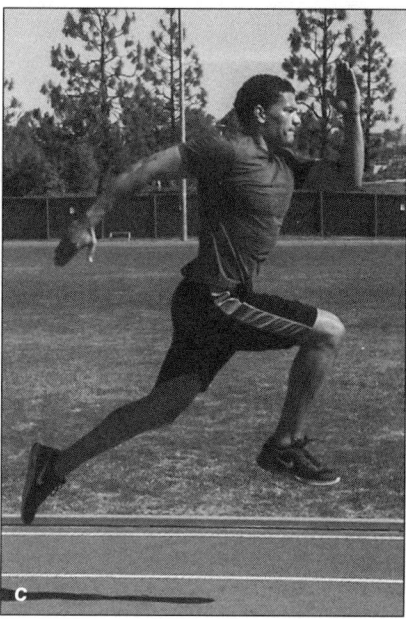

23

Single-Leg Bounds

Purpose

To increase hip extension and flexion strength, improve ankle-muscle stiffness, and enhance leg power and stride length.

Procedure

- Get a slow running start and begin hopping on a single leg (see figure *a-c*).
- Work on recovery mechanics similar to sprint mechanics (heel to gluteus, high knee, pawing action as the leg prepares to jump again).
- Measure improvement by comparing the distance covered in a given number of hops over different sets.

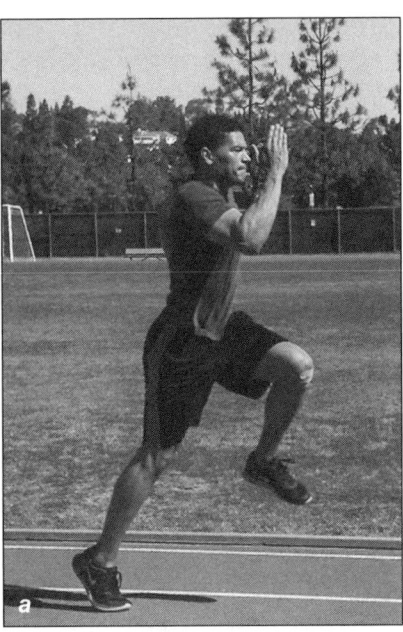 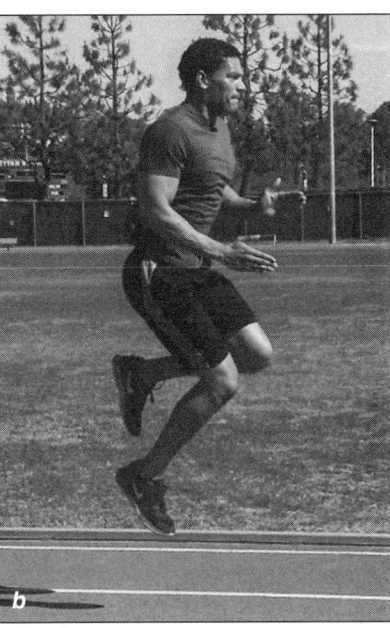 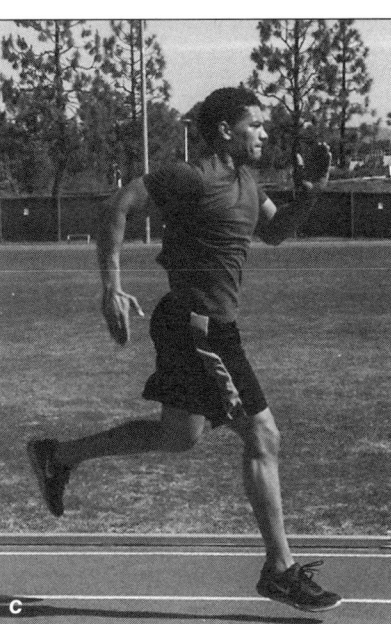

24

Quick Feet Into Acceleration

Purpose

To combine a high-cadence stride frequency drill into acceleration runs.

Procedure

- Move forward in an upright tall position with knees up and toes up, using aggressive arm drive (see figure *a-c*).
- Emphasize stride frequency *not* horizontal speed.
- After 5 to 10 yards or meters of quick feet, without pausing lean the torso forward and then accelerate for 5 to 10 more yards or meters.
- Keep the torso tight and erect throughout; emphasize powerful steps, and attempt to get the feet off of the ground as fast as possible. Use powerful arm drive emanating from the shoulders.

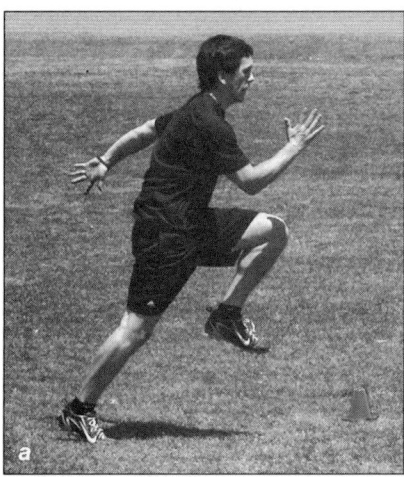 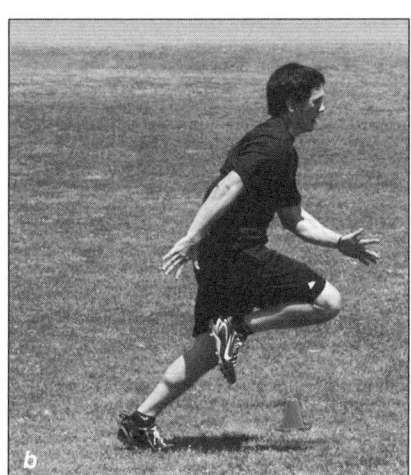 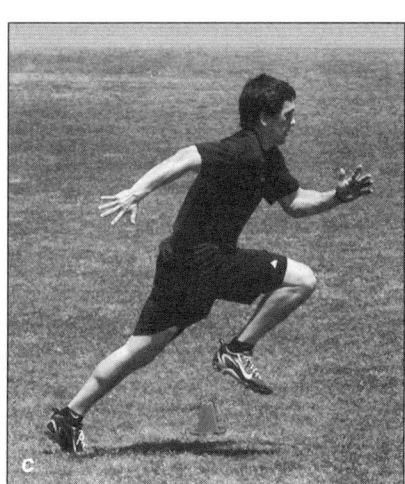

25
Straight-Leg Bound Into Acceleration

Purpose
To incorporate an acceleration technique drill into an acceleration run of 5 to 10 yards or meters.

Procedure
- Run explosively while keeping the legs straight and the feet dorsiflexed (see figure *a-c*).
- Emphasize fast ground contacts with the ball of the foot, and spring forward while keeping tall posture and without leaning back.
- After 5 to 10 yards or meters of straight-leg bounding, without pausing, lean the torso forward and then accelerate for 5 to 10 more yards or meters.
- Keep the torso tight and erect throughout; emphasize powerful steps, and attempt to get the feet off of the ground as fast as possible. Use powerful arm drive emanating from the shoulders.

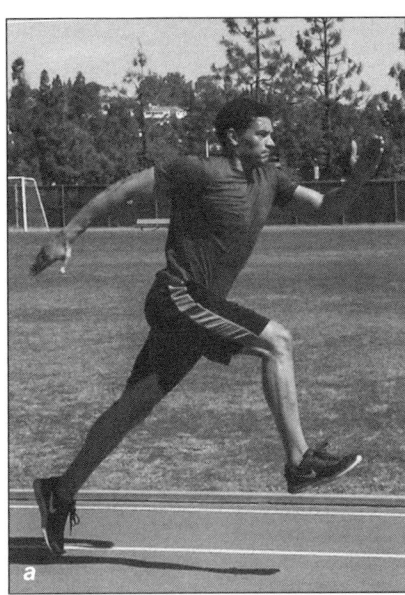 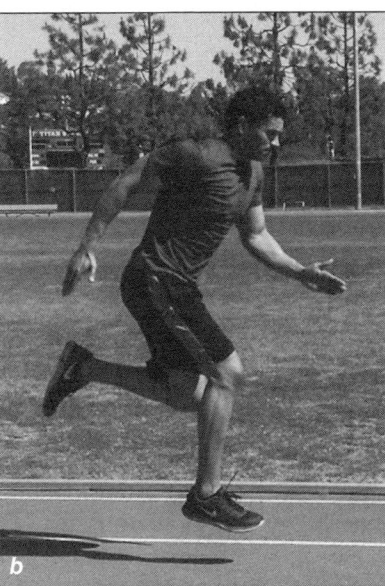 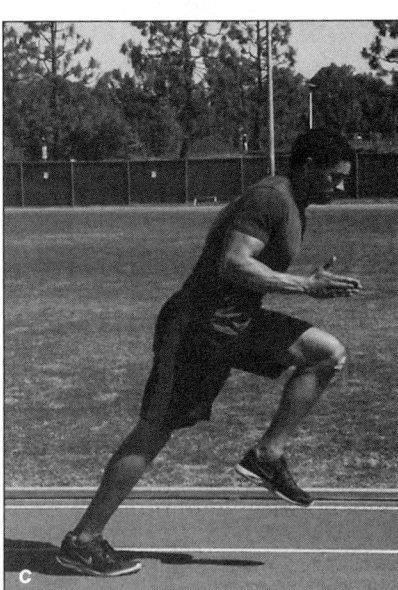

26

 # Bound Into Acceleration

Purpose
To combine a plyometric exercise that enhances acceleration capabilities with an acceleration sprint of 10 to 15 yards or meters.

Procedure
- After 10 to 15 yards or meters of bounding, without pausing, break into a full acceleration sprint for an additional 10 to 15 yards or meters (see figure *a-c*).
- Keep the torso tight and erect throughout; emphasize powerful steps, and attempt to get the feet off of the ground as fast as possible. Use powerful arm drive emanating from the shoulders.

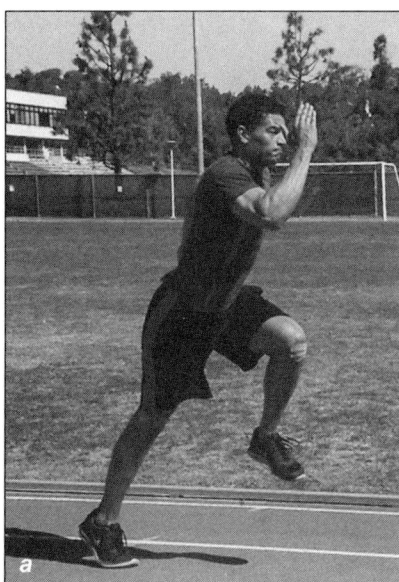 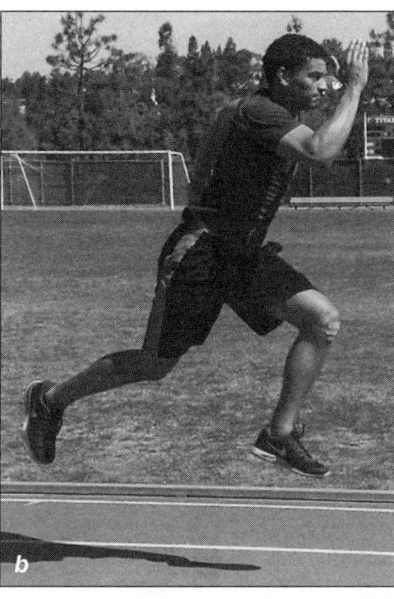 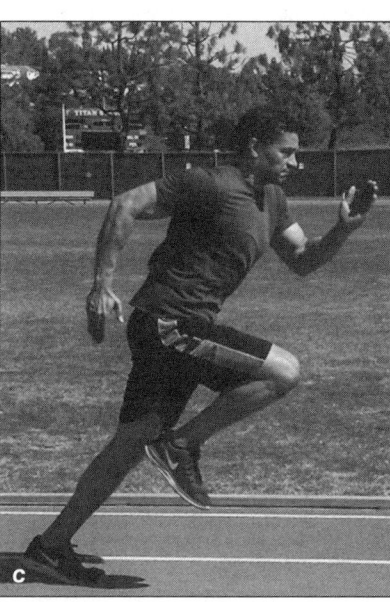

27
▶ Broad Jump Into Acceleration

Purpose
To combine a linear explosive jumping exercise with a short acceleration run.

Procedure
- Stand up straight with feet between hip- and shoulder-width apart.
- Drop into a squat position and aggressively swing the arms back (see figure *a*).
- Swing the arms through, extending the knees and hips to jump forward (see figure *b*).
- Land on either leg (not both) in a tight position (see figure *c*).
- Continue without pausing to accelerate as fast as possible for 5 to 10 yards or meters.

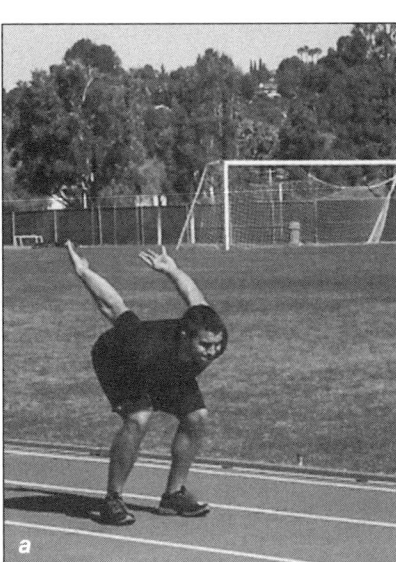
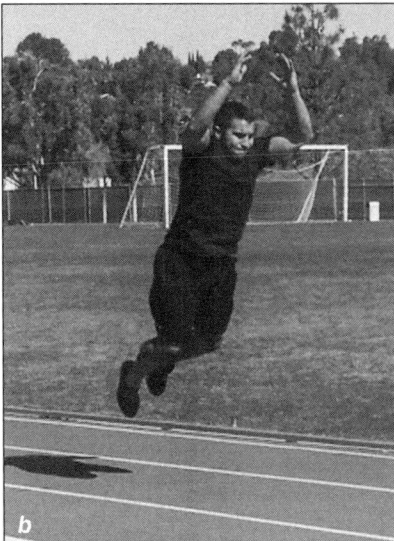
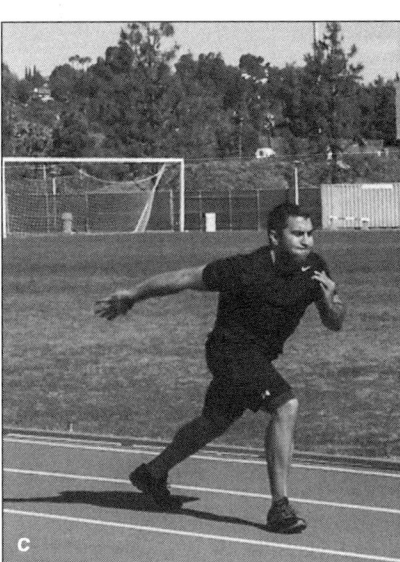

28

Mountain Climber Into Acceleration

Purpose

To enhance starting and acceleration capabilities.

Procedure

- Assume a push-up position with the arms straight and the body in a straight line from head to ankles.
- Without changing the posture of the torso, raise the right knee toward the chest (see figure *a*).
- Pause momentarily, and then return to the starting position and repeat with the left leg (see figure *b*); that is one repetition.
- Do three repetitions in succession, and then without pausing, accelerate forward as fast as possible for 5 to 10 yards or meters (see figure *c* and *d*).

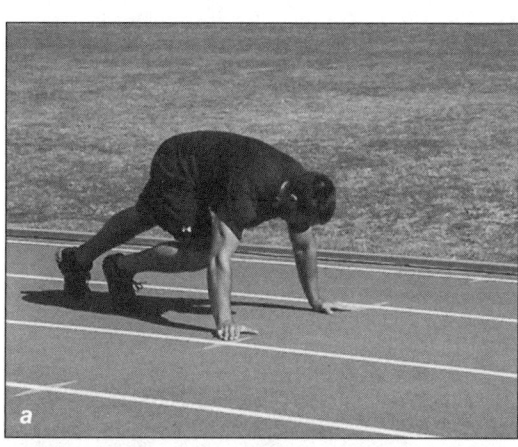
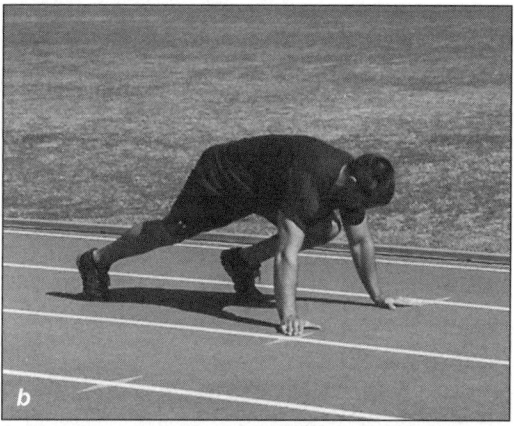
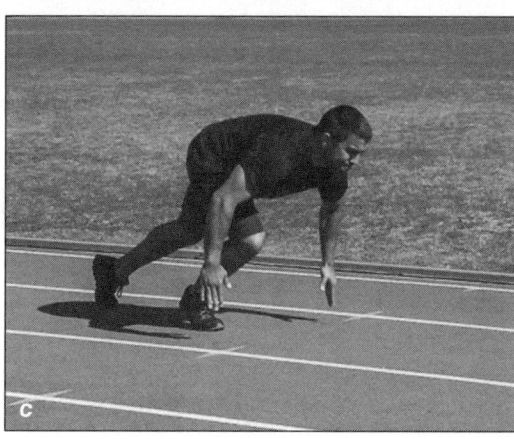
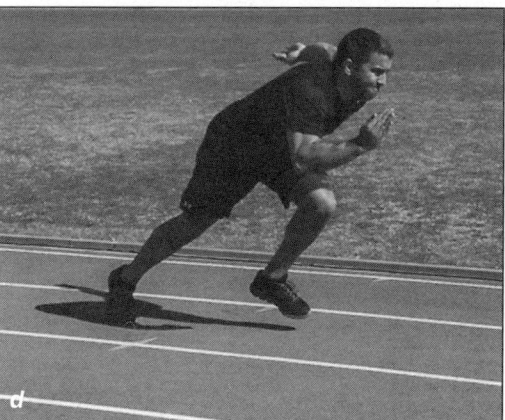

29

Light Sled Pull

SPEED

Purpose

To enhance running strength and power and improve stride length.

Procedure

- Attach a weighted sled or car tire to yourself and drag approximately 5 to 15 meters (see figure).
- Emphasize proper sprinting mechanics.
- Do not make the sled so heavy that altered acceleration mechanics are needed to pull it.
- Do not exceed 10 to 13 percent of your body weight with the sled; a heavier sled pull is not recommended for younger athletes.

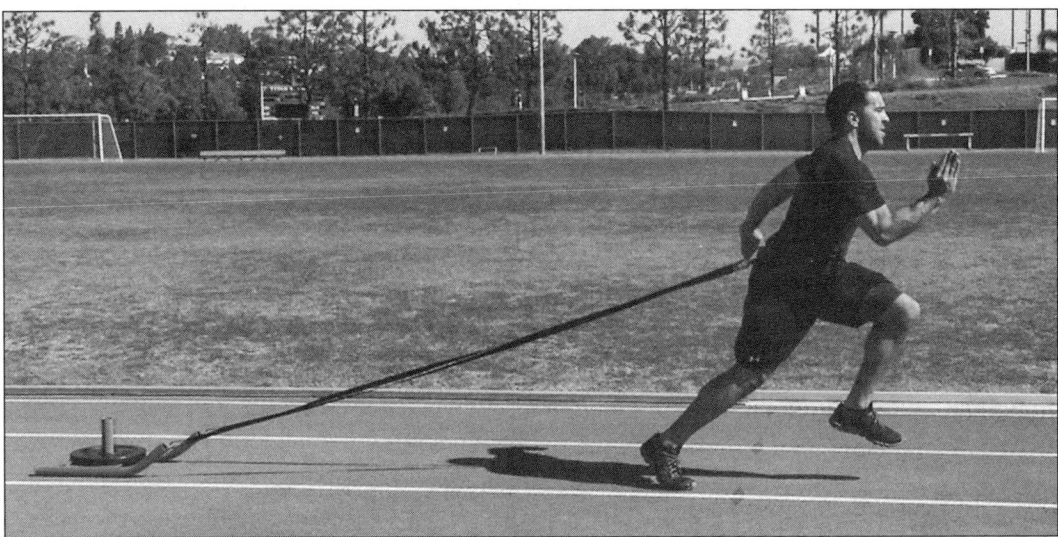

30

Heavy Sled Pull

Purpose

To enhance starting power and stride length.

Procedure

- Attach a weighted sled to yourself, which you then drag during a 15- to 20-yard (14 to 18 m) acceleration run (see figure).
- Emphasize an explosive start and acceleration mechanics.
- Recommended for fully mature athletes; do not exceed 30 percent of your body weight.

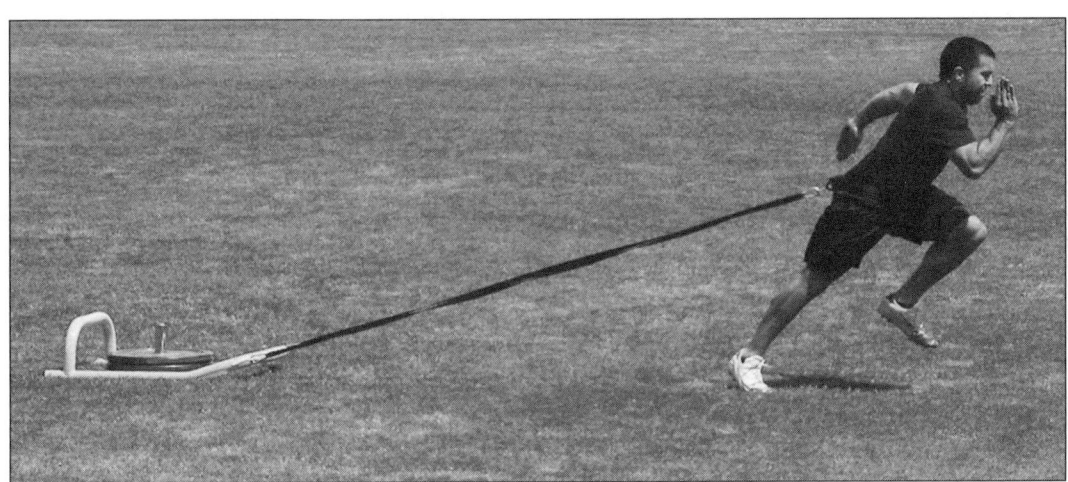

31
Uphill Acceleration Runs

Purpose
To enhance starting power and improve stride length during acceleration.

Procedure
- Use a hill with an incline of 20 to 35 degrees.
- Take 4- to 8-second runs up the hill.
- Count your strides, and mark your spot at your chosen time.
- Try to beat the distance with fewer strides in subsequent timed runs.

32
Stadium Stairs

Purpose
To enhance starting power and stride length.

Procedure
- Run up stadium stairs or bleachers for 4 to 8 seconds.
- Keep posture tight and straight.
- Use aggressive arm swing with quick, powerful steps.

Variation
Wear a weighted vest.

PARTNER-ASSISTED ACCELERATION DRILLS

33

 Resist From Front

Purpose
To enhance starting power and stride length.

Procedure
- You can be resisted during the first 8 to 10 strides by a partner.
- Your partner is situated in front of you with his hands on your shoulders (see figure *a*).
- Drive forward (maintaining a tight body posture) against the mild resistance of your partner (see figure *b*).
- Without notice, the partner quickly steps to the side and you continue to accelerate for another (±) 5 to 10 yards or meters.
- The drill ends after 8 to 10 strides.

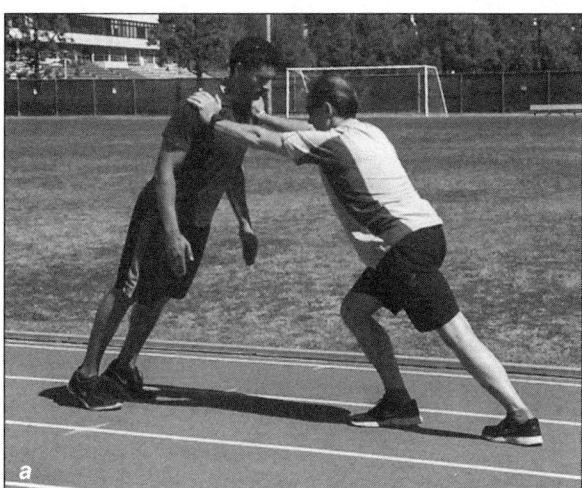
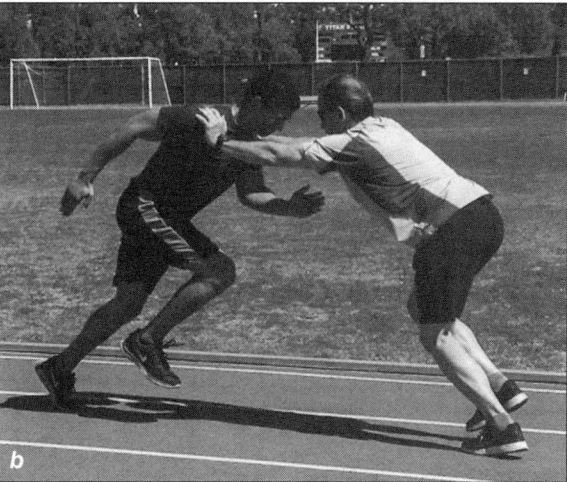

34 Resist From Behind

Purpose
To enhance starting power and stride length.

Procedure
- A partner is situated behind you with his hands on your waist (see figure *a*).
- During the first 8 to 10 strides, your partner will provide resistance, backpedaling and holding your waist as you drive forward (see figure *b*).
- Your partner will then quickly let go, allowing you to continue accelerating.

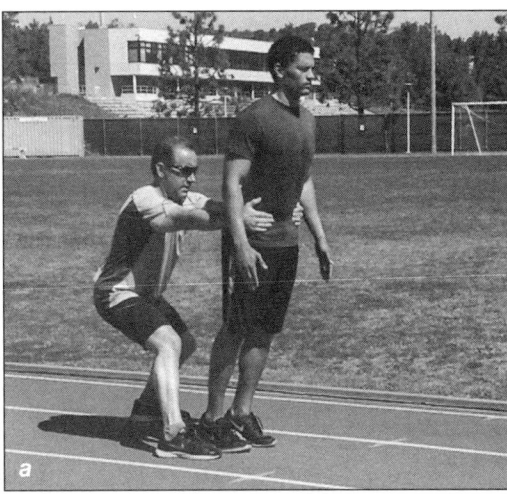
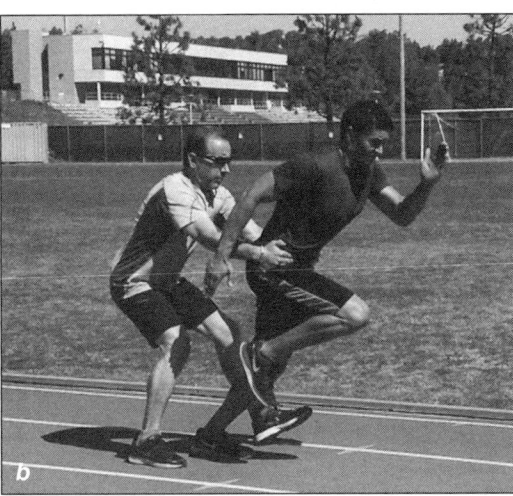

35

Face and Chase

Purpose

To add a competitive component to the partner-resisted starts.

Procedure

- Your partner is situated in front of you with his hands on your shoulders (see figure *a*).
- Your partner resists you for 5 to 10 yards or meters; then without notice, your partner drop-steps, turns 180 degrees, and sprints for another 10 yards or meters (see figure *b*).
- Your objective is to catch your partner before he reaches the finish line about 15 to 20 yards or meters in front of where you both started.

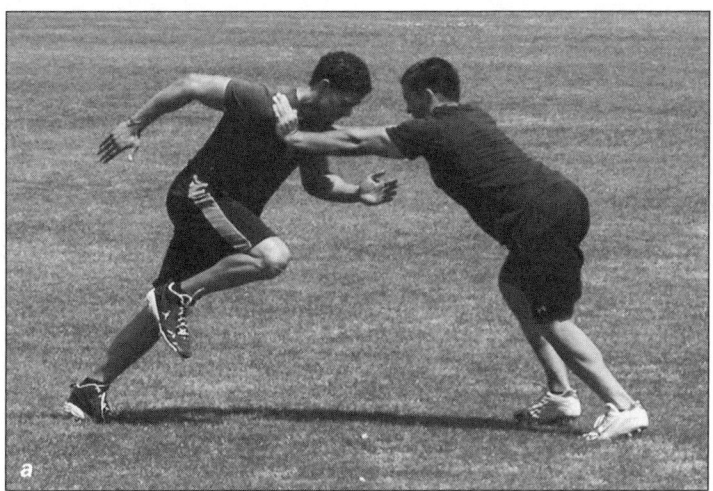

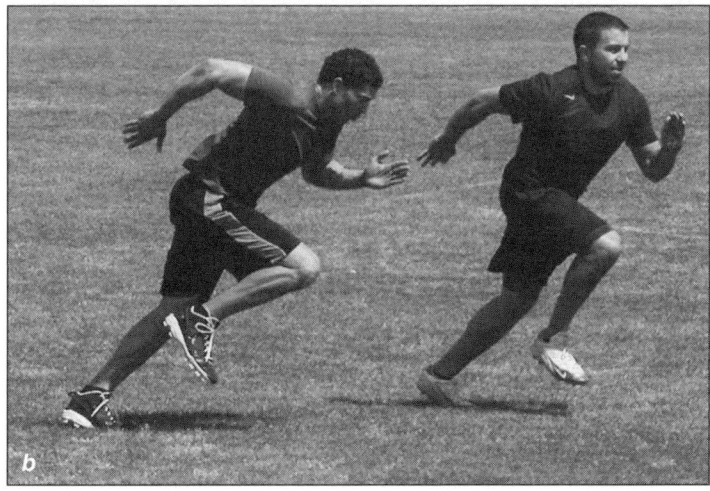

36

 Harness Pull

Purpose

To increase acceleration.

Procedure

- You are connected by a harness and handle system that allows your partner to gently resist you as you accelerate over 15-20 yards or meters (see figure).

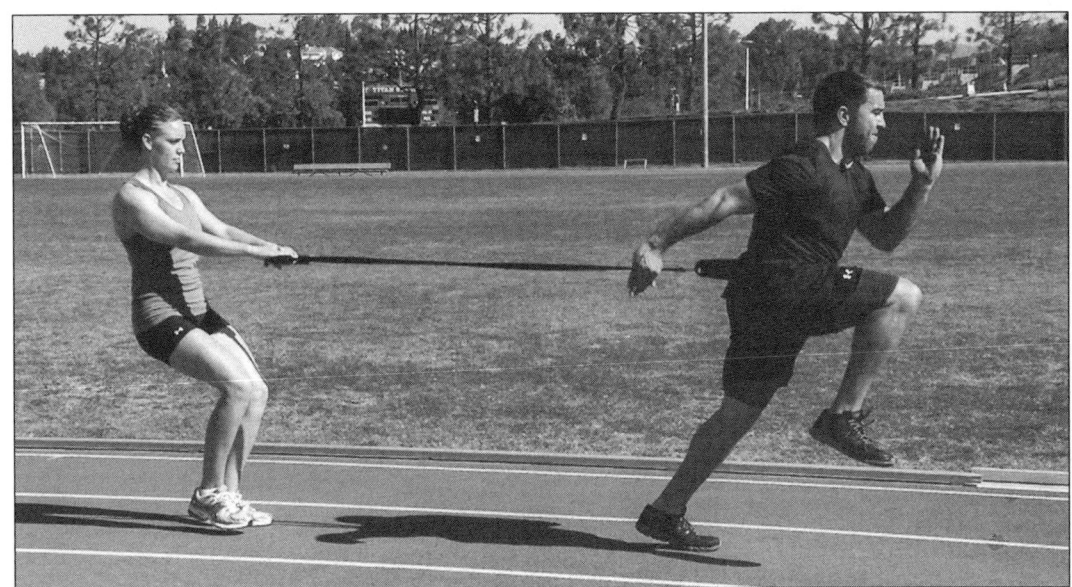

37

Bullet Belt

Purpose

To teach quick transitions in speed and enhance stride frequency of acceleration.

Procedure

- A bullet belt allows you to be held by a partner while you are attempting to accelerate until enough force is applied to the belt so that the Velcro strip holding it to you breaks (see figure *a* and *b*).
- There are several techniques used to release the accelerating athlete, including the rip and the pop methods.

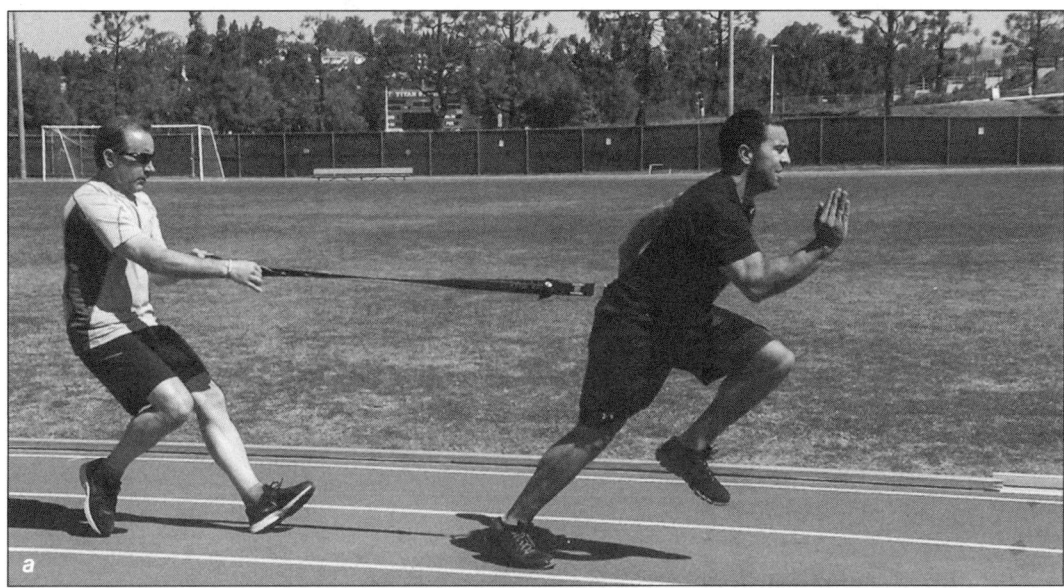

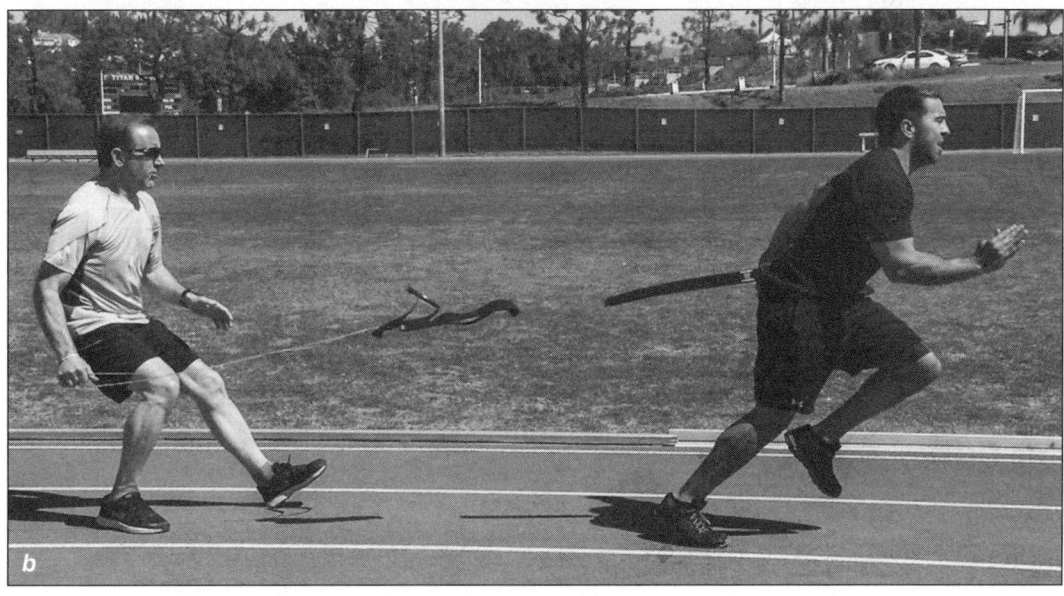

38 Partner-Assisted Tubing Acceleration

Purpose

To improve quick leg recovery in the first few steps and enhance stride frequency during acceleration.

Procedure

- You and your partner are attached at the waist by a 10- to 20-yard (9 to 18 m) piece of rubber tubing.
- Your partner lines up at a distance 15 to 25 yards or meters from you, the assisted athlete (see figure *a*).
- Get into the ready position of your choice, and at the signal to begin, explode for 10 to 20 yards or meters with the aid of the rubber tubing (see figure *b*).
- For longer acceleration runs, your partner can run at the signal to begin providing continued assistance for a longer duration.

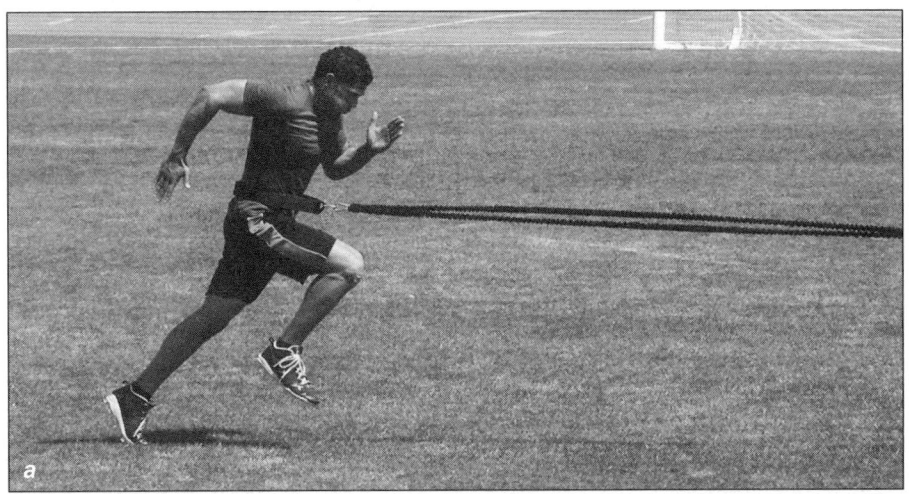

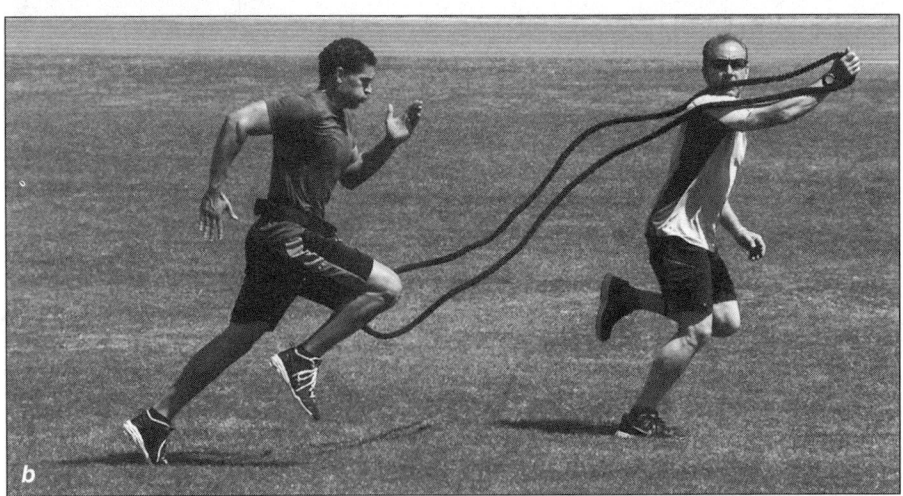

START DRILLS

39

Start From Staggered Two-Point Stance

Purpose

To enhance two-point start capabilities.

Procedure

- Start in a slightly crouched position with slight flexion at the hips and knees (see figure *a*).
- The front foot should be pointed straight ahead and the majority of weight distributed to the forefoot.
- The trail leg should be pointed straight ahead, the majority of weight on the forefoot, and positioned about hip-width apart and at the heel of the front foot.
- Drive out of the stance, with the trail leg punching forward and the same-side arm driving backward, while attempting to step forward in a straight line (see figure *b*).

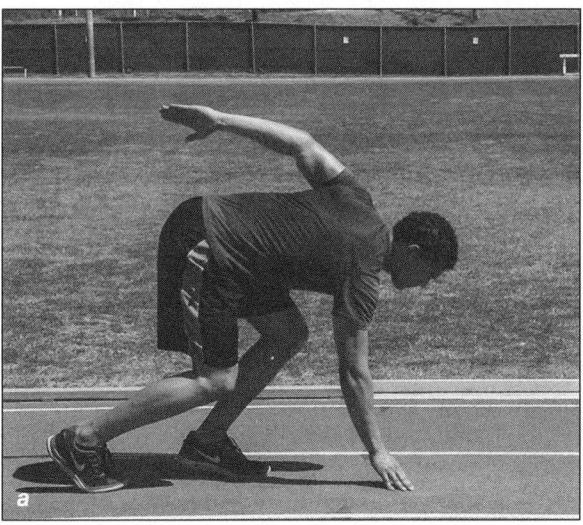 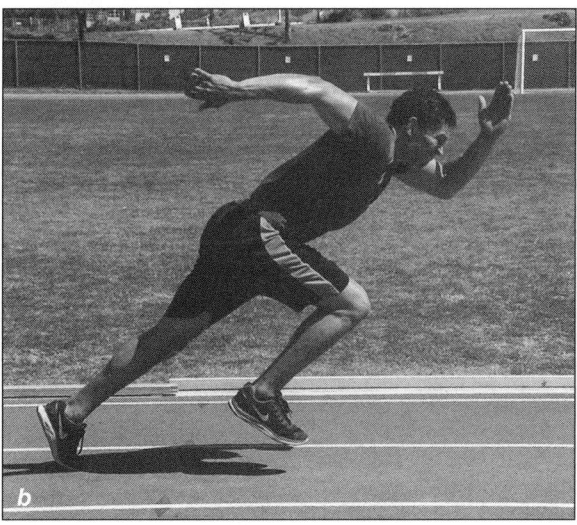

40

Start From Parallel Two-Point Stance

Purpose

To maximize starting capabilities from a parallel stance position, which is common to many nontrack sports.

Procedure

- Start in an athletic position, with the knees and hips slightly flexed and the feet pointed straight ahead and shoulder-width apart or slightly wider (see figure *a*).
- With one foot, quickly punch the ground slightly behind your center of mass (see figure *b*).
- Simultaneously, keeping the torso and body tight, lean the shoulders forward and use aggressive arm action to explosively step forward (see figure *c*).
- Try to step quickly directly behind your starting position so that all forward momentum occurs in a straight line.
- This quick back step, or rhythm step, utilizes the stretch–shortening cycle to enhance powerful starts from stationary or near-stationary positions.

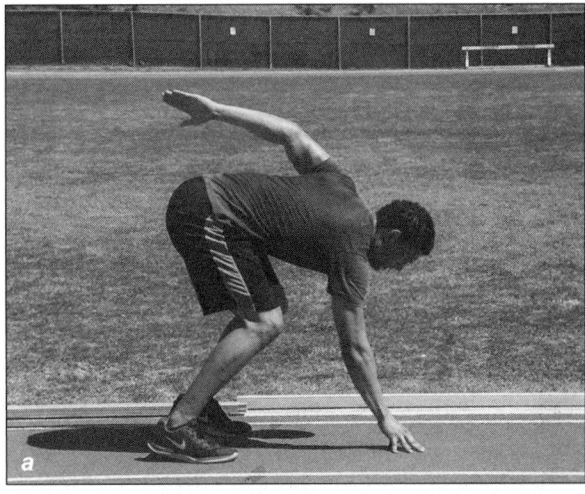

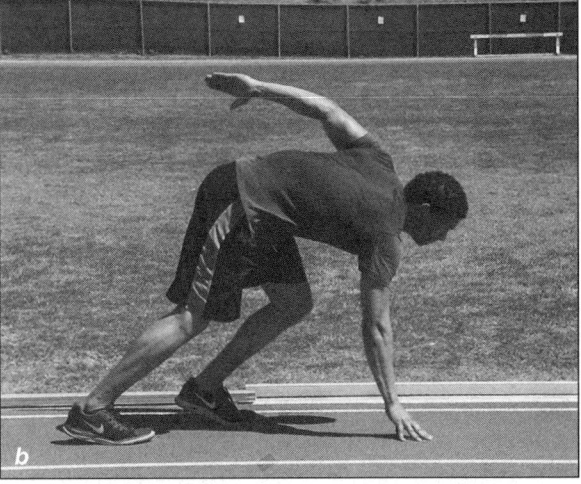

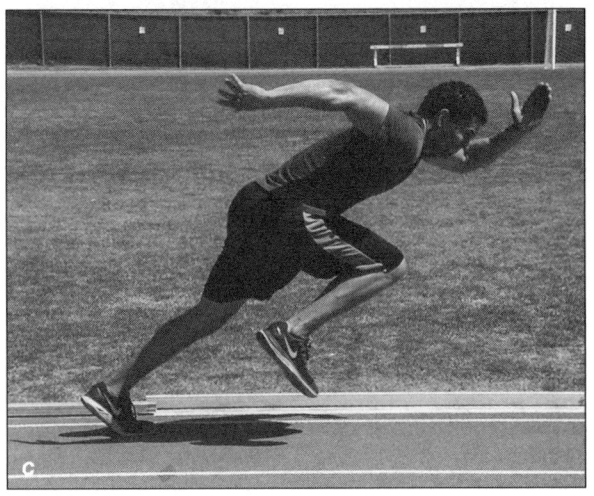

41

Falling Starts

Purpose
To enhance quick leg turnover at the start and teach the proper acceleration lean.

Procedure
- Stand with the feet together and lean forward until your balance is lost (see figure *a* and *b*).
- At this point, accelerate at full speed to catch yourself (see figure *c*).
- Run 20 to 30 yards or meters.

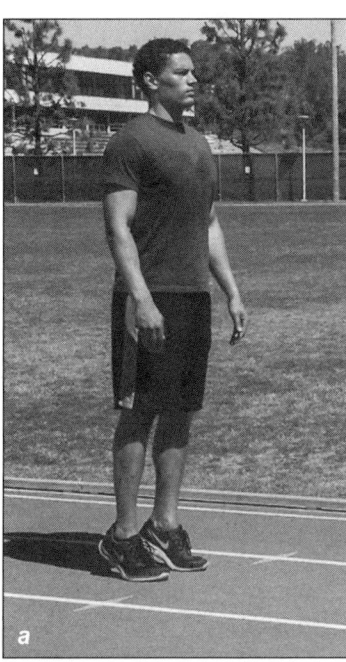
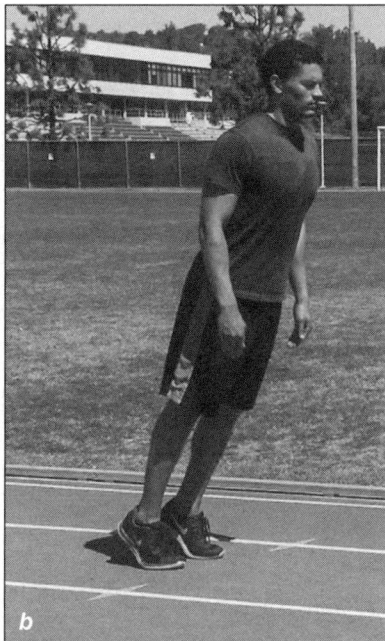
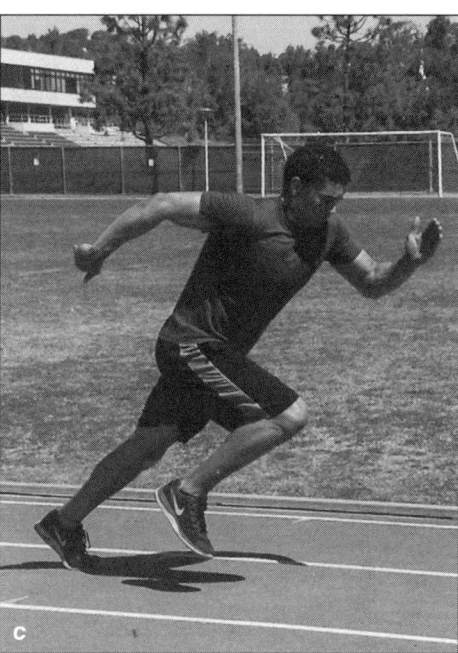

42

30-Yard Flying Start

Purpose
To test and build on transition from slow run to full acceleration.

Procedure
- Start with a light jog over about 5 yards.
- Once you hit the start line, accelerate as hard as you can over 30 yards.

43 Medicine Ball Shovel Toss

Purpose
To assist an athlete's starting capabilities.

Procedure
- Beginning on the knees, place a medicine ball on the ground directly in front of you (see figure *a*).
- Keeping the shoulders slightly protracted (back), chest out and in a tight position, position the shoulders slightly in front of the medicine ball.
- With arms fully extended and relaxed, toss the medicine ball as far as possible by quickly extending the hips and trunk (see figure *b*).
- Catch yourself in a push-up position.

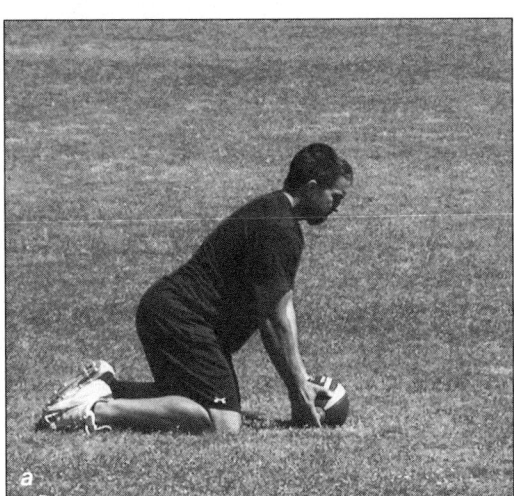 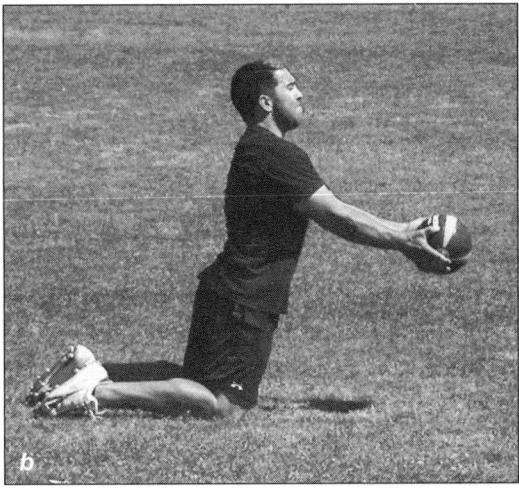

44 Medicine Ball Scoop Toss

Purpose

To develop the triple extension of the ankle, knee, and hip joints required for powerful starts.

Procedure

- Start in a squat position with a medicine ball on the ground between your legs.
- Grasp the medicine ball on either side, with fingers spread apart.
- Extend the arms, keeping the head up and the torso in a tight position (see figure *a*).
- Thrust the hips forward and move the shoulders upward while maintaining full extension of the arms (see figure *b*).
- With an underhand toss or scoop, try to lift the body and the medicine ball as high as possible (see figure *c*).
- Let the medicine ball drop to the ground.

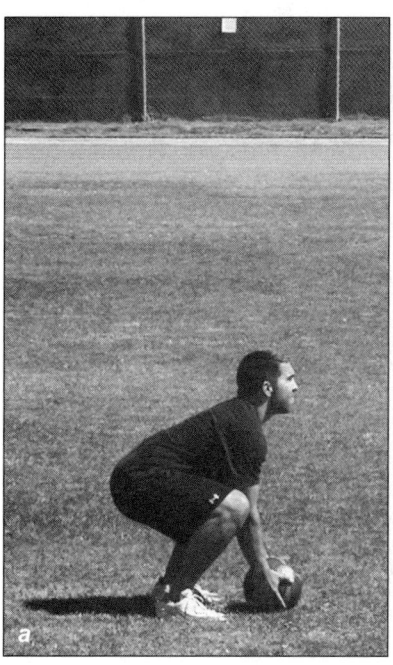
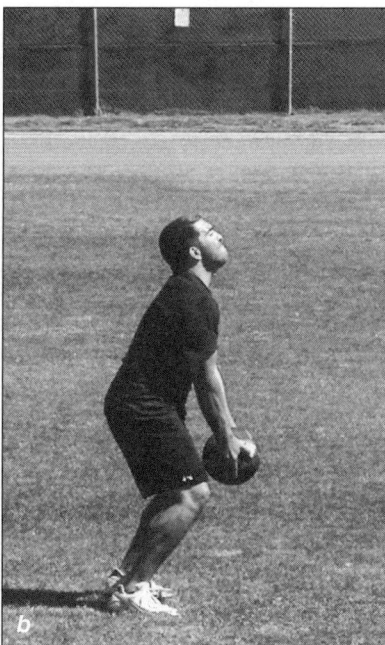
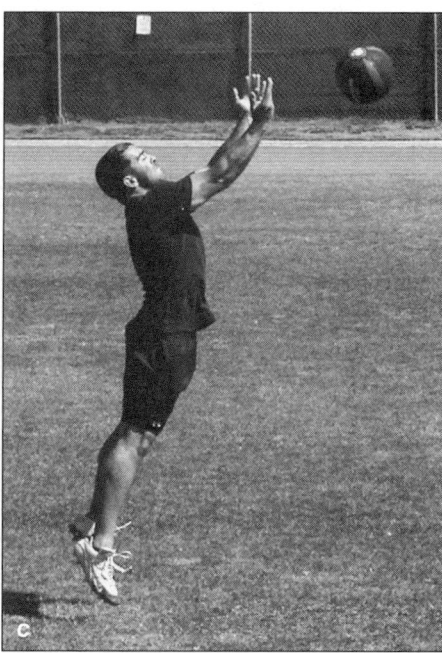

MAXIMAL VELOCITY DRILLS

45

Abbreviated B March

Purpose

To improve hip-extension mechanics and enhance hamstring firing.

Procedure

- Perform a B-movement march using perfect posture and arm action, where the recovery leg's knee achieves a position as high as possible (above parallel to the ground).
- Bring the knee on the recovery leg high, and keep it fully flexed while keeping the ankle close to the gluteus and dorsiflexed (see figure *a*).
- Allow the recovering leg to extend in front of you after a high knee raise (see figure *b*).
- Paw down and drive the hips through (see figure *c*).

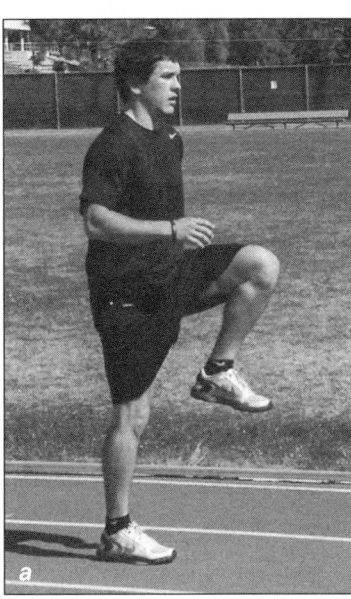
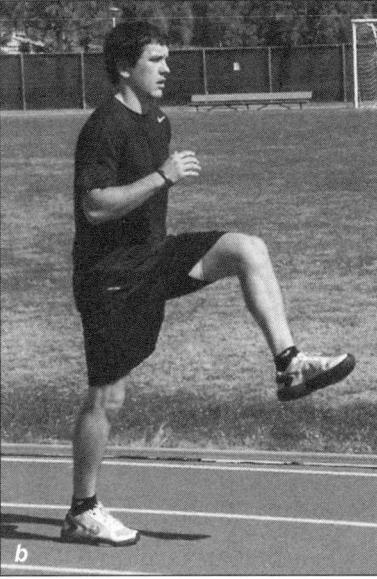
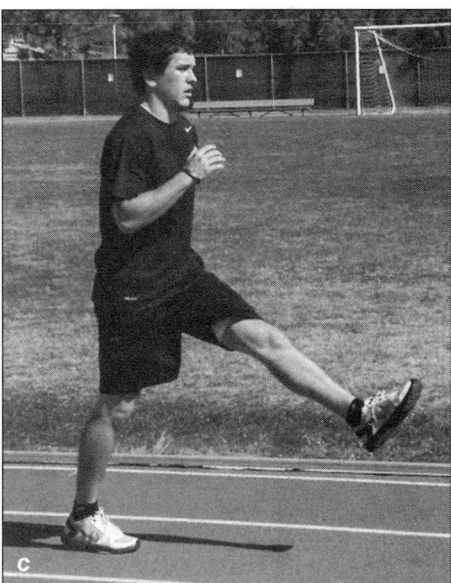

46
 Abbreviated B Skip

Purpose
To increase stride length and frequency, enhance hamstring and hip performance, and improve muscle stiffness at the ankle complex.

Procedure
- Perform the B leg movement while skipping where the recovery leg's knee blocks, or stops, as high as possible.
- Emphasize pawing, and drive the hips through.

47
 Galloping

Purpose
To promote good hip projection and back-leg push-off and improve lead-leg mechanics and proper pawing, or leg-cycle, mechanics.

Procedure
- Begin in a staggered stance position.
- Without changing foot position, skip forward using a basic step hop pattern.
- Gallop, keeping the trailing ankle locked to emphasize a spring-loaded landing and takeoff.

48

Paw Drill (Cycling)

Purpose
To train top-speed mechanics.

Procedure
- Extend one arm and lean against a partner so the outside leg can swing freely (see figure *a*).
- While keeping the torso stationary, cast the outside leg forward in a whiplike fashion (see figure *b* and *c*).
- At foot strike, the ball of the foot should land directly under or slightly in front of the center of mass, similar to using a pawing motion.

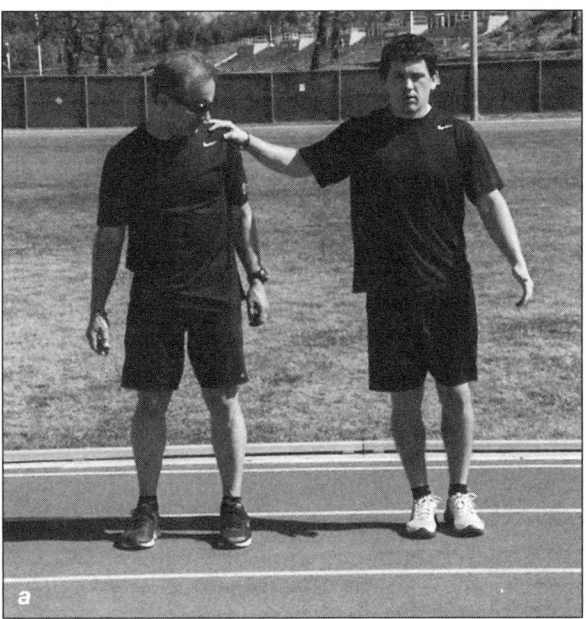

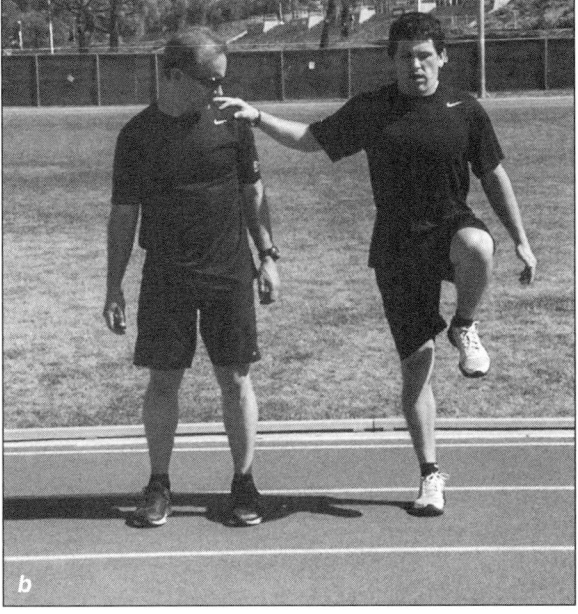

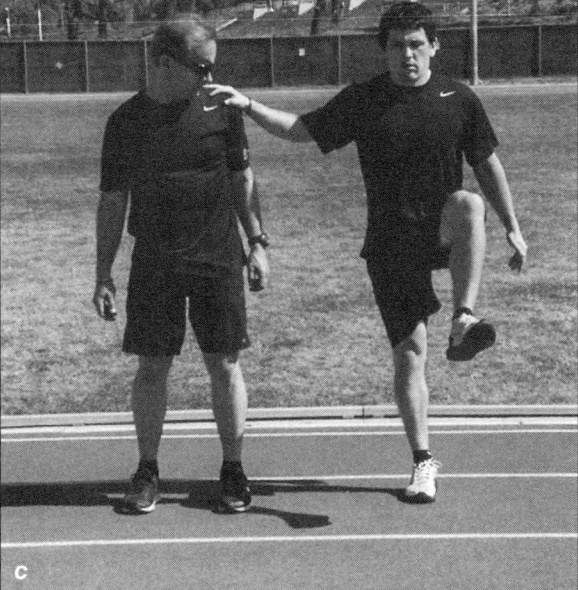

49 Single-Leg Fast Leg

Purpose
To emphasize stride mechanics during maximal velocity.

Procedure
- Run forward and on every third stride, cycle the right leg through in a similar manner to the B march.
- After completing the set distance, repeat the drill using the left leg.

50 Alternating Fast Leg

Purpose
To emphasize stride mechanics during maximal velocity. The single-leg fast leg drill should be mastered before moving on to this progression.

Procedure
- This drill is performed in a similar manner to the single-leg fast leg drill. However, rather than cycling a single leg, the athlete cycles in an alternating fashion.
- Perform three successive pawing actions on the right leg, then alternate and repeat using the left leg.
- Focus on performing a fast, cyclical, "A" motion, while shuffling and keeping the heel close to the buttocks during recovery.
- Block over the opposite leg knee with the lead leg.
- Repeat for 20-30 meters.

51

Continuous Fast Leg

Purpose

To emphasize stride mechanics during maximal velocity. The alternating fast leg drill should be mastered before moving on to this progression.

Procedure

- This drill is performed in a similar manner to the alternating fast leg drill. However, the athlete cycles the legs through one after the other, similar to a B march.
- Perform successive pawing actions using the same leg.
- Focus on performing a fast, cyclical, "A" motion, while shuffling and keeping the heel close to the buttocks during recovery.
- Block over the opposite leg knee with the lead leg.
- Repeat for 20-30 meters.

52

Run-Through

Purpose

To enhance stride frequency while strengthening hip flexors and improving lower-body ambidexterity.

Procedure

- Set 8 to 10 6- to 12-inch (15 to 32 cm) hurdles about 3 feet (91 cm) apart.
- Run through the hurdles with emphasis on quick "knee-up/toe-up" and a quick heel-to-gluteus recovery.
- Perform the exercise with a two-foot strike between each hurdle or run faster with a one-foot strike between hurdles.
- Maintain the same lead leg through the drill.

53

Hurdle Fast Legs

Purpose
Enhance stride frequency while strengthening hip flexors and improving lower-body ambidexterity.

Procedure
- Stagger 8- to 10-inch (15 to 32 cm) hurdles so that half line up with the right leg and the other half line up with the left leg.
- The hurdle pattern should be a hurdle for the left leg followed by one for the right leg with the hurdles 3 feet (91 cm) apart; repeat the pattern.
- The leg sequence entails hurdling the left foot over the left hurdle then taking two steps to the next hurdle for the right foot.

54

Split-Squat Jumps

Purpose
Increase hip power and stride length.

Procedure
- Start in a lunge position.
- Jump straight into the air and return to the original position.
- Repeat without pausing.
- The knee closest to the ground should never touch the ground.
- Your hands are placed on either side of your head near the ears or may be used in unison to drive upward with each jump.
- Repeat for the other leg.

Variation
- *Alternating split-squat jumps*: On each jump, the legs switch positions and the other leg is in front of you at ground contact.

55

Uphill to Flat Contrast Speed Runs

Purpose

To enhance running strength and power and improve stride length.

Procedure

- Gravity provides resistance on uphill runs.
- Emphasize perfect maximal speed mechanics.
- Do not exceed a 3-degree incline if the goal is to develop maximal running speed.
- Higher inclines are more appropriate for acceleration mechanics and will be discussed later.

56

Downhill Speed Runs

Purpose

To increase top-end speed and stride frequency.

Procedure

- Gravity provides assistance on downhill runs.
- Emphasize perfect maximal speed mechanics.
- You can exceed a 3- to 7-degree decline if your goal is to develop maximal running speed, but be aware that overstriding will result in deceleration and interfere with your speed development.
- Perform this drill on a grass surface rather than on asphalt to prevent injury if you fall.

57

Downhill to Flat Contrast Speed Runs

Purpose

To increase top-end speed and stride frequency.

Procedure

- Position yourself 10 to 20 yards or meters above the bottom of the hill.
- Quickly build up to near-maximal speed by the time you are about 5 yards or meters above the bottom of the hill.
- Continue to increase speed as you transition to flat ground.
- Try to maintain supramaximal speed through the transition and on to the flat ground (for about 2 to 3 seconds), running for an additional 10 to 15 yards or meters.

58

Parachute Running

Purpose

To enhance running strength and power and improve stride length.

Procedure

- Wear a belt with a small parachute attached by a cord. Have a partner hold the parachute behind you.
- Start running (see figure). The parachute deploys in zero to four steps, depending on wind conditions and the parachute model, and provides extra air resistance.

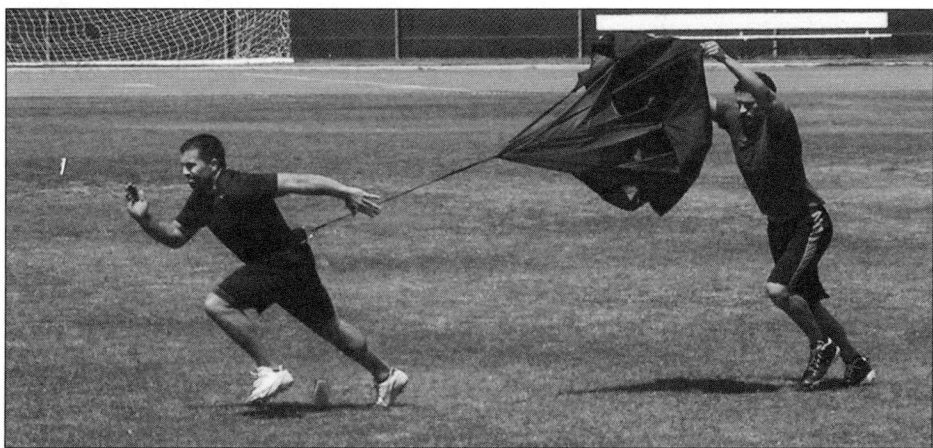

59
Contrast Parachute Running

Purpose
To enhance stride length of start and turnover at top speed and increase starting speed and transition to top speed.

Procedure
- Attach a parachute to yourself, which is to be dragged behind you during the run.
- Emphasize proper speed mechanics.
- After a buildup and 10 to 20 yards or meters of near-maximal running, release the Velcro belt to allow for unresisted running.
- You should feel an overspeed sensation over the next 10 to 20 yards or meters.

60
Sand Running

Purpose
To increase stride length and hip strength.

Procedure
- Sprinting on the beach in loose sand makes sprinting more difficult and can provide good resistance training.
- It also provides increased proprioception to the locomotive environment.

Speed is one of the most highly sought after attributes in all of sport. The key to developing explosive speed is mastering basic speed mechanics in the start, in the acceleration phase, and while transitioning into maximal velocity. Furthermore, participating in a properly structured strength and conditioning program that includes resistance training and plyometric exercise can augment an athlete's physiological capabilities by improving muscle quality and developing greater explosiveness. By addressing these components, an athlete will have the greatest opportunity to maximize his genetic potential and perform at his best.

Chapter 5

Agility Training

John F. Graham

Agility can be defined by the abilities and skills necessary to make explosive changes in direction and speed. It is a necessary skill for athletes in just about any field or court athletic endeavor. Agility generally refers to two distinct forms of motor function. It is fundamental to the capacity to explosively start, accelerate, change direction, and reaccelerate while maintaining body control and minimizing the loss of speed. In this regard, agility is essential in athletics because movements are often initiated from a variety of body alignments. Therefore, athletes need to be able to react with explosive power and quickness from these alignments in bursts of less than 10 yards or meters before making a change of direction. Agility may also refer to the ability to synchronize two or more sport-specific skill tasks concurrently, such as when a quarterback avoids would-be tacklers when scrambling while also looking downfield for a pass receiver (Cissik and Barnes 2011; Halberg 2001).

Many athletes and coaches believe agility is established principally by genetics and hence is challenging to improve or enhance to any considerable degree. Coaches often become enamored with an athlete who possesses natural physical attributes—physical size, strength, vertical and horizontal power, ideal body composition, and so on—that are associated with a successful performance. However, these attributes alone will not guarantee success in sports that require agility.

Unfortunately, because of the focus placed on physical characteristics, off-season programs often revolve around strength training and conditioning. Agility and speed development at sport-specific speeds are ignored or receive limited attention during small blocks of time in the preseason. However, agility involves essential neural adaptations that can be developed only over time with many repetitions (Brown and Khamoui 2012). It takes athletes weeks and months to see improvements in speed and agility. Thus, agility training should be regarded as an integral component of the annual training program. The movement abilities and sport-specific movements that occur at high velocities during athletics have minimal time to be improved if they are not attended to throughout the off-season. There is a direct correlation between increased agility and timing, rhythm, and movement (Cissik and Barnes 2011; Costello and Kreis 1993; Plisk 2008).

Considerable research regarding the physical training of athletes has resulted in a number of changes to how athletes are instructed, prepared, and trained. These changes have resulted in a newfound concentration on how agility training is designed and implemented, which has led to the evolution of faster, stronger, and better-conditioned athletes. The key to improving agility is to minimize the loss of speed when shifting an athlete's center of gravity. Drills that require rapid changes of direction forward, backward, vertically, and laterally will help improve agility as well as coordination by training the body to make these changes in movement more quickly (Arthur and Bailey 1998). This chapter provides an extensive account of how agility training generates these gains.

Why do athletes need agility training? Sport coaches often have difficulty applying the benefits gained from strength, power, and metabolic training and conditioning to sport performance. Even for the athlete who will never make a move like Michael Jordan and bring the viewing audience to its feet, agility training provides the benefits of neuromuscular adaptation and improved athleticism.

Neuromuscular Adaptation

Agility training may be the most efficient way to address the neuromuscular demands of effectively performing sport-specific skills since it most closely resembles the intensity, duration, and recovery time found in sport performance (Cissik and Barnes 2011). The inclusion of agility training in an annual training cycle is critical for translating comprehensive strength and conditioning work into gains in the athletic arena.

Improved Athleticism

The primary effect of agility training is increased body control, which results from a concentrated kinesthetic awareness. In other words, it focuses on the intricacies of controlling small motor transitions in the neck, shoulder, back, hip, knee, and ankle joints for the best postural alignment. This enhances the athlete's sense of control, allowing her to move faster. In this respect, agility training can also prove central to developing the confidence of athletes discouraged by their performance, in particular those with little coordination. Agility training enables athletes to learn more about themselves.

Designing Agility Programs

When designing an agility program to enhance athletic performance, a strength and conditioning coach should incorporate forms of training that emphasize these components: acceleration, coordination, deceleration, dynamic balance, energy system utilization, power, and strength.

Acceleration

Acceleration is measured by the change in velocity per unit of time. It plays a central role in going from a stationary position to top speed and then quickly increasing speed again on making a directional change. Having the ability to accelerate quickly could certainly mean the difference between, for example, a running back's getting through a hole in the line or being tackled.

Coordination

Coordination involves the ability to control and process multiple muscle movements in order to perform athletic skills (Cissik and Barnes 2011). It entails the smooth interplay of different muscle groups. Nearly all human movement occurs through multiple joints and muscles working in a coordinated fashion in order to accomplish a given task.

Deceleration

Deceleration refers to the ability to decrease speed or come to a stop from a maximal or near-maximal speed. It is the key to slowing the body down to a speed at which one can change direction quickly and then reaccelerate. Deceleration can occur in a number of ways, from slowing within one or more footfalls to backpedaling, shuffling, or using a crossover step. In all these situations, it involves eccentric muscle actions. It places a good deal of stress on the joints and is a main cause of injury among athletes.

Dynamic Balance

Dynamic balance is the ability to maintain control over the body while in motion. When the body is in motion, an athlete gains feedback through the use of sight, kinesthetic awareness, and perturbations made by the nervous system that allow him to adjust his center of gravity (Cissik and Barnes 2011). Agility is closely aligned with balance in that it requires athletes to regulate shifts in the body's center of gravity while undergoing postural deviation (Brittenham 1996).

Energy System Utilization

All three energy systems (phosphagen, glycogen, and oxidative) are always activated; however, the type of exercise will influence which of these energy systems is predominant. The phosphagen and glycolytic energy systems do not require oxygen and are therefore referred to as anaerobic energy systems; the oxidative energy system does require oxygen and is referred to as the aerobic energy system (Hoffman 2012). Since most activities in sport requiring agility generally are restricted to short bursts of explosive activity (5 to 10 seconds), the phosphagen system should be the primary energy system trained (Brown and Khamoui 2012). The phosphagen energy system is predominantly used during maximal effort, short-duration exercise of less than 15 seconds (Hoffman 2012).

Power

Power may well be the single most essential component of training. It refers to the rate at which work is done (force × velocity). The faster an athlete gets from one point to another, the greater the power. So power can be increased by improving speed.

Strength

Strength refers to the maximal force a muscle or muscle group can generate at a specified velocity (Harman 2008a; Murphy and Forney 1997). When an athlete is in contact with an opponent, the combination of the force applied on the athlete by an opponent and the athlete's own body weight together act as resistance (Cissik and Barnes 2011). Research has demonstrated a strong correlation between lower body strength and agility. The more emphasis placed on strength within a given sporting activity, the greater the need for strength training.

When designing an agility training program for athletes, a number of design variables should be considered. A brief description of these variables follows.

- *Drill selection*: Drills are chosen based on four factors—movement patterns of the sport, work intervals (considering distance and time), rest intervals (will vary according to training objectives), and complexity (Cissik and Barnes 2011).
- *Duration*: The distance or time of the work interval
- *Equipment*: Once the athlete is able to demonstrate proper technique at sport-specific speeds, implements such as balls, resistance bands, sport cords, or other athletes can increase the complexity of the drill. Technique suggestions on how to increase the complexity of the drill are included.
- *Frequency*: The number of training sessions performed in a given week. During the off-season, athletes should perform an agility training workout twice per week and once per week in-season.
- *Intensity*: The speed at which the drill is performed. If the drill is timed, then intensity is the distance covered.
- *Recovery*: The time between repetitions. Recovery between repetitions should be based on the complexity of the skill and the metabolic demands of the sport.
- *Repetition*: The execution of one complete movement skill
- *Sequence*: Drills that are the most technical, require the highest power output, and are most similar to the demands of the sport should be performed first.
- *Set*: A group of agility drills and relief intervals
- *Training factors*: Factors such as medical history, the age of the athlete, physical maturity level of the athlete, sport skill level, training experience, present fitness levels, and plyometric and strength training experience and level must be considered.
- *Volume load*: The amount of exercise performed per agility program. As an example, the athlete may perform four drills on the agility ladder two times each.

PERFECTING AGILITY DRILLS

When instructing athletes on the execution of agility exercises, it is critical to focus on the following: initial speed and direction, decrease or increase in speed (or both), redirection of movement, and final speed and direction (Plisk 2008). Perfecting the technique of the drill is of utmost importance. Drills performed sloppily because the speed cannot be controlled do the athlete no good.

Agility Training Drills

The following types of drills should be included in an agility training program:

- *Line drills*: Drills conducted in a linear fashion that incorporate change of direction, footwork, reaction time, acceleration, deceleration, stopping ability, conditioning, transitions between skills, and cutting ability
- *Cone drills*: Drills that incorporate change of direction, footwork, reaction time, acceleration, deceleration, stopping ability, conditioning, transitions between skills, and cutting ability while using cones
- *Agility ladder drills*: Drills that require the use of an agility ladder to enhance coordination, lower body quickness, balance, and footwork quickness
- *Bag drills*: Drills that require the use of bags to enhance change of direction, quick foot action, flexibility, high knee action, and lateral movement
- *Backpedal drills*: Drills that incorporate backpedal movements with change of direction, reaction time, acceleration and deceleration
- *Mini-hurdle drills*: Drills that enhance lateral explosive change of direction through the use of mini-hurdles

LINE DRILLS

61

Pro Agility (20-Yard Shuttle)

Purpose
To develop change of direction, footwork, and reaction time.

Procedure
- Start in a two-point stance, straddling the starting line.
- Turn to the right, sprint, and touch a line 5 yards or meters away with your right hand.
- Turn back to the left, sprint 10 yards or meters, and touch the far line with your left hand.
- Turn back to the right, and sprint 5 yards or meters through the starting line to the finish.

Variations
- Perform different biomotor skills on each leg of the line drill.
- Pick up a ball placed at each line.

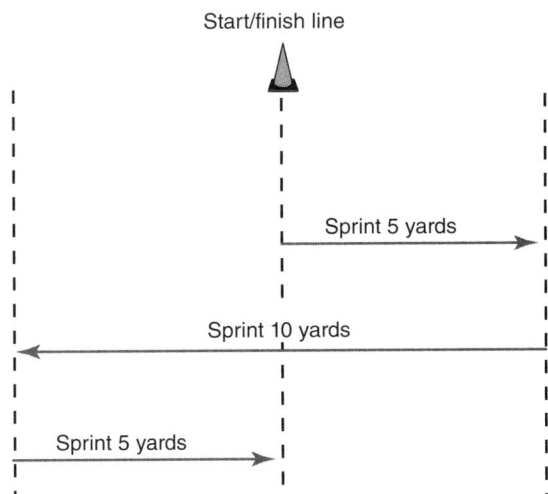

Squirm

Purpose

To develop footwork and reaction time.

Procedure

- Start in a two-point stance.
- Sprint forward 5 yards or meters.
- Rotate 360 degrees and sprint another 5 yards or meters.
- Rotate 360 degrees and sprint another 5 yards or meters.
- Sprint right or left for 10 yards or meters.

Variations

- Put your right hand down on the ground during the first 360 and your left hand down on the ground during the second 360.
- Vary the distance.
- Make turns on command by the coach.
- Use various biomotor skill combinations throughout the drill.

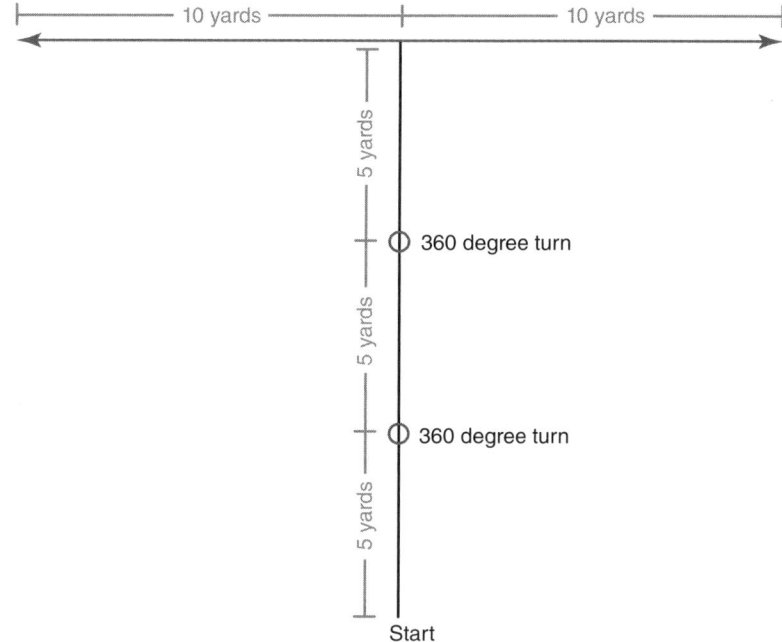

63
40-Yard Line Sprint

Purpose
To develop agility and conditioning

Procedure
- Start in a two-point stance on the starting line.
- Sprint 5 yards or meters to the first line, touch the line with your right hand, return to the starting line, and touch it with your left hand.
- Sprint 10 yards or meters to the second line, touch the line with your right hand, return to the starting line, and touch it with your left hand.
- Sprint 5 yards or meters to the first line, touch the line with your right hand, and return to the starting line.

Variations
- Combine biomotor skills during each leg of the drill.
- Start the drill from various positions (e.g., lying, sitting).
- Add tumbling to each turn.

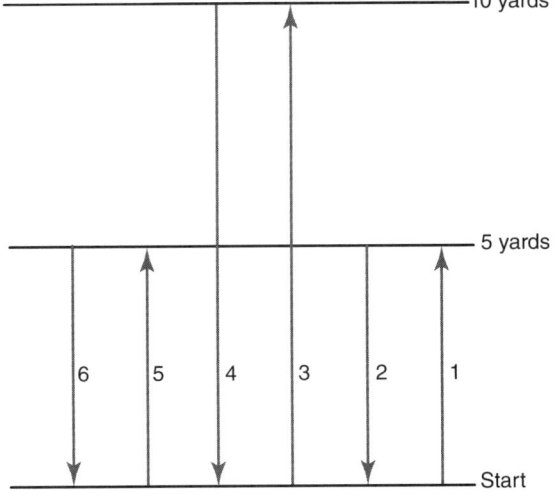

64
60-Yard Line Sprint

Purpose
To develop agility and conditioning.

Procedure
- Sprint forward 5 yards or meters to the first line and touch it with either hand.
- Turn and go back to the starting line.
- Sprint forward 10 yards or meters to the second line and touch it with either hand.
- Turn and go back to the starting line.
- Sprint forward 15 yards or meters to the third line and touch it with either hand.
- Turn and go back through the finish line.

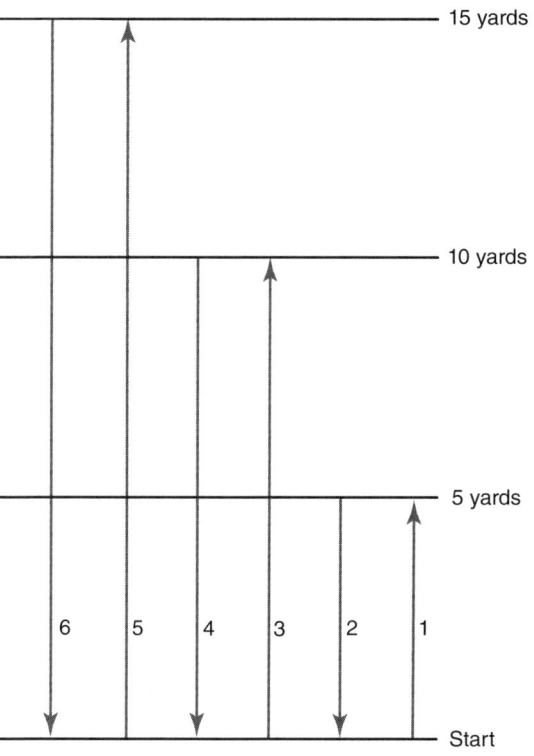

65
30-Yard T Drill

Purpose
To develop agility, conditioning, flexibility in the abductors and adductors, and strength.

Procedure
- Sprint forward 5 yards or meters to a marked spot on the ground.
- Side shuffle to the right, and touch a line 5 yards or meters away with the right hand.
- Shuffle back to the left 10 yards or meters, and touch the far line with your left hand.
- Shuffle back to the right 5 yards or meters to the marked spot.
- Touch the marked spot with either foot, and backpedal through the starting line to the finish.

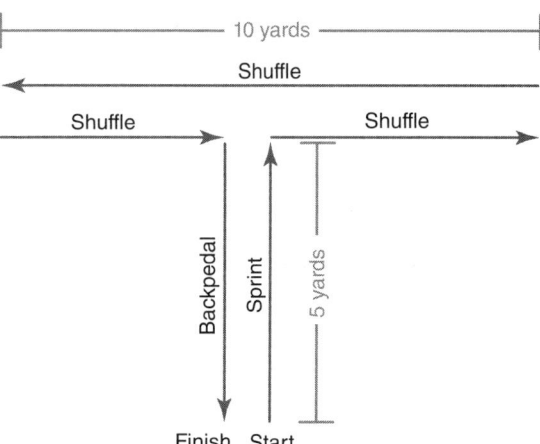

66

40-Yard Line Shuffle

Purpose

To develop agility, conditioning, flexibility in the abductors and adductors, and strength.

Procedure

- Start in a two-point stance, straddling the starting line.
- Shuffle 5 yards or meters to the first line, touch the line with the right foot, shuffle back to the starting line, and touch it with the left foot.
- Shuffle 10 yards or meters to the second line, touch the line with right foot, shuffle back to the starting line, and touch it with the left foot.
- Shuffle 5 yards or meters to the second line, touch the line with the right foot, and shuffle back to the starting line.

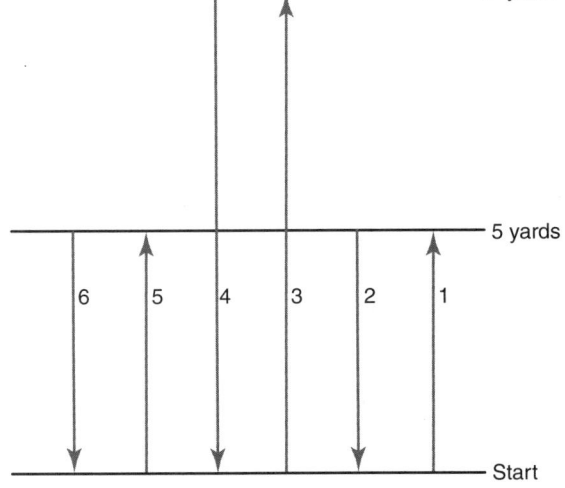

67

40-Yard Line Backpedal to Sprint

Purpose

To develop agility, change of direction, and conditioning.

Procedure

- Start in a two-point stance with your back to the starting line.
- Backpedal 5 yards or meters to the first line, touch the line with either foot, sprint back to the starting line, and touch it with either foot.
- Backpedal 10 yards or meters to the second line, touch the line with either foot, sprint back to the starting line, and touch it with either foot.
- Backpedal 5 yards or meters to the first line, touch the line with either foot, and sprint back to the starting line.

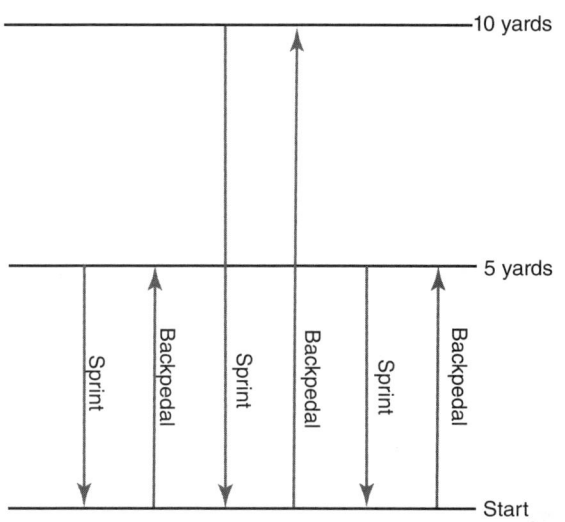

68

40-Yard Line Backpedal Turn 180 Degrees and Sprint

Purpose

To develop agility, change of direction, and conditioning.

Procedure

- Start in a two-point stance with your back to the starting line.
- Backpedal 10 yards or meters, pivot to the right 180 degrees, sprint 10 more yards or meters, and touch the line with either foot.
- Backpedal 10 yards or meters, pivot to the left 180 degrees, and sprint 10 yards or meters to the starting line.

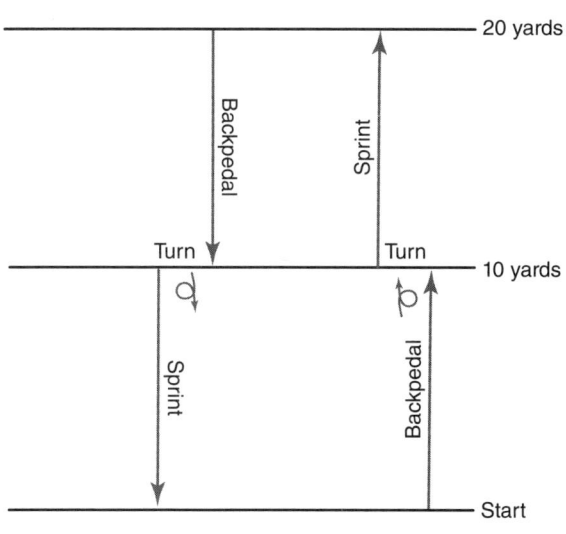

69

55-Yard Line Sprint to Backpedal

Purpose
To develop acceleration and stopping ability.

Procedure
- Sprint forward 10 yards or meters.
- Backpedal 5 yards or meters.
- Sprint forward 10 yards or meters.
- Backpedal 5 yards or meters.
- Sprint forward 10 yards or meters.
- Backpedal 5 yards or meters.
- Sprint forward 10 yards or meters.

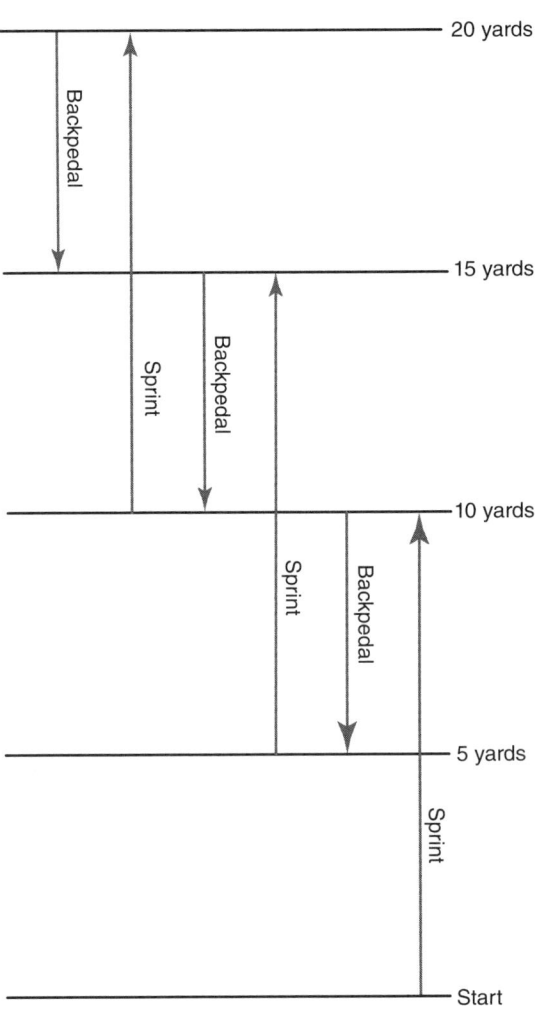

70

100-Yard Line Shuttle

Purpose

To develop change of direction, footwork, and reaction time.

Procedure

- Start in a two-point stance on the starting line.
- Sprint 5 yards or meters to the first line, touch the line with your right hand, return to the starting line, and touch it with your left hand.
- Sprint 10 yards or meters to the second line, touch the line with your right hand, return to the starting line, and touch it with your left hand.
- Sprint 15 yards or meters to the first line, touch the line with your right hand, return to the starting line, and touch it with your left hand.
- Sprint 20 yards or meters to the second line, touch the line with your right hand, return to the starting line, and touch it with your left hand.

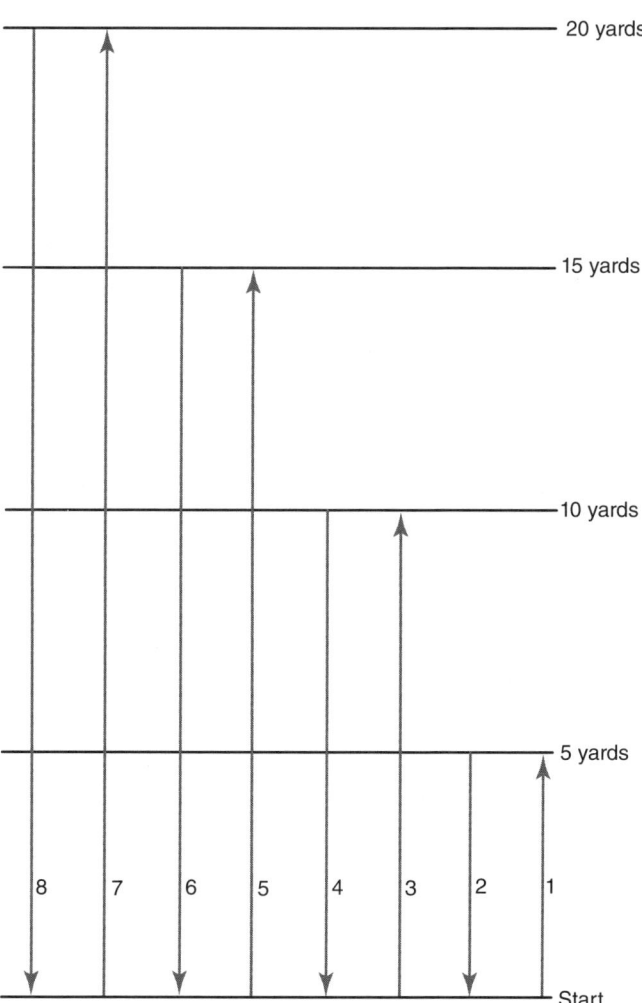

71
30-yard Backpedal to Sprint

Purpose

To develop change of direction and reaction.

Procedure

- Start in a two-point stance with your back toward starting line.
- Backpedal 5 yards or meters to the first line and sprint to the starting line.
- Backpedal 10 yards or meters to the second line and sprint to the starting line to finish.

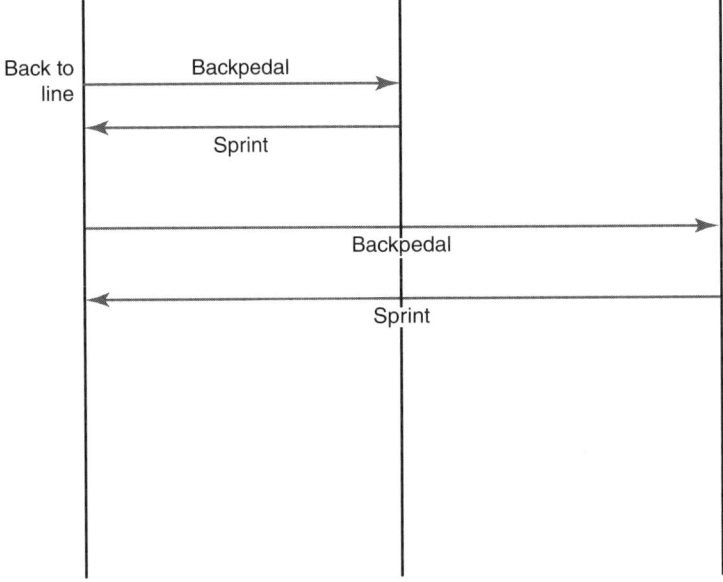

72

90-Degree Backpedal With Turn

Purpose
To develop change of direction and reaction.

Procedure
- Start in a two-point stance with your back toward the starting line.
- Backpedal 10 yards or meters to the line.
- Turn at a 90-degree angle and sprint 10 yards or meters to the right or left.

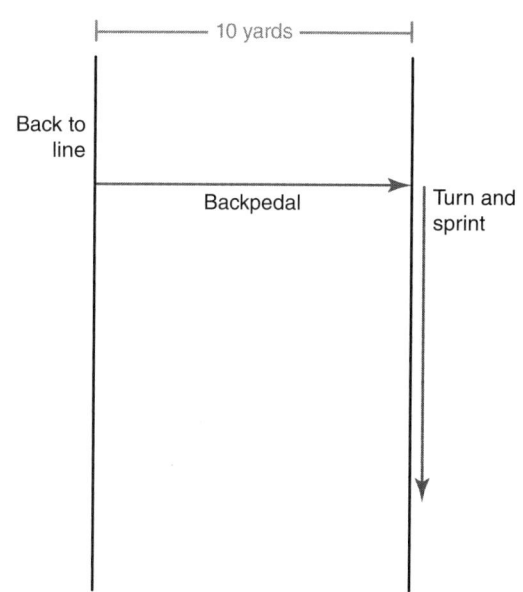

73

45-Degree Backpedal With Turn

Purpose
To develop change of direction and reaction.

Procedure
- Start in a two-point stance with your back toward the starting line.
- Backpedal 10 yards or meters to the line.
- Reverse direction and sprint at a 45-degree angle to the right or left.

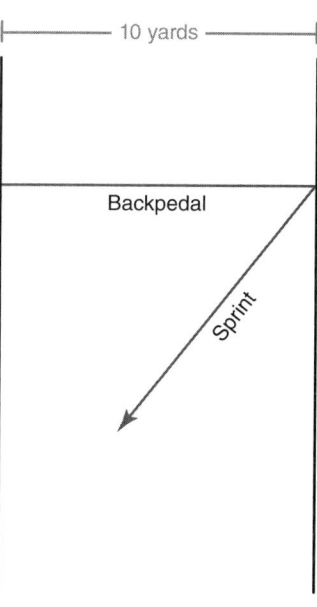

74

Post–Corner

Purpose
To develop change of direction and acceleration after a turn.

Procedure
- Backpedal 10 yards or meters to the line.
- Turn and accelerate at a 45-degree angle forward for 20 yards or meters right or left.

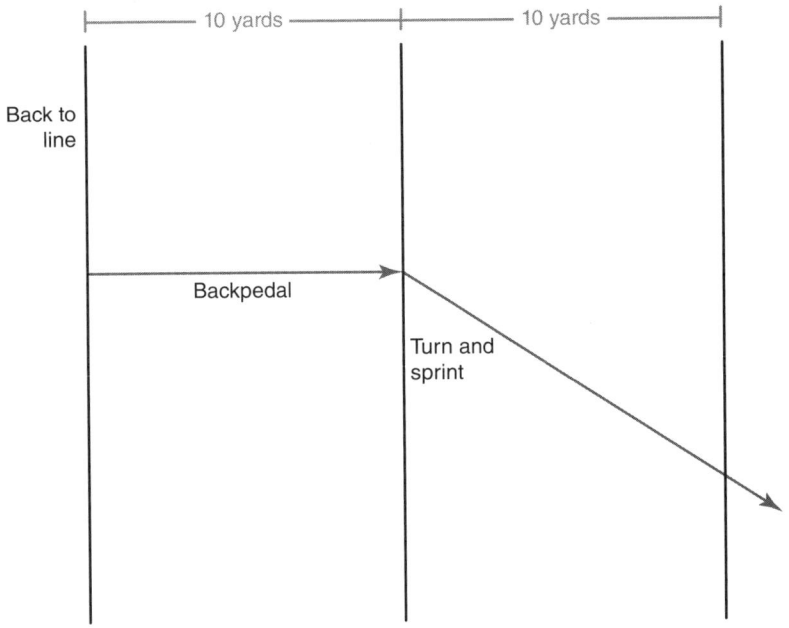

75

Post–Corner–Post

Purpose

To develop change of direction, reaction, and acceleration after a turn.

Procedure

- Backpedal 10 yards or meters to the line.
- Turn and accelerate at a 45-degree angle forward for 10 yards or meters.
- Turn in the opposite direction and accelerate at a 45-degree angle forward for 10 yards or meters.

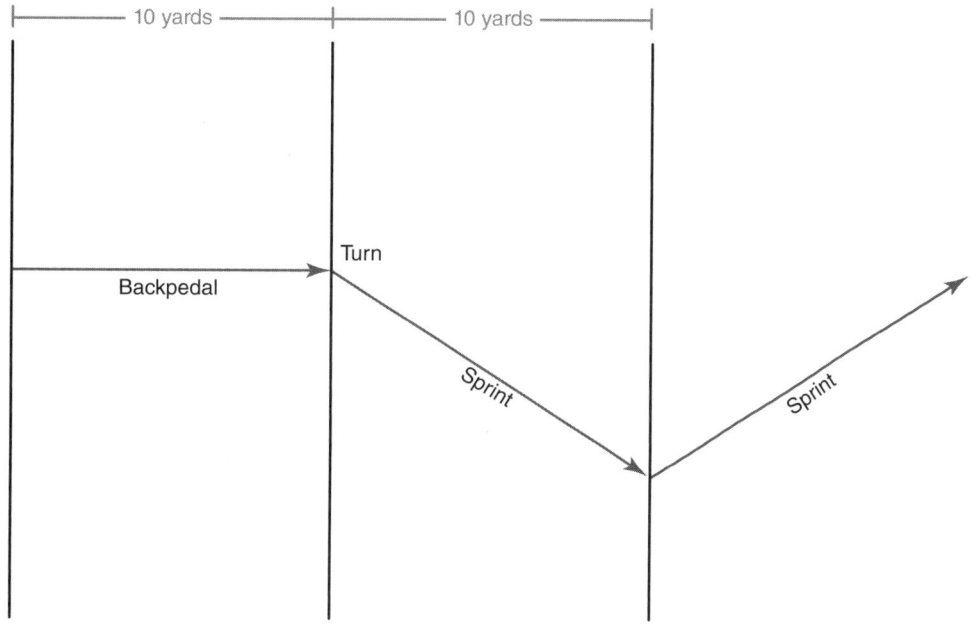

76

Comeback

Purpose

To develop change of direction and reaction.

Procedure

- Start in a two-point stance with your back toward the starting line.
- Backpedal 10 yards or meters to the line.
- Sprint forward 10 yards or meters, concentrating on accelerating.

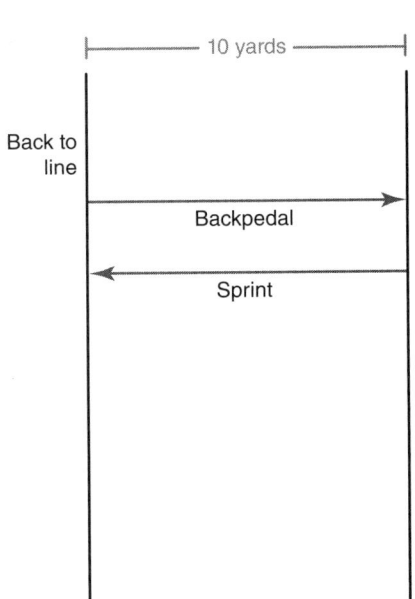

77

Crossover Skipping

Purpose

To develop explosive crossover mechanics for direction changes; enhance explosive contralateral hip flexion and extension

Procedure

- Start in a two-point stance.
- Begin skipping laterally to your left along a line, crossing the right leg over the left.
- Emphasize left-hip extension and right-hip flexion.
- Rotate the hips to the left as the right leg goes over and in front of the left.
- Keep the shoulders square to the front.

78

Crossover Run

Purpose
To loosen up the foot and ankle by gently pushing off instep

Procedure
- Run forward 20 yards stepping one foot over the center line of the body landing on instep.
- Continue crisscrossing your feet as though over a line.
- Return to start by performing the same movement backward.

79

Double-Side Forward Jump

Purpose
To develop agility, balance, and quickness.

Procedure
- Stand with both feet shoulder-width apart on one side of a 20-yard (18 m) line (see figure *a*).
- Hop back and forth over the line, emphasizing quickness as you move forward (see figure *b* and *c*).
- Continue the movement pattern for the entire length of the line.

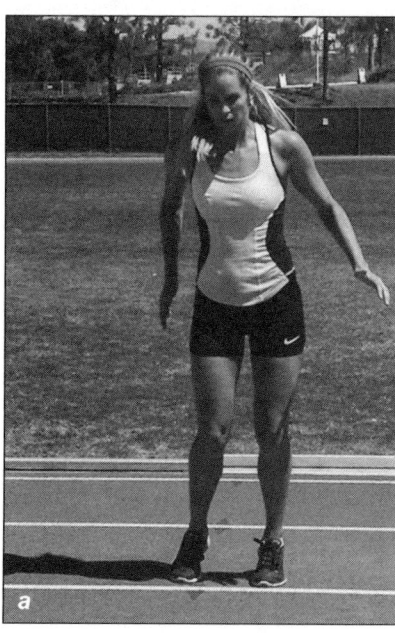
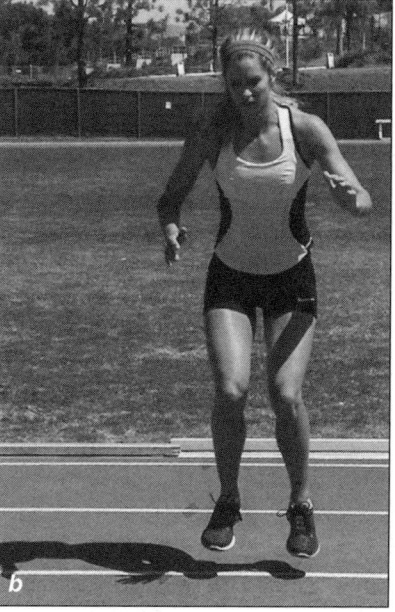
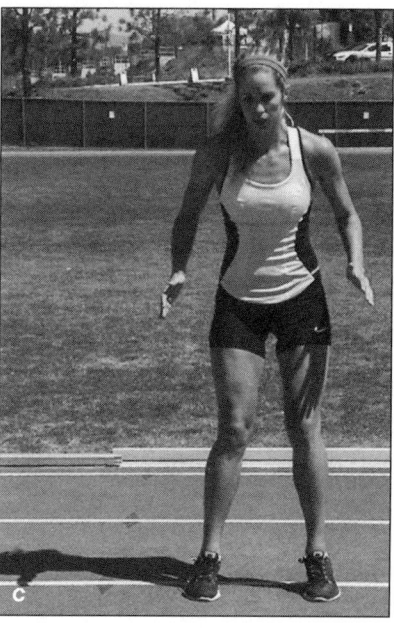

80
Single-Side Forward Hop

Purpose
To develop agility, balance, leg strength, and quickness.

Procedure
- Start on one foot on one side of a 20-yard (18 m) line (see figure *a*).
- Hop back and forth over the line on one foot, emphasizing quickness as you move forward (see figure *b* and *c*).
- At 10 yards (9 m), switch feet without stopping.
- Continue the movement pattern until you reach the end of the line.

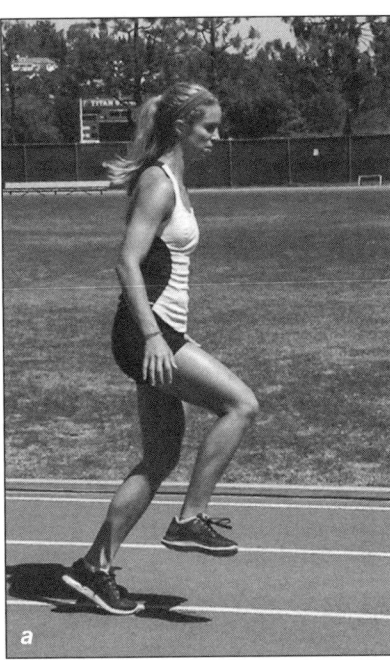
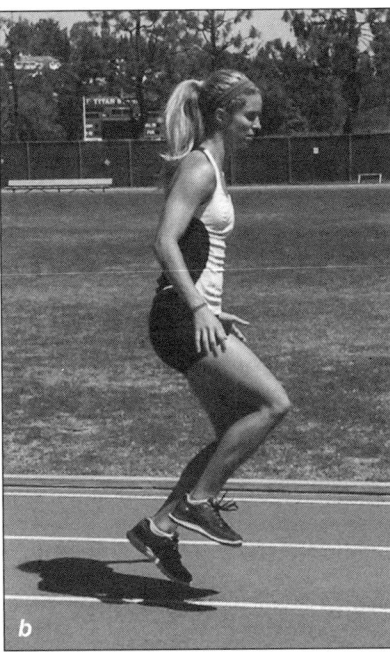
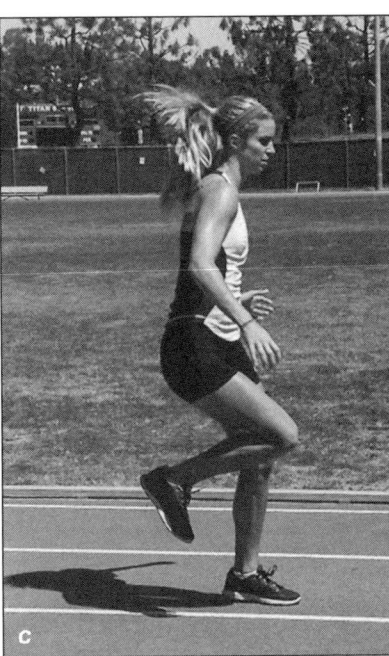

81

Lateral Shuffle

Purpose

To develop agility, balance, lateral movement, and quickness.

Procedure

- Stand with both feet shoulder-width apart, sideways on a 20-yard (18 m) line (see figure *a*).
- Quickly shuffle down the line (see figure *b-d*).
- As you reach the end of the line, quickly reverse directions.

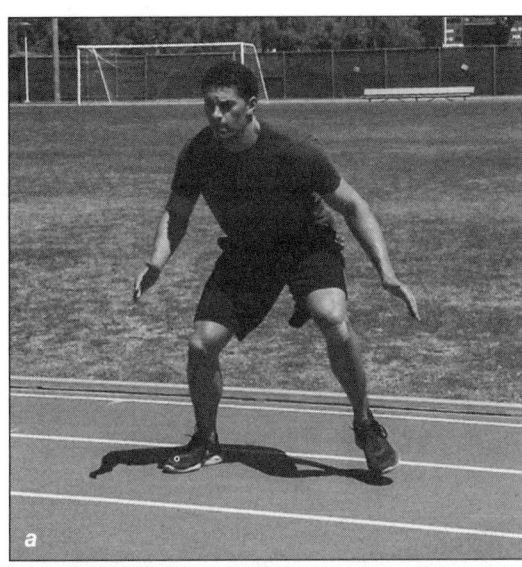
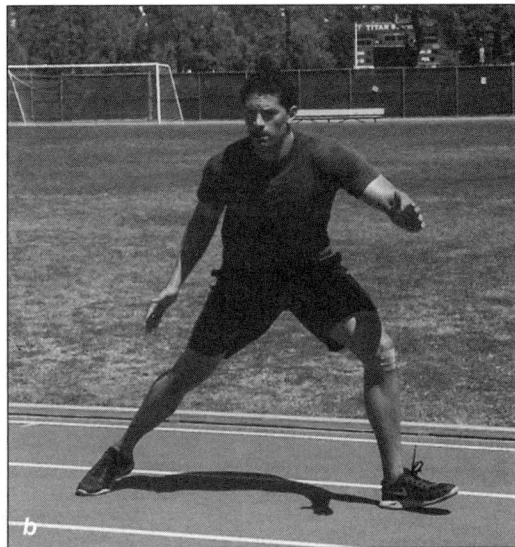
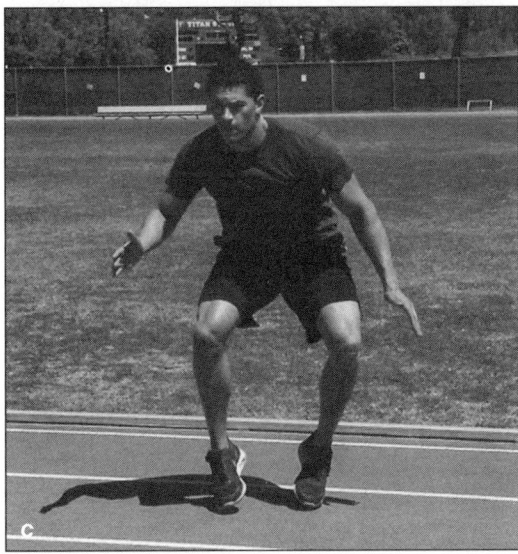
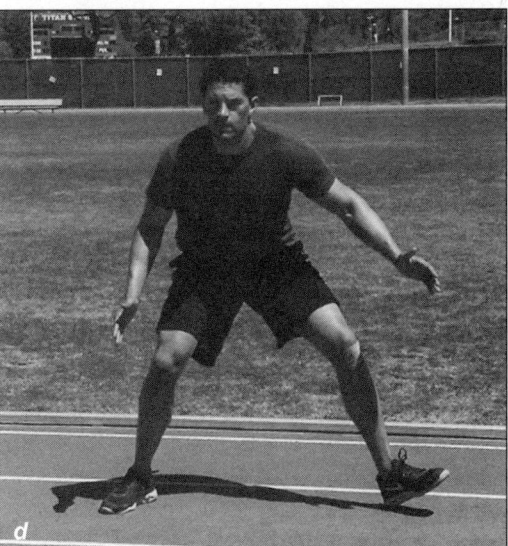

82

Ali Shuffle

Purpose
To develop agility, balance, coordination, and quickness.

Procedure
- Stand straddling a 20-yard (18 m) line.
- Do the Ali shuffle as you move laterally down the line—one foot goes forward of the line as one foot stays behind the line (see figure *a-c*).
- As you reach the end of the line, quickly reverse directions.

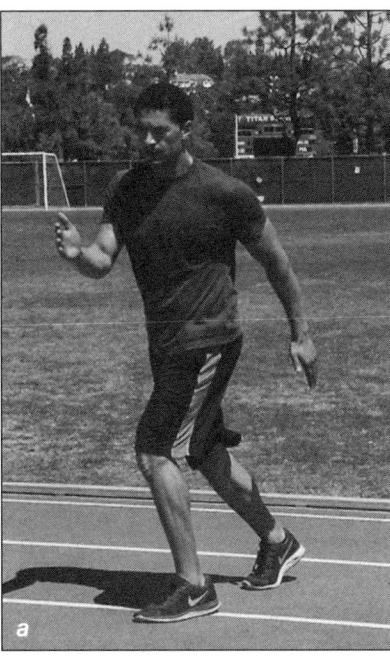 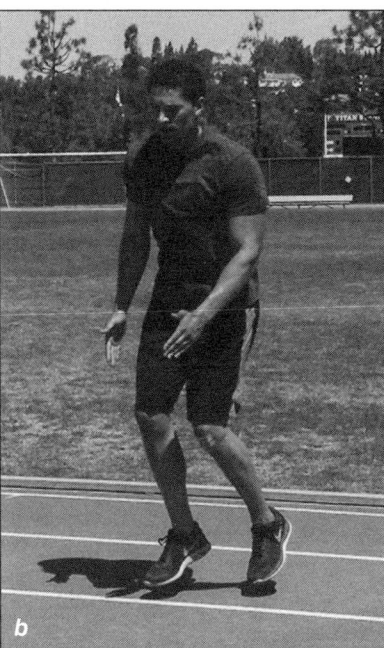 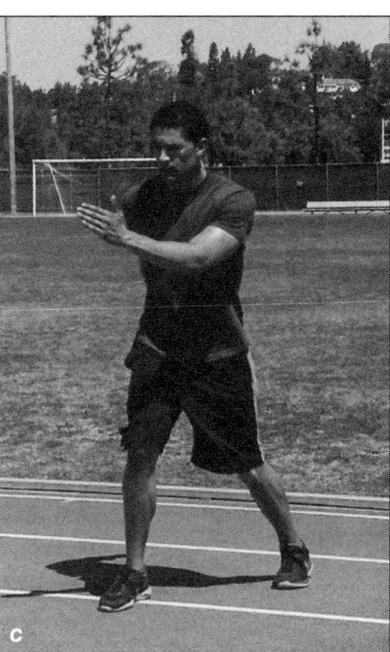

83
Scissors Step

Purpose
To develop agility, balance, coordination, and quickness.

Procedure
- Stand straddling a 20-yard (18 m) line, with feet on each side of the line (see figure *a*).
- Perform a scissors step as you move forward down the line—the feet cross over each other to the front and back. The feet should be crossed on both sides of the line (see figure *b* and *c*).
- Switch the feet each time you jump into the air.
- As you reach the end of the line, quickly turn around and reverse directions.

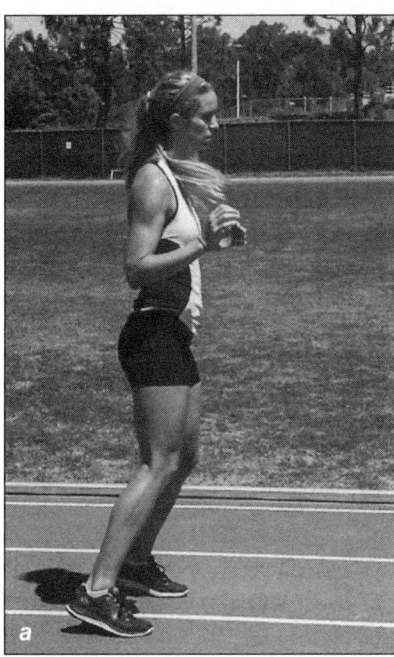 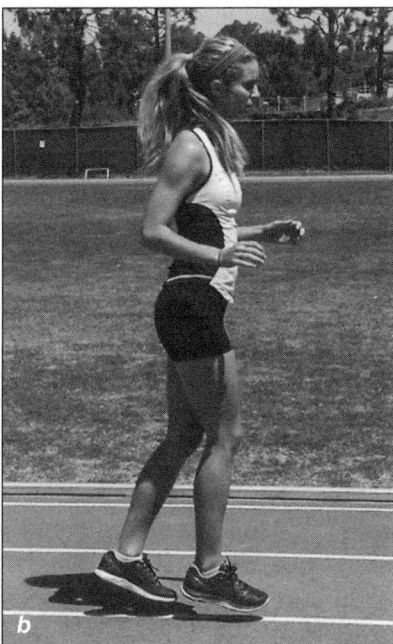 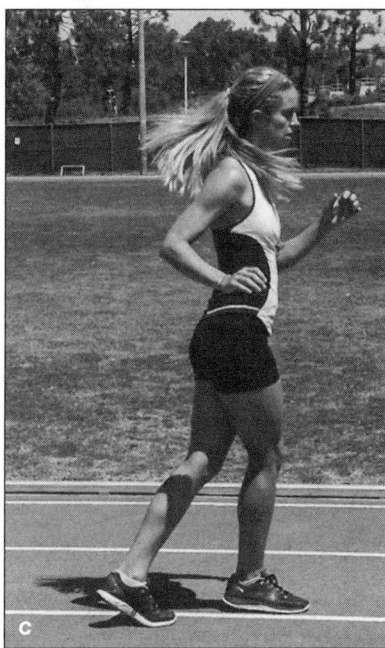

84
180-Degree Line Turn

Purpose

To develop agility, balance, hip flexibility, and quickness.

Procedure

- Straddle a 20-yard (18 m) line facing the direction the drill originates from.
- Jump a half turn so that both feet are straddling the line facing the direction the drill is going as you move forward (see figure *a*).
- Continue repeating the half turns until you reach the end of the line (see figure *b* and *c*).
- At the end of the line, reverse directions and repeat the drill.

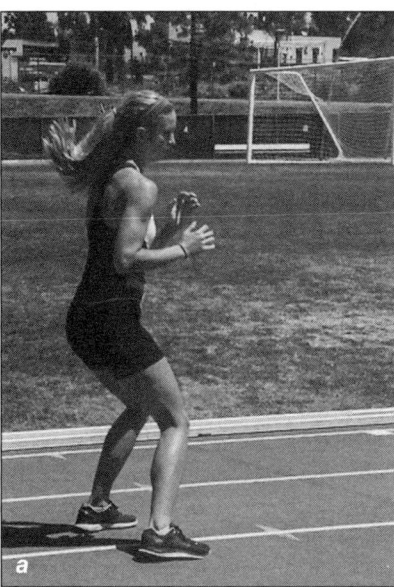 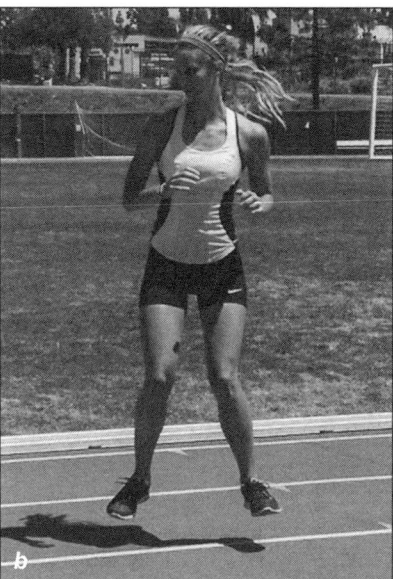 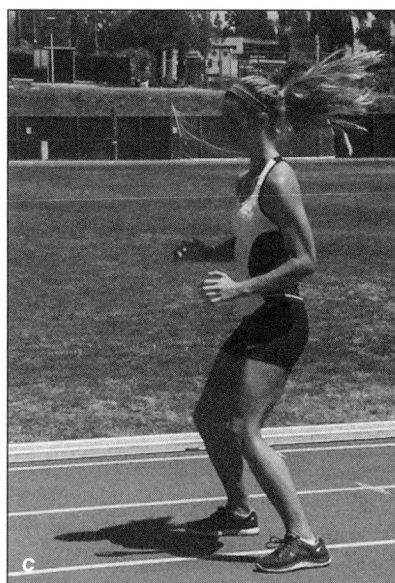

CONE DRILLS

85

15-Yard Turn Drill

Purpose

To improve ability to change direction, flexibility in hips, and footwork.

Procedure

- Start in a two-point stance.
- Sprint forward 5 yards (4.6 m) to cone 1 and make a sharp right turn around it.
- Sprint to cone 2, located 5 yards (4.6 m) to the right of the start and diagonal from the first cone, and make a left turn around it.
- Sprint 5 yards (4.6 m) through the finish.

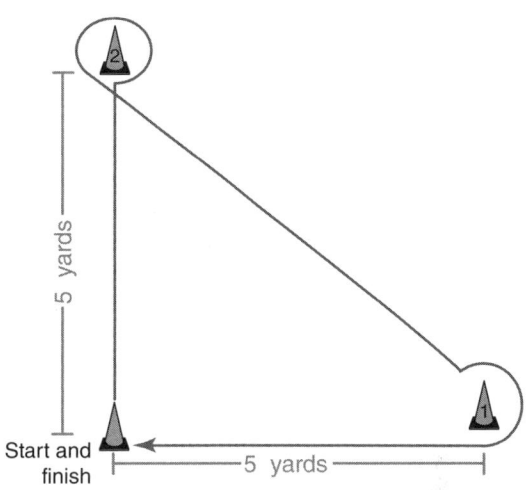

Variations

- Place the inside hand on the ground when making turns.
- Change the distance to the cones.
- Make turns on command, not at the cones.

86

20-Yard Square

Purpose

To improve change of direction and body position, transitions between skills, and cutting ability.

Procedure

- Cones are set up in a square.
- Start in a two-point stance.
- Sprint 5 yards or meters to the first cone and make a sharp right cut.
- Shuffle right 5 yards or meters and make a sharp cut back.
- Backpedal 5 yards or meters to the next cone and make a sharp left cut.
- Left shuffle through the finish.

Variations

- Start from different positions (e.g., lying, four-point stance).
- Change the distance between the cones to the appropriate distance for the sport and energy system.
- Change the skills of each leg to meet specific needs.
- Cut with the inside or outside leg; cut on the outside of the cone; or circle around the cones.
- Put the inside hand on the ground during turns.
- Catch a ball on the cut.

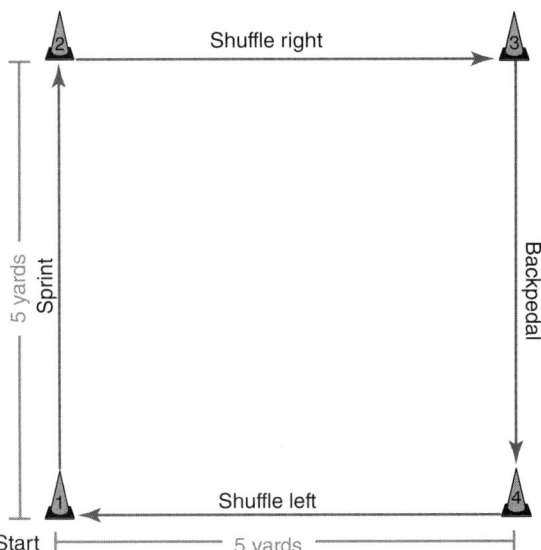

X-Pattern Multiskill

Purpose

To improve transitional movement and cutting ability.

Procedure

- Cones are set up in a square and the drill is run in an X formation.
- Start in a two-point stance.
- Sprint 10 yards or meters to cone 1.
- At cone 1, sprint diagonally 14 yards or meters to cone 2.
- Backpedal 10 yards or meters to cone 3.
- At cone 3, sprint diagonally 14 yards or meters to cone 4.

Variations

- Start from different positions (e.g., lying, four-point stance).
- Change the distance between the cones to the appropriate distance for the sport and energy system.
- Change the skills of each leg to meet specific needs.
- Cut with the inside or outside leg, cut on the outside of the cone, or circle around the cones.
- Put the inside hand on the ground during turns.
- Perform an additional skill, such as dribbling, while performing the drill.

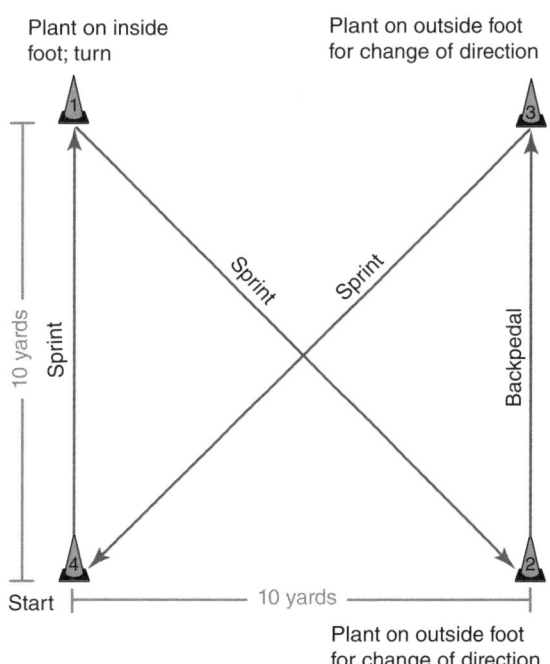

Z-Pattern Run

Purpose
To improve transitional movement and turning ability.

Procedure
- Position six cones on two lines 5 yards or meters apart such that the cones on line 1 are at 0, 10, and 20 yards or meters, and the cones on line 2 are at 5, 15, and 25 yards or meters.
- Start in a two-point stance.
- Sprint diagonally 5 yards or meters to cone 1, plant the outside foot, and run around the cone.
- Continue to sprint diagonally to each cone, running around each one.

Variations
- Start from different positions (e.g., lying, four-point stance).
- Change the distance between the cones to the appropriate distance for the sport and energy system.
- Change the skills of each leg to meet specific needs.
- Cut with the inside or outside leg.
- Cut on the outside of the cone, or circle around the cones.
- Put the inside hand on the ground during turns.
- Once cones are completed, run down the field while performing a skill such as dribbling.

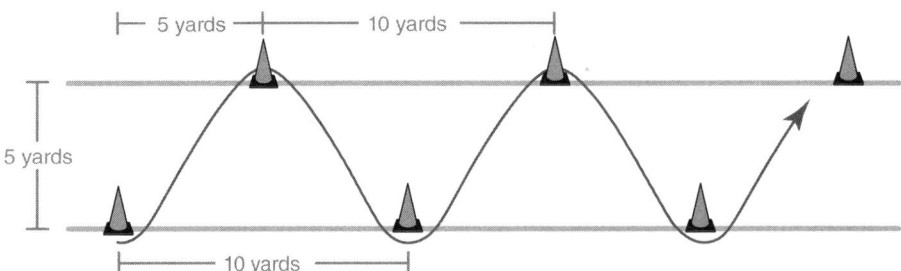

89

40-Yard Square Carioca

Purpose
To develop change of direction, flexibility in the hips, and footwork.

Procedure
- Cones are set up 10 yards apart in a square.
- Start in a two-point stance.
- Begin on the right side of the square, and sprint forward 10 yards or meters.
- At cone 1 make a reverse pivot.
- Carioca 10 yards or meters to the next cone.
- Reverse pivot and backpedal 10 yards or meters to the next cone.
- Reverse pivot and carioca 10 yards or meters to the finish.

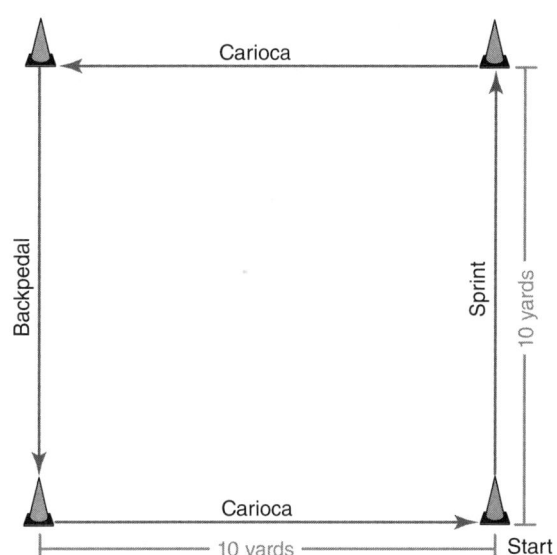

90

40-Yard Square Shuffle

Purpose
To develop flexibility, footwork, and strength in groin area.

Procedure
- Cones are set up 40 yards apart in a square.
- Start in a two-point stance.
- Start on the right side of the square, and sprint forward 10 yards or meters.
- At cone 1 make a reverse pivot and shuffle 10 yards or meters to the next cone.
- Reverse pivot and backpedal 10 yards or meters to the next cone.
- Reverse pivot and shuffle to the finish.

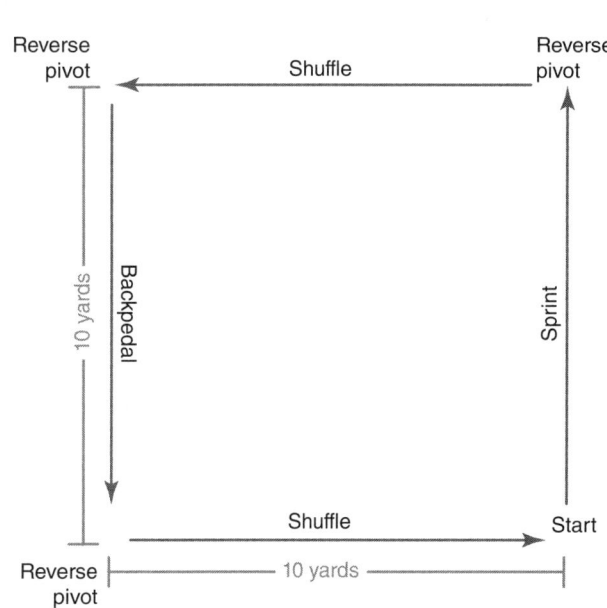

91

X-Pattern Backpedal Sprint

Purpose
To improve backpedaling, change of direction, and footwork.

Procedure
- Cones are set up in a square and drill is run in an X formation.
- Start in a two-point stance.
- Start on the right side of the square, and backpedal 10 yards or meters to cone 1.
- At cone 1 sprint diagonally 14 yards or meters to cone 2.
- Backpedal 10 yards or meters to cone 3.
- At cone 3 sprint diagonally 14 yards or meters to cone 4.

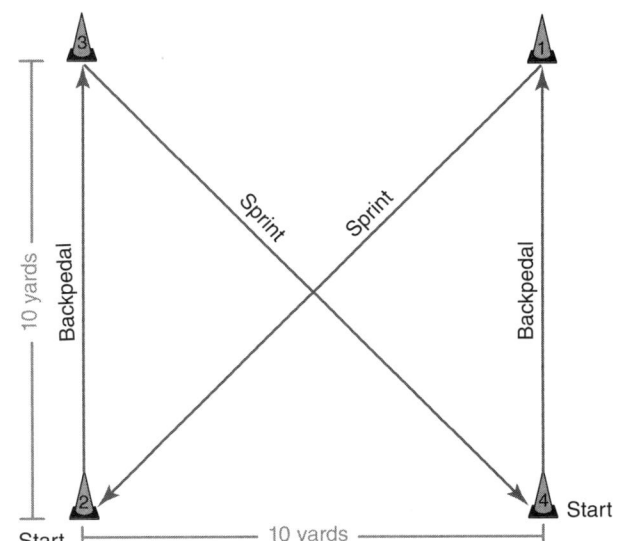

92

X-Pattern Sprint to Backpedal

Purpose
To improve change of direction and footwork.

Procedure
- Set up cones in a square formation.
- Start in a two-point stance.
- Start on the right side of the square, and sprint forward 10 yards or meters.
- Backpedal diagonally 14 yards or meters.
- Sprint 10 yards or meters forward.
- Backpedal diagonally 14 yards or meters to finish.

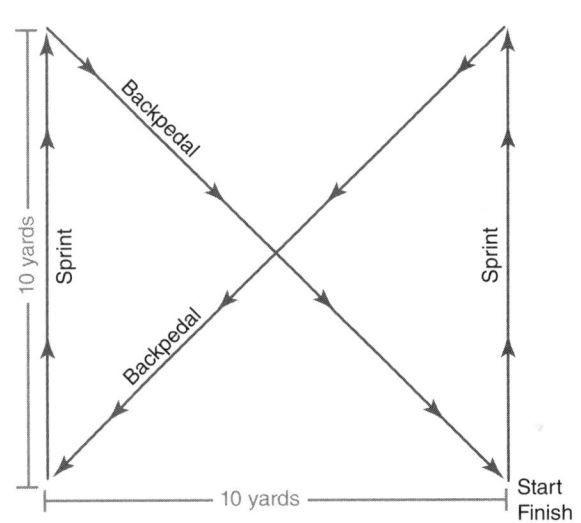

93

Cone Spin

Purpose
To develop flexibility in the legs and hips, foot speed, footwork, and quickness.

Procedure
- Cones are set up 10 yards or meters apart in a square.
- Start at one corner in a two-point stance.
- Sprint 10 yards or meters to cone 1 and rotate 360 degrees on the right hand.
- Sprint 10 yards or meters to cone 2 and rotate 360 degrees on the left hand.
- Sprint 10 yards or meters to cone 3 and rotate 360 degrees on the right hand.
- Sprint 10 yards or meters to cone 4 and rotate 360 degrees on the left hand.

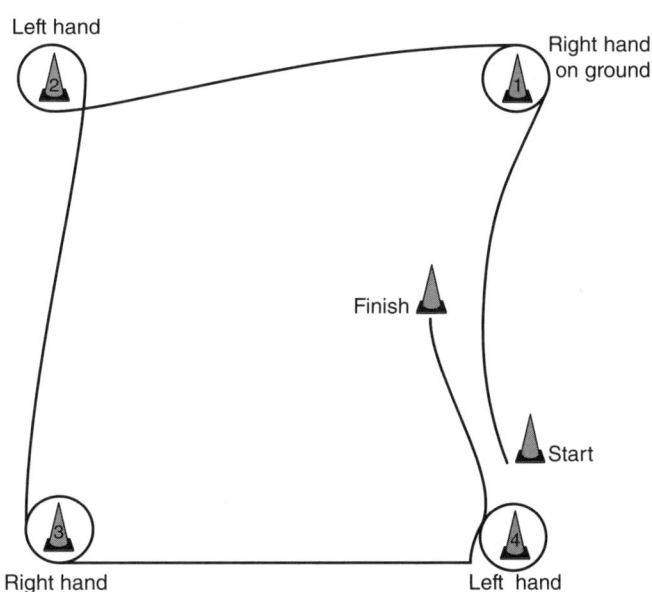

94

Sprint–Shuffle–Backpedal–Break

Purpose
To develop acceleration, change of direction, deceleration, and footwork.

Procedure
- Set up cones in a square formation.
- Start in a two-point stance.
- Sprint 10 yards or meters to cone 1.
- Drive off the left foot using a side step, and shuffle 10 yards or meters right to cone 2.
- At cone 2 backpedal 10 yards or meters to cone 3.
- At cone 3, plant the left foot and sprint at a 45-degree angle to the right for 10 yards.

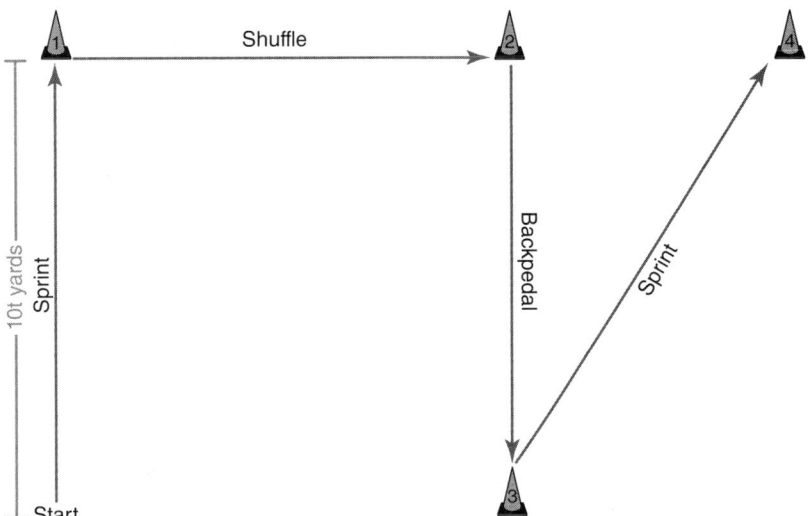

95
Z-Pattern Cuts

Purpose

To develop foot quickness.

Procedure

- Position six cones on two lines 5 yards or meters apart such that the cones on line 1 are at 0, 10, and 20 yards or meters and the cones on line 2 are at 5, 15, and 25 yards or meters.
- Start in a two-point stance.
- Sprint diagonally 5 yards or meters to cone 1, plant the outside foot, and cut sharply to cone 2.
- Continue to sprint diagonally 5 yards or meters to each cone, planting the outside foot and using a side step to cut hard.

96
Cone Zigzag

Purpose

To develop footwork and quickness.

Procedure

- Start in a two-point stance facing a row of 10 cones, each cone 1 yard or meter apart.
- Quickly step forward diagonally with the right foot to the right of cone 1 and then slide the left foot to the right foot.
- Lead with the left foot to the left side of the next cone, and then slide the right foot to the left foot.
- Zigzag through all the cones quickly and explosively.

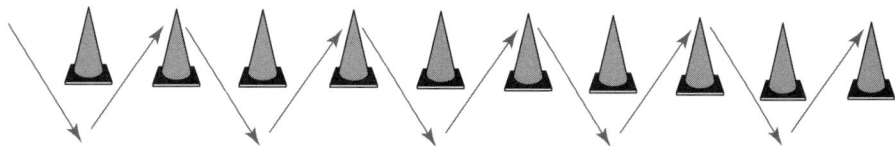

97

Backward Zigzag

Purpose

To develop coordination and foot quickness.

Procedure

- Start in a two-point stance with your back to a row of 10 cones, each cone 1 yard or meter apart.
- Step diagonally backward, leading with the left foot to the left of cone 1 and sliding the right foot to the left foot.
- Step diagonally backward with the right foot to the right of the next cone, sliding the left foot to the right foot.
- Repeat the action through all the cones.

98

Combo Zigzag

Purpose

To improve change of direction, coordination, and foot quickness.

Procedure

- Start in a two-point stance with your back to cone 1 in a row of 10 cones, each 1 yard or meter apart.
- Step diagonally backward, leading with your left foot facing cone 2 and sliding your right foot toward your left foot.
- Repeat going in the opposite direction.
- Continue this pattern for all 10 cones.

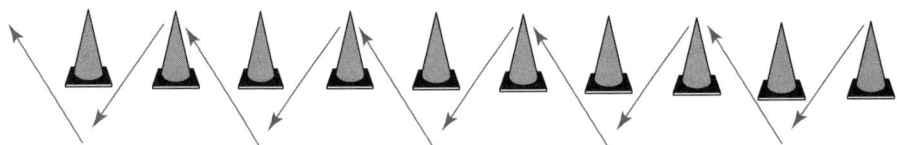

99
Sprint–Sprint–Backpedal

Purpose
To develop change of direction and foot quickness.

Procedure
- Start in a two-point stance.
- Sprint from cone 1 to cone 2.
- Make a quick backshoulder turn and sprint back to cone 1.
- Backpedal from cone 1 to cone 3.
- Sprint from cone 3 back to cone 1.

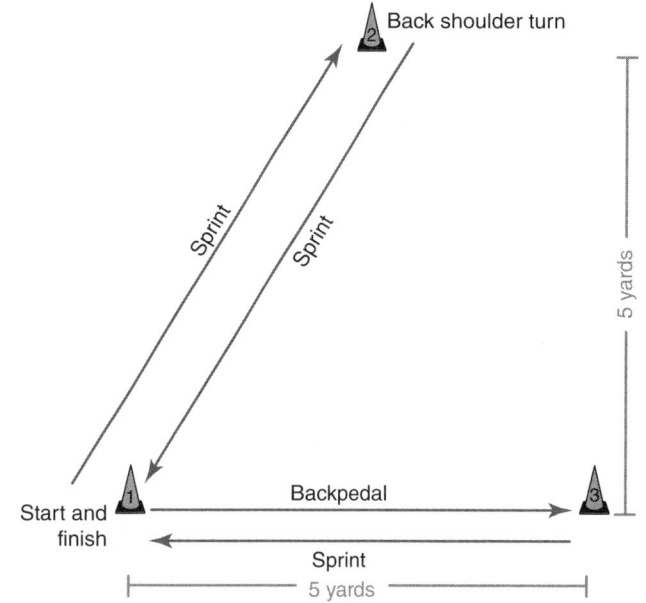

100
Z-Pattern Diagonal Shuffle

Purpose
To develop flexibility, footwork, and strength in the groin area.

Procedure
- Start in a two-point stance at cone 1.
- Perform a lateral shuffle diagonally to cone 2.
- Cut hard off outside foot and shuffle diagonally to cone 3.
- Repeat procedure through all of the cones.

Variation
- Alternate between sprints and diagonal shuffles.

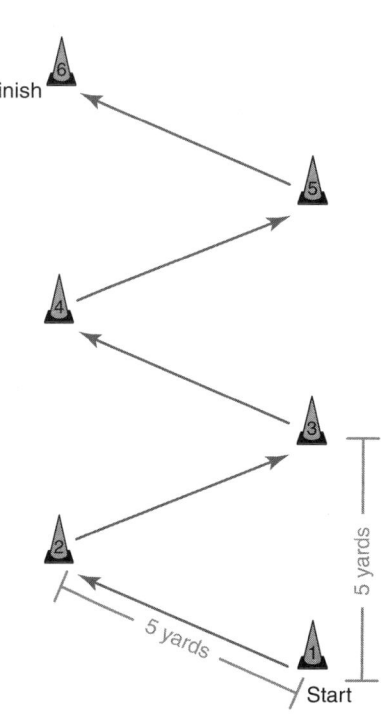

101
S-Pattern Run

Purpose

To develop foot quickness.

Procedure

- Place two cones on two different lines 5 yards or meters apart such that the cones on the right line are 5 yards or meters and 10 yards or meters from the starting line and the cones on the left line are 7.5 yards or meters and 12.5 yards or meters from the start.
- Start in a two-point stance on the left line.
- Sprint diagonally to slightly in front of cone 1 on the right, place your right hand on top of the cone, and spin 360 degrees.
- Sprint diagonally to slightly ahead of cone 1 on the left, place your left hand on top of the cone, and spin 360 degrees.
- Repeat the procedure to each side before sprinting diagonally 5 yards or meters to finish the drill.
- Begin the movement at a controlled pace until you acquire the proprioception and balance needed, and then progressively increase speed.

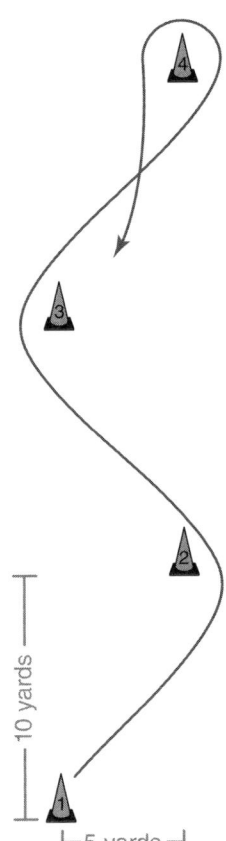

102

20-Yard Rectangle

Purpose

To improve change of direction and body position, transitions between skills, and cutting ability.

Procedure

- Start in a two-point stance at cone 1.
- Sprint 8 yards to cone 2.
- Make a hard back shoulder spin and left lateral shuffle 2 yards to cone 3.
- Sprint from cone 3 to cone 4.
- Mark hard right cut at cone 4 and lateral shuffle to cone 1.

Variations

- Start from different positions (e.g., seated, lying, four-point stance).
- Change the distance between the cones to the appropriate distance for the sport and energy system.
- Change the skills of each leg to meet specific needs.
- Cut with the inside or outside leg.
- Cut on the outside of the cone, or circle around the cones.
- Put the inside hand on the ground during turns.

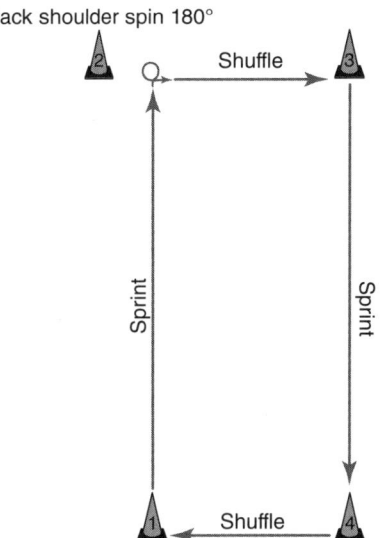

103

Triangle Drill

Purpose

To develop acceleration, stopping ability, and body control.

Procedure

- Place three cones in an upside-down triangle such that cones 2 and 3 are 5 yards or meters apart and cone 1 is in the middle, 5 yards or meters in front.
- Run from cone 1 to cone 2.
- Touch cone 2 and run back to cone 1.
- Touch cone 1 and run to cone 3.
- Touch cone 3 and run back to cone 1.

Variations

- Use shuffling, backpedaling, or combinations.
- Perform the drill for time.

104

Sprint–Shuffle–Sprint

Purpose

To develop acceleration, stopping ability, lateral acceleration, and body control.

Procedure

- On command, sprint forward 5 yards or meters.
- Shuffle 5 yards or meters to the right or left.
- Sprint forward 5 yards or meters.
- Maintain a low center of gravity, keeping the knees and hips bent while shuffling.
- Move the feet as quickly as possible while shuffling.

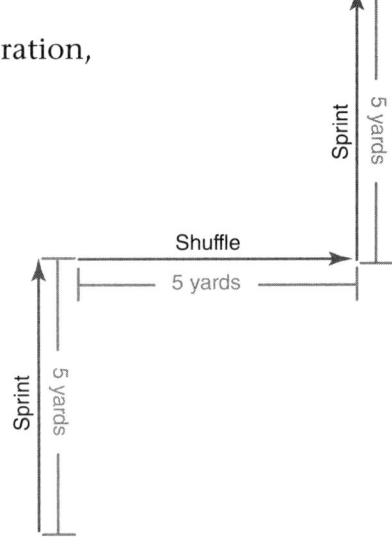

105

Side Shuffle–Angled Shuffle–Sprint

Purpose

To develop controlled change of direction.

Procedure

- Side shuffle 5 yards or meters to cone 1.
- Angle shuffle 5 yards or meters to the right.
- Angle shuffle 5 yards or meters to the left.
- Sprint diagonally to the right 5 yards or meters.
- Side shuffle 5 yards or meters to the left.

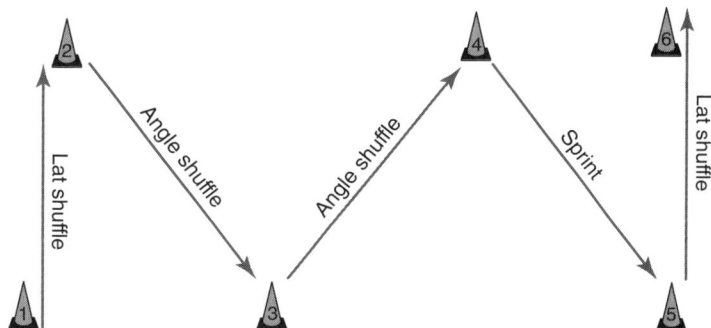

106

M-Shuffle Drill

Purpose

To develop effective transitions between movements and body control.

Procedure

- Begin by angle sliding to the right for 10 yards or meters to cone 1.
- Angle slide to the left for 10 yards or meters to cone 2.
- Angle slide to the right for 10 yards or meters to cone 3.
- Angle slide to the left for 10 yards or meters to cone 4.

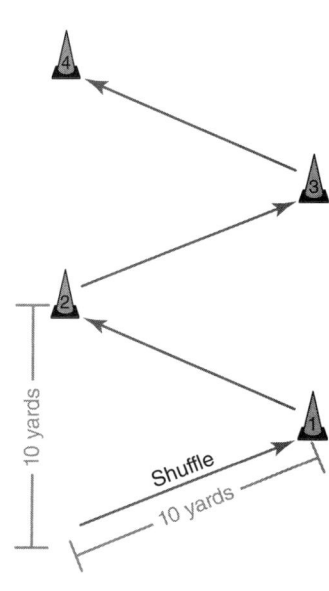

107

W-Pattern Sprint to Quick Step Carioca

Purpose

To develop acceleration and stopping ability.

Procedure

- Set up cones such that three cones are lined up 5 yards or meters apart in a straight line along a goal line, end line, or baseline.
- Place a cone 7 yards or meters in front of and between cones 1 and 2 and another in front of and between 2 and 3.
- Start at one end of the W at cone 1 and sprint to cone 2.
- Perform a low quick step carioca to cone 3.
- Sprint to cone 4 and continue this sequence for the remaining cones.

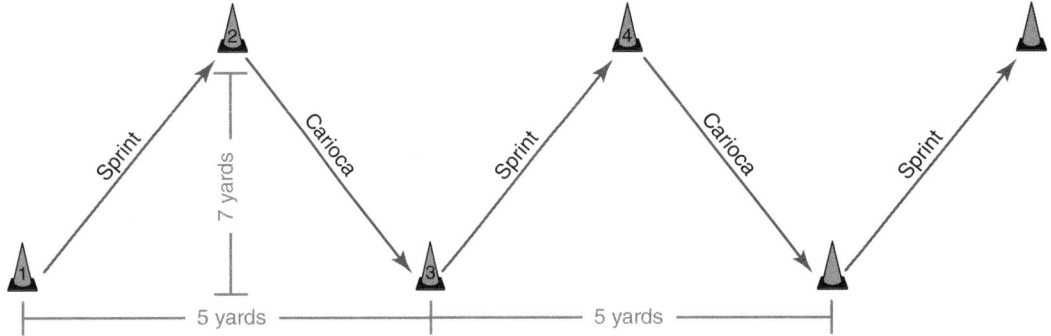

108
Diamond Shuffle

Purpose
To develop lateral acceleration, stopping ability, and a low athletic stance.

Procedure
- Start at the center cone and assume a low center of gravity, with the knees and hips bent, a flat back, and the eyes up.
- Shuffle to cone 2 and then shuffle back to the center cone.
- Proceed around the pattern until all cones have been reached.
- Touch each cone with the outside hand.
- Keep the head up and eyes forward, using peripheral vision to locate the cones.

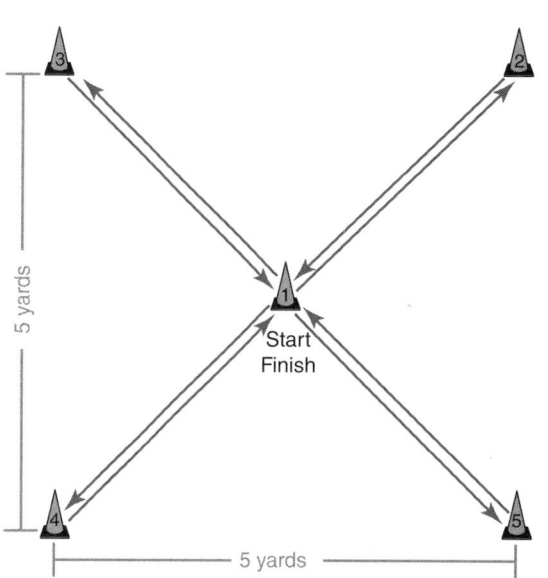

109
Backpedal–Shuffle–Sprint

Purpose
To develop acceleration, stopping ability, lateral acceleration, the crossover step, and body control.

Procedure
- Backpedal 5 yards or meters to cone 1.
- Shuffle 5 yards or meters to the left or right.
- Execute the crossover step, and then sprint 5 yards or meters.
- Maintain a low center of gravity, keeping the knees and hips bent while shuffling.
- Move the feet as quickly as possible while shuffling.

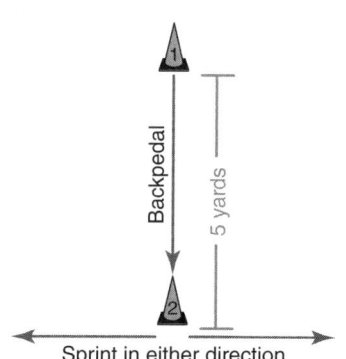

110

Forward Run With Lateral Shuffle

Purpose

To develop controlled change of direction and integrate two movement patterns.

Procedure

- Begin by sprinting 10 yards or meters from cone 1 diagonally to cone 2.
- Shuffle laterally 10 yards or meters to the left to cone 3.
- Sprint 10 yards or meters diagonally to cone 4.
- Shuffle laterally 10 yards or meters to the right after passing cone 4 to cone 5.
- Keep the head up and eyes forward, using peripheral vision to locate the cones.

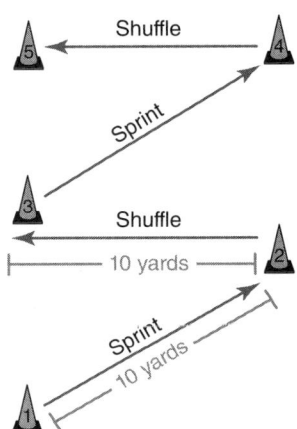

111

15-Yard Z Drill

Purpose

To develop change of direction, flexibility in the hips, and footwork.

Procedure

- Set up cones in a Z formation.
- Start in a two-point stance.
- Sprint forward 5 yards or meters to cone 1 and make a right turn around it by putting the right hand on the ground to pivot.
- Sprint to cone 2 (located 5 yards or meters to the right of the start and diagonal from cone 1), and make a left turn by putting the left hand on the ground.
- Sprint 5 yards or meters forward through the finish.

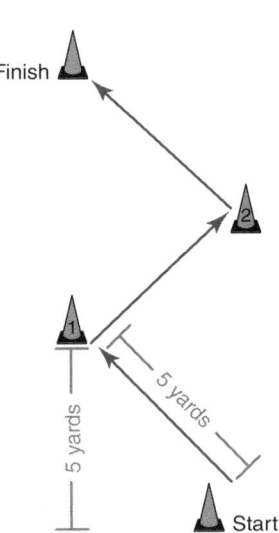

112
40-Yard Square Multiskill

Purpose
To improve change of direction and body position, transitions between skills, and cutting ability.

Procedure
- Position four cones in a square 10 yards or meters apart such that cone 1 is on the starting line, cone 2 is 10 yards or meters straight ahead, cone 3 is 10 yards or meters to the left of cone 2, and cone 4 is 10 yards or meters to the left of cone 1.
- Start in a ready position at cone 1.
- Make two consecutive trips around the lane—one counterclockwise and one clockwise.
- On "Go," sprint forward from cone 1 to cone 2.
- Upon reaching cone 2, bear-crawl to the left until you reach cone 3.
- Backpedal from cone 3 to cone 4.
- Bear-crawl to the right from cone 4 to cone 1.
- Upon reaching the starting point, repeat the drill, going in the opposite direction.

Variation
Repeat the drill, but this time sprint, single-leg hop, and backpedal.

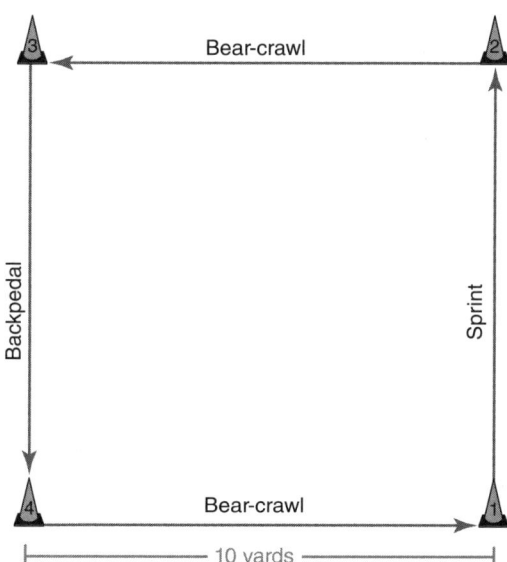

113
Snake Drill 1

Purpose

To improve change of direction and body position, transitions between skills, and cutting ability.

Procedure

- Position four cones in a square 10 yards or meters apart such that cone 1 is on the starting line, cone 2 is 10 yards or meters straight ahead, cone 3 is 10 yards or meters to the left of cone 2, and cone 4 is 10 yards or meters to the left of cone 1. Cone 5 should be placed in the middle of the square.
- Start in a ready position between cone 1 and cone 2.
- Sprint forward around cone 2.
- Sprint diagonally around cone 5.
- Sprint diagonally around cone 3.
- Sprint forward around cone 4.
- Sprint diagonally around cone 5.
- Sprint diagonally around cone 1.
- Sprint from cone 1 to midway between cone 1 and cone 2.

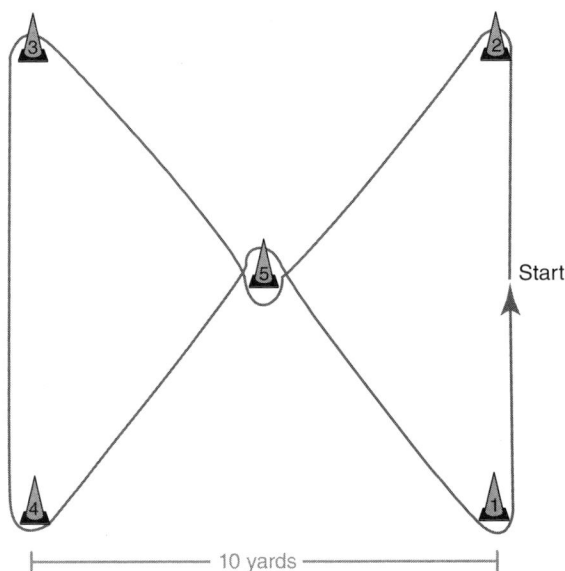

114

Snake Drill 2

Purpose

To improve change of direction and body position, transitions between skills, and cutting ability.

Procedure

- Place seven cones in a straight line 5 yards or meters apart. Place cones 5 yards or meters in front of cones 2, 4, and 6.
- Without crossing over with your feet, shuffle to the right from cone 1 to cone 2.
- Plant your right foot and drive forward to the cone 5 yards or meters in front of cone 2. Sprint around the cone and diagonally to cone 3.
- Without crossing over with your feet, shuffle to the right from cone 3 to cone 4.
- Plant your right foot and drive forward to the cone 5 yards or meters in front of cone 4. Sprint around the cone and diagonally to cone 5.
- Without crossing over with your feet, shuffle to the right from cone 5 to cone 6.
- Plant your right foot and drive forward to the cone 5 yards or meters in front of cone 6. Sprint around the cone and diagonally to cone 7.
- Perform the drill in both directions for one repetition.

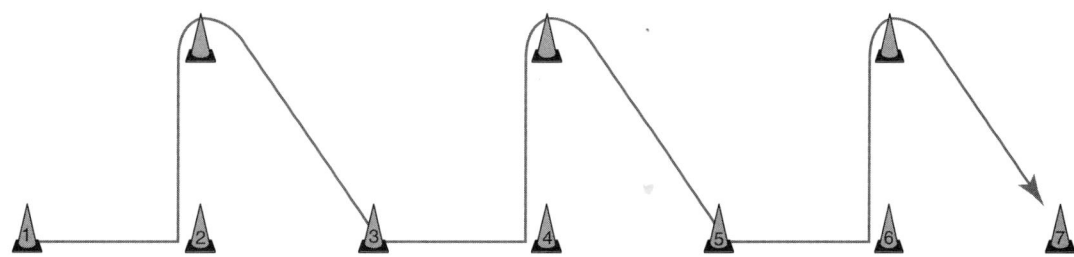

115

V Drill

Purpose

To improve change of direction and body position, transitions between skills, and cutting ability.

Procedure

- Place three cones to form a 45-degree angle. Cone 1 will be on the starting line, and cones 2 and 3 will be 10 yards or meters to the left and right respectively and 10 yards or meters forward.
- Sprint diagonally forward to the left to cone 2.
- Plant your left foot and backpedal back to cone 1.
- Without pause, sprint diagonally forward to the right to cone 3.
- Plant your right foot and backpedal back to cone 1.
- A sprint and backpedal in both directions are one repetition.

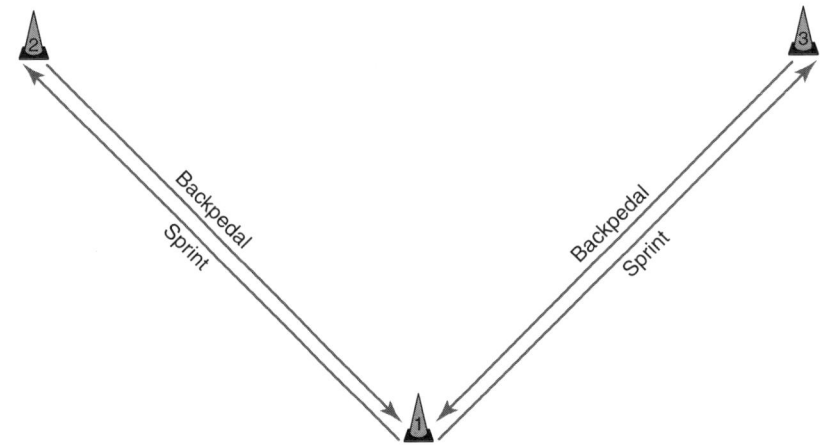

116

A Movement

Purpose

To improve change of direction and body position, transitions between skills, and cutting ability.

Procedure

- Place five cones in an A shape such that cone 1 and cone 5 are 10 yards or meters apart on the starting line. Cones 2 and 3 are 5 yards or meters in front of 1 and 5 and 5 yards or meters apart. Cone 4 is 5 yards or meters in front of and between 2 and 3.
- Sprint from cone 1 to cone 2.
- Shuffle from cone 2 to cone 3.
- Shuffle back from cone 3 to cone 2.
- Sprint from cone 2 to cone 4.
- Backpedal from cone 4 to cone 5.

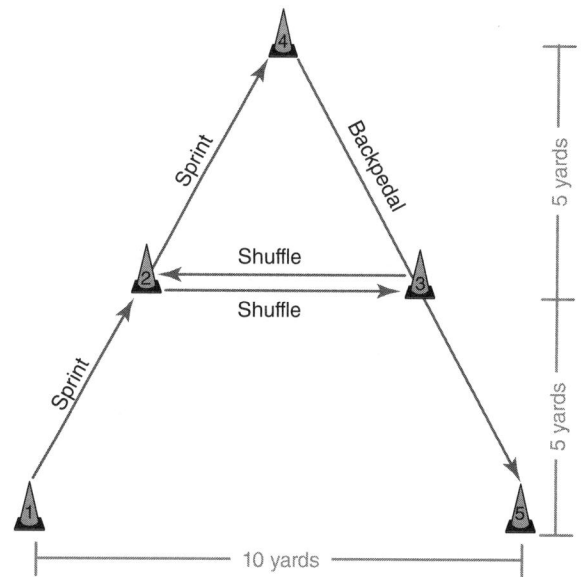

Variation

Perform an additional skill, such as dribbling, while performing the drill.

117

E Movement

Purpose
To improve change of direction and body position, transitions between skills, and cutting ability.

Procedure
- Place six cones in an E shape such that cone 1 and cone 2 are 10 yards or meters apart on the starting line. Cones 3 and 4 are 5 yards or meters in front of 1 and 2, and cones 5 and 6 are 5 yards or meters in front of 3 and 4.
- Shuffle from cone 1 to cone 2.
- Sprint from cone 2 to cone 3.
- Shuffle from cone 3 to cone 4.
- Shuffle back from cone 4 to cone 3.
- Sprint from cone 3 to cone 5.
- Shuffle from cone 5 to cone 6.
- Shuffle back from cone 6 to cone 5.
- Backpedal from cone 5 to cone 2.
- Shuffle from cone 2 to cone 1.

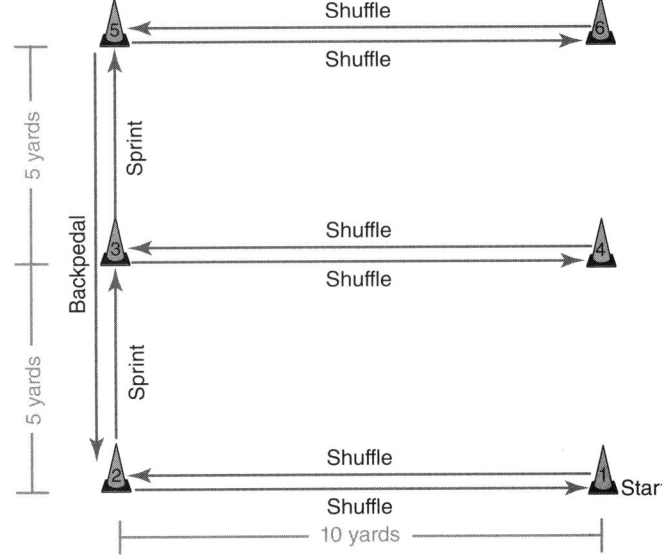

Variation
Perform an additional skill, such as dribbling, while performing the drill.

118

F Movement

Purpose
To improve change of direction and body position, transitions between skills, and cutting ability.

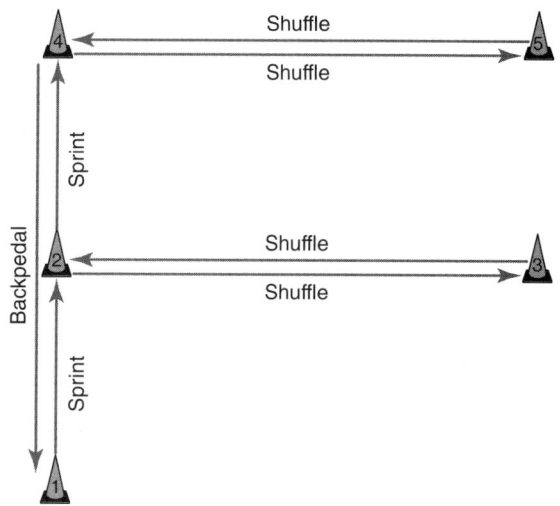

Procedure
- Place five cones in an F shape such that cone 1 is on the starting line. Cone 2 is 5 yards or meters in front of cone 1, and cone 3 is 5 yards or meters to the right of cone 2. Cones 4 and 5 are 5 yards or meters in front of 2 and 3.
- Sprint from cone 1 to cone 2.
- Shuffle from cone 2 to cone 3.
- Shuffle back from cone 3 to cone 2.
- Sprint from cone 2 to cone 4.
- Shuffle from cone 4 to cone 5.
- Shuffle back from cone 5 to cone 4.
- Backpedal from cone 4 to cone 1.

Variation
Perform an additional skill, such as dribbling, while performing the drill.

119

H Movement

Purpose

To improve change of direction and body position, transitions between skills, and cutting ability.

Procedure

- Place six cones in an H shape such that cone 1 is on the starting line. Cone 2 is 5 yards or meters in front of 1, and cone 3 is 5 yards or meters to the right of cone 2. Cones 4 and 5 are 5 yards or meters in front of 2 and 3. Cone 6 is 5 yards or meters to the right of cone 1.
- Sprint from cone 2 to cone 4.
- Backpedal from cone 4 to cone 2.
- Shuffle from cone 2 to cone 3.
- Sprint from cone 3 to cone 5.
- Backpedal from cone 5 to cone 6.
- Sprint from cone 6 to cone 3.
- Shuffle back from cone 3 to cone 2.
- Backpedal from cone 2 to cone 1.

Variation

Perform an additional skill, such as dribbling or catching, while performing the drill.

120
Star Drill

Purpose
To improve change of direction and body position, transitions between skills, and cutting ability.

Procedure
Position four cones in a square 10 yards or meters apart such that cone 1 is on the starting line, cone 2 is 10 yards or meters straight ahead, cone 3 is 10 yards or meters to the left of cone 2, and cone 4 is 10 yards or meters to the left of cone 1. Cone 5 should be placed in the middle of the square.

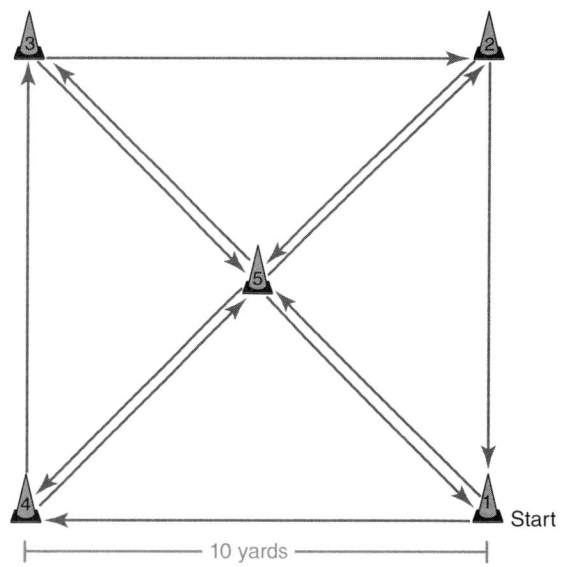

Variation
Additional combinations are as follows:
Sprint–Shuffle–Backpedal; Sprint–Carioca–Shuffle; Sprint–Carioca–Backpedal; Sprint–Backpedal–Carioca; Sprint–Shuffle–Carioca; Sprint–Bear-Crawl–Shuffle; Sprint–Bear-Crawl–Backpedal; Sprint–Backpedal–Bear-Crawl; and Sprint–Shuffle–Bear-Crawl

121
Multidirectional Skipping

Purpose
To improve quickness and coordination in locomotive mechanics.

Procedure
- Set up any size area with cones.
- Skip in various directions inside the cones while continuing to face a target in front of you.
- While skipping, respond to commands or cues to change your direction, using forward, backward, and side skipping.

Variations
- Increase the amplitude of your skip and lower the number of reps.
- Concentrate on the first skip after the command to change direction.
- Add a sprint or skill on command.

122

Figure-Eight Cone Drill

Purpose
To improve the ability to change direction and reaction time.

Procedure
- Position two flat cones 5 to 10 yards (4.6 to 9 meters) apart.
- Start in a two-point stance.
- Run a figure eight between cones, placing your inside hand on each cone while you make the turn.

Variations
- Change the distance between cones.
- Change the radius of the turns.
- Start the drill from various positions (for example, lying, sitting, a four-point stance, and so on).

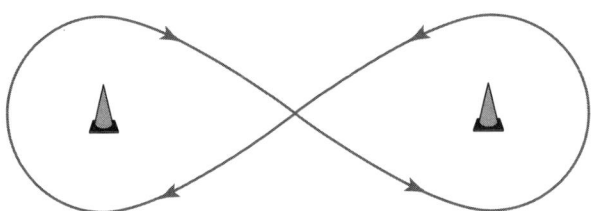

AGILITY LADDER DRILLS

123

Icky Shuffle

Purpose
To enhance coordination and improve lower body quickness.

Procedure
- Start on the left side of the ladder.
- Take a lateral step with the right foot and place it in the first square; the left foot follows the right foot inside the first square of the ladder.
- Take a lateral step with the right foot to the right side of the ladder, and then advance the left foot to the next square in the ladder.
- Bring the right foot to the square the left foot is in.
- Take a lateral step to the left side of the ladder, and advance the right foot to the next square in the ladder.
- Repeat the pattern forward and backward.

Variation
To add complexity to all ladder drills, look up during the drill and avoid looking at your feet.

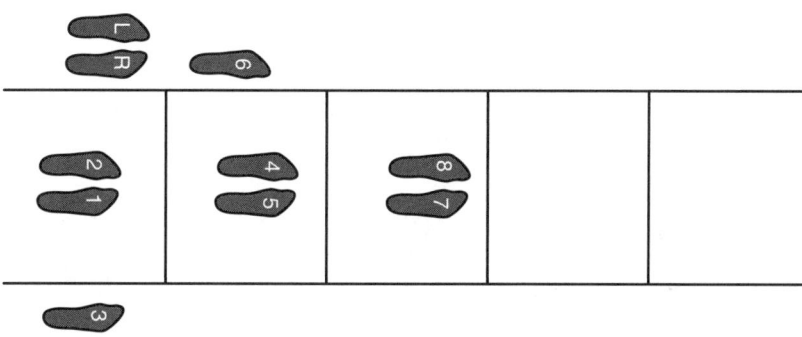

124

In–Out Shuffle

Purpose

To develop agility, balance, coordination, and quickness.

Procedure

- Start in a two-point stance.
- Begin standing sideways to the ladder, with the ladder in front of you.
- Step with the left foot straight ahead into the first square.
- Follow with the right foot into the first square.
- Step back and diagonally with the left foot until it is in front of the second square.
- Follow with the right foot until it is in front of the second square.
- Repeat this sequence throughout the ladder.
- Each foot hits every box.

Variations

- Perform the same pattern with each foot in a separate box.
- Use every other box, and increase the lateral step.
- Perform the drill backward (i.e., start with the ladder behind you).
- Add an additional skill, such as passing, while peforming the drill.

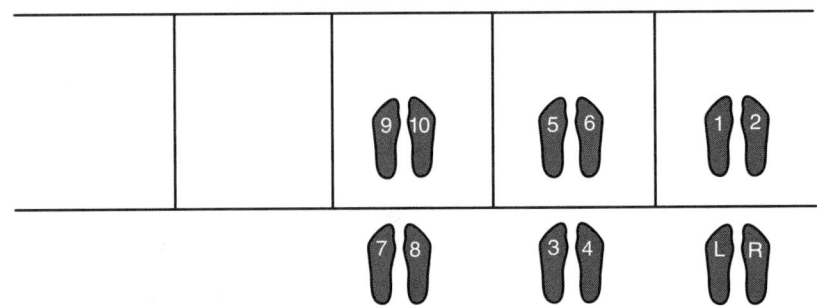

125
180-Degree Ladder Turn

Purpose
To develop agility, balance, hip flexibility, and quickness.

Procedure
- Start in a two-point stance, straddling the first rung of the ladder (see figure *a*).
- With both feet, jump and turn 180 degrees to land straddling the next rung (see figure *b* and *c*).
- Continue repeating the half turns into every square through the agility ladder.

Variation
Perform the drill while facing perpendicular to the ladder.

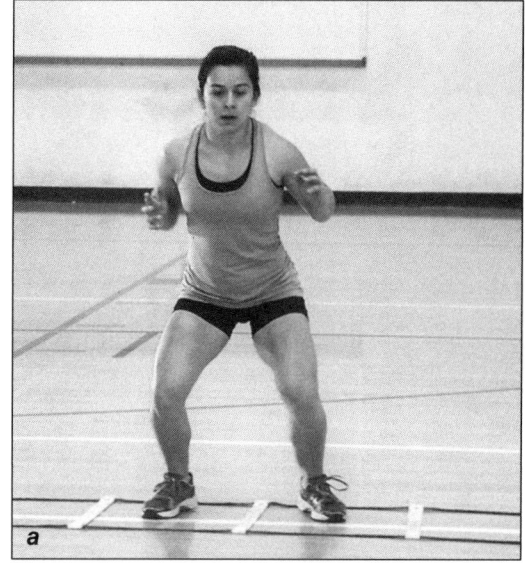

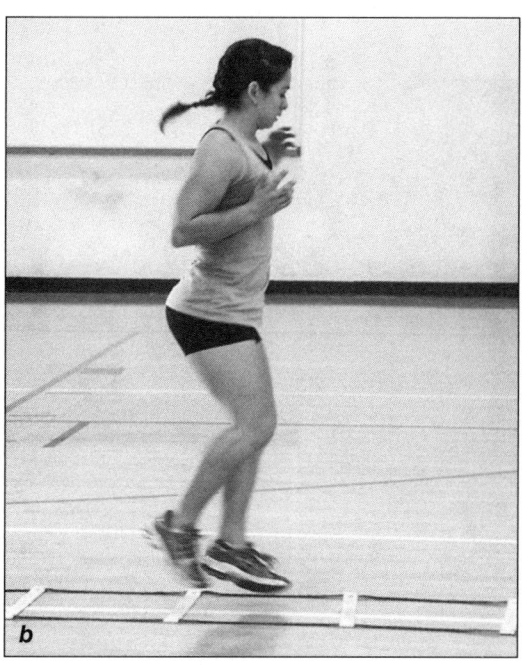

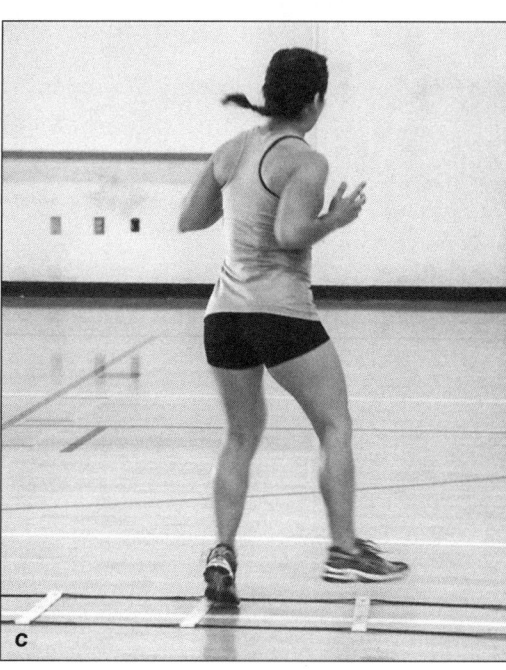

126

Every Hole

Purpose
To develop balance, flexibility, footwork, and high knee action.

Procedure
- Start in a two-point stance.
- Sprint forward using high knee and good arm action.
- Hit the alternate foot in each square of the ladder (see figure *a-c*).

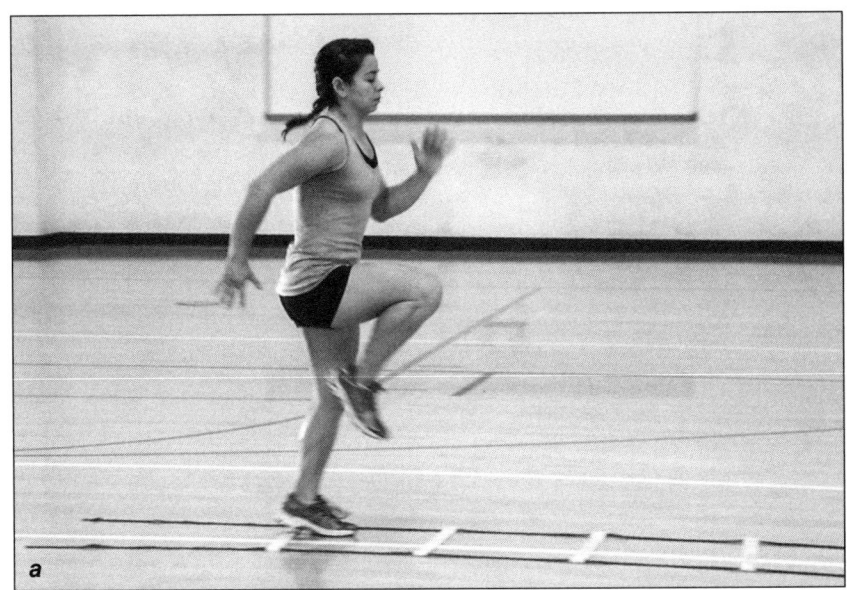
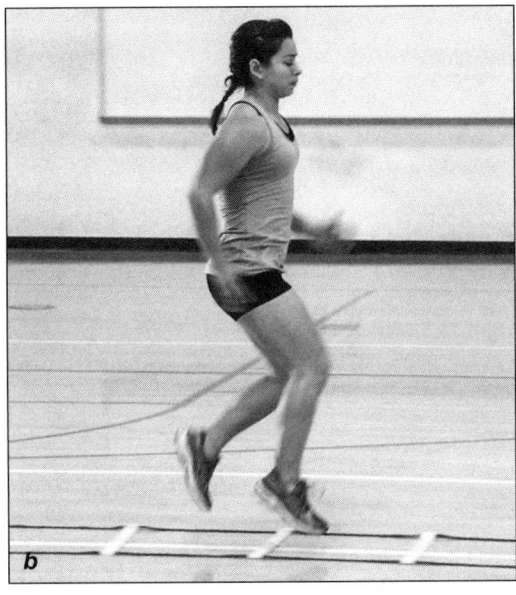
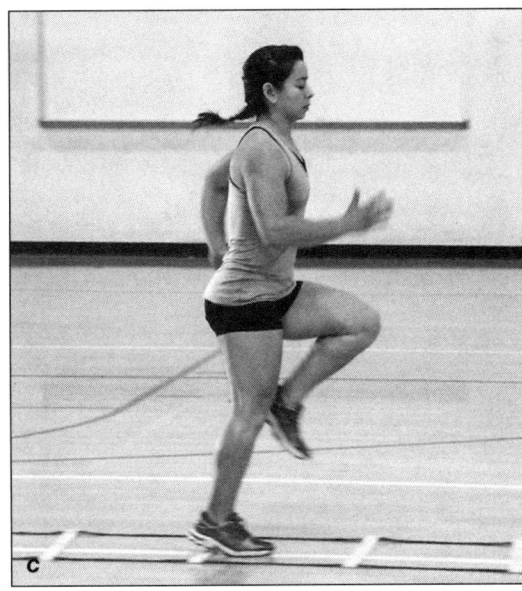

127

Double Step

Purpose

To develop balance, flexibility, foot quickness, and high knee action.

Procedure

- Start in a two-point stance.
- Sprint forward using high knee and good arm action.
- The right foot and left foot hit in each square through the ladder (see figure *a-c*).

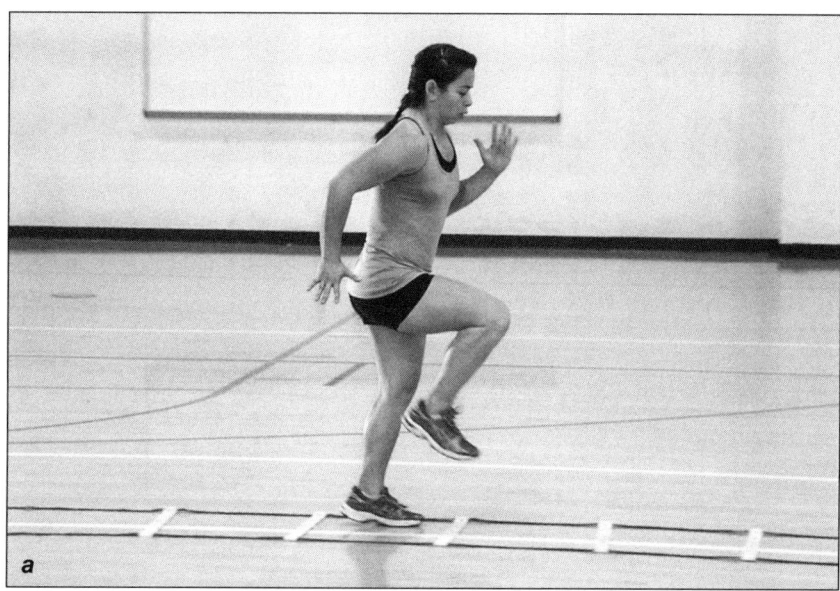

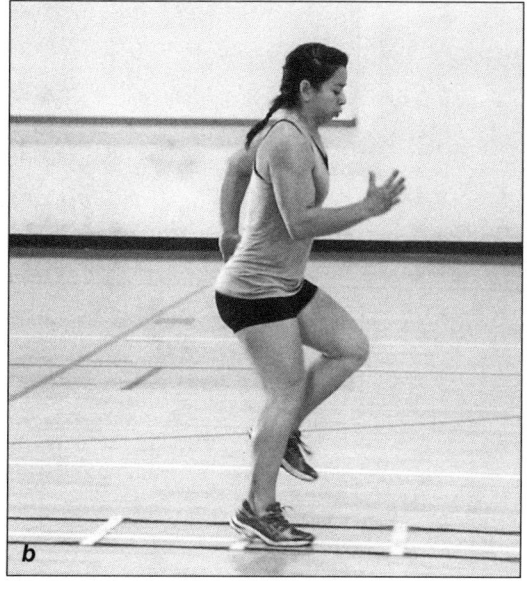 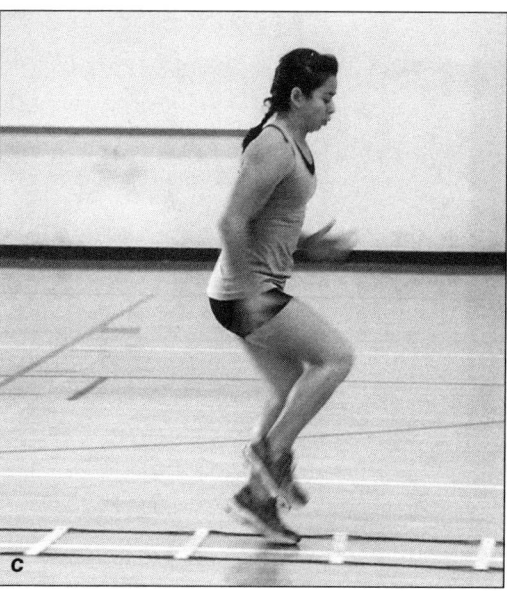

128
Carioca

Purpose

To develop balance, flexibility in the hips, footwork, and peripheral vision.

Procedure

- Start in a two-point stance.
- Begin standing sideways at one end of the ladder.
- Step with the right foot into the first square.
- Cross the left foot into the second hole. The left foot should cross in front of the right foot.
- Step with the right foot into the third square. The right foot should cross behind the left foot.
- The left foot crosses over in front of the right foot into the next square.
- Repeat this sequence through the ladder (see figure *a-c*).
- Emphasize a high knee step when crossing over in front.

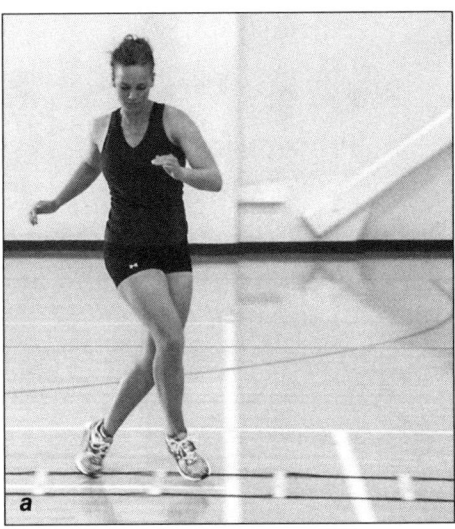

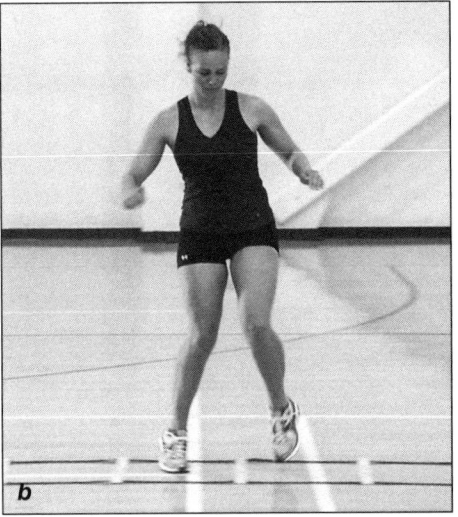

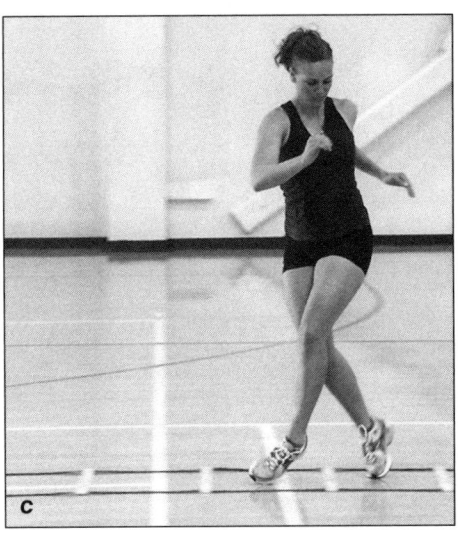

129

Ladder Side Step

Purpose

To develop balance, flexibility, footwork, and peripheral vision.

Procedure

- Start in a two-point stance.
- Sprint laterally through the agility ladder using high knee and good arm action.
- Hit the alternating foot in each square of the ladder (see figure *a* and *b*).

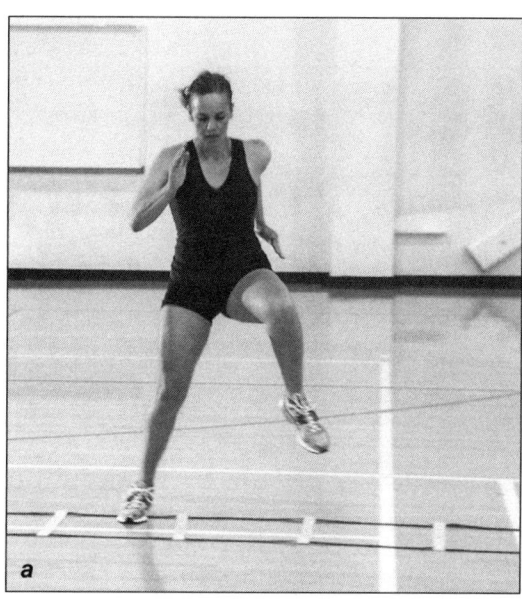 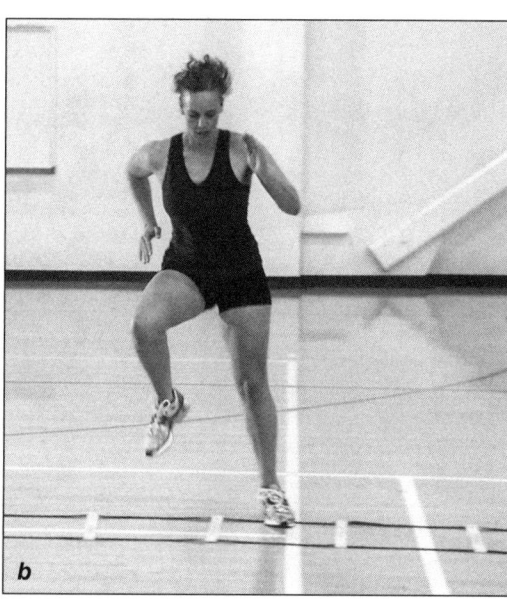

130

Ladder Side Step With Double Step

Purpose
To develop balance, flexibility, foot quickness, and peripheral vision.

Procedure
- Start in a two-point stance.
- Sprint laterally through the agility ladder using high knee and good arm action.
- Hit each foot in every square of the ladder (see figure *a-c*).

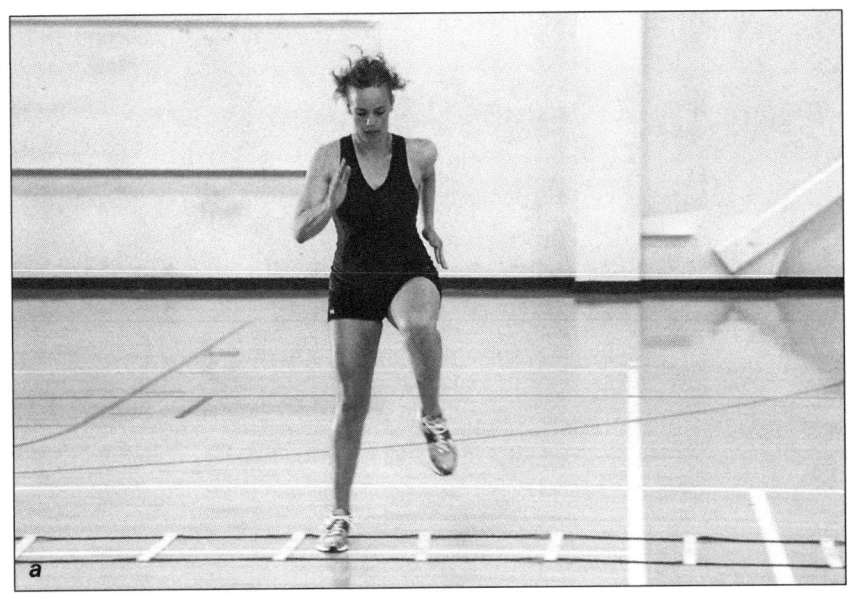
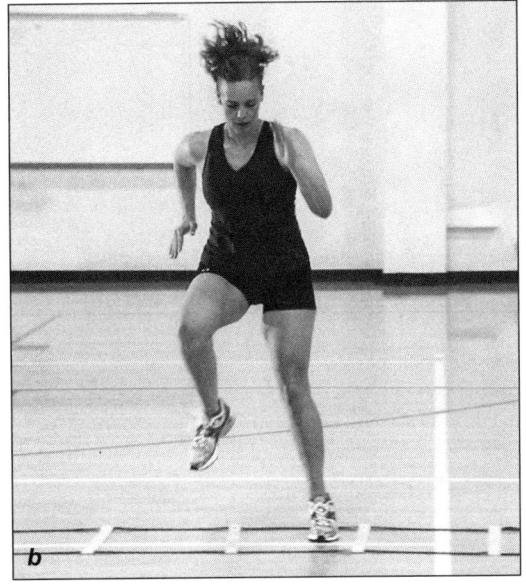
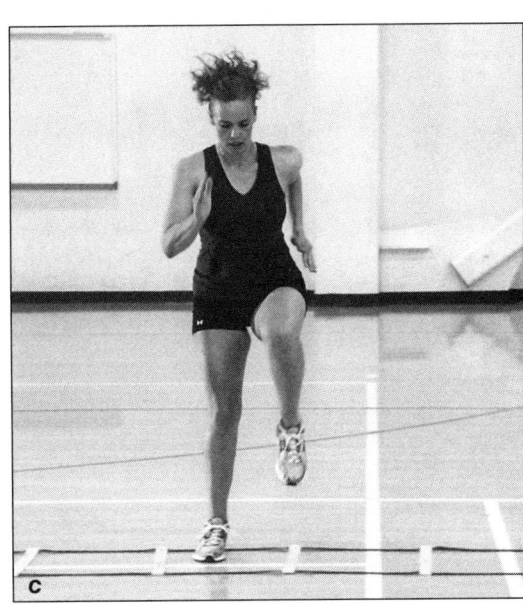

131

Slalom Jump

Purpose
To develop agility, balance, coordination, and quickness.

Procedure
- Start in two-point stance straddling the side strap with left foot in the box and right foot out.
- Jump across the ladder to straddle the opposite side strap with right foot in the box and left foot out.
- Continue down the ladder in this sequence (see figure *a-c*).

Variation
Perform the drill on one leg as you become more experienced.

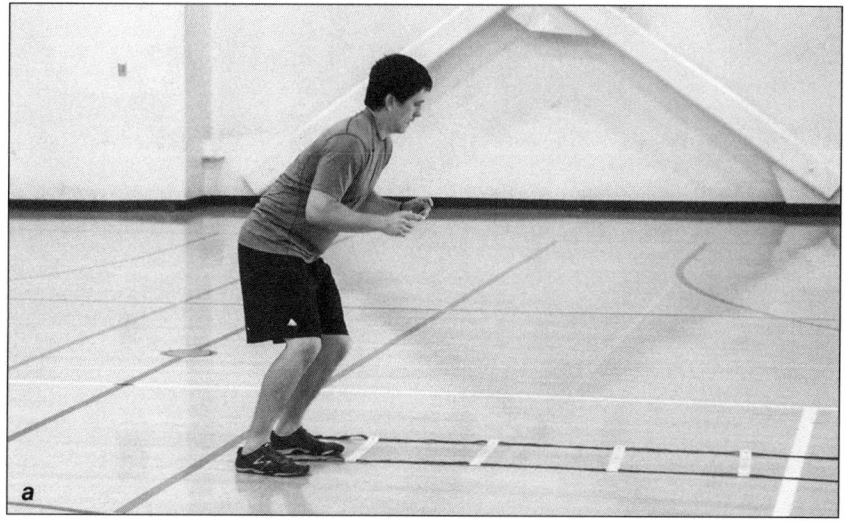

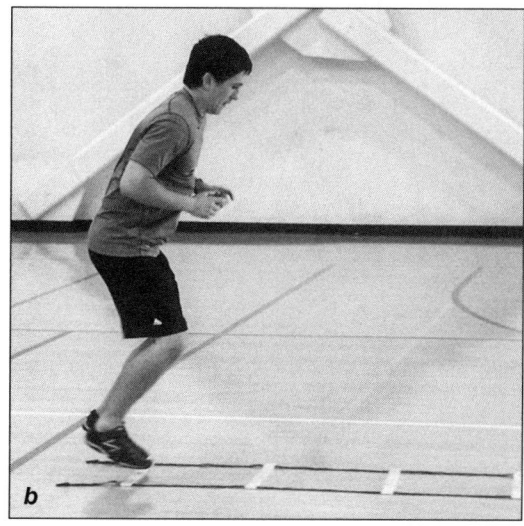
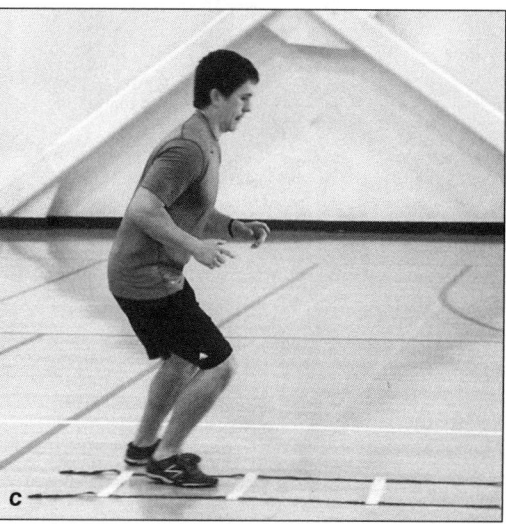

132

Twist Jump

Purpose
To develop agility, balance, coordination, hip flexibility, and quickness.

Procedure
- Start in a two-point stance.
- Keeping both feet together, perform a series of quarter-turn jumps (see figure *a-c*).
- The direction of the feet for each jump is as follows: straight ahead, right, straight ahead, left, straight ahead, and so on.
- This drill forces you to rotate the hips with each jump.

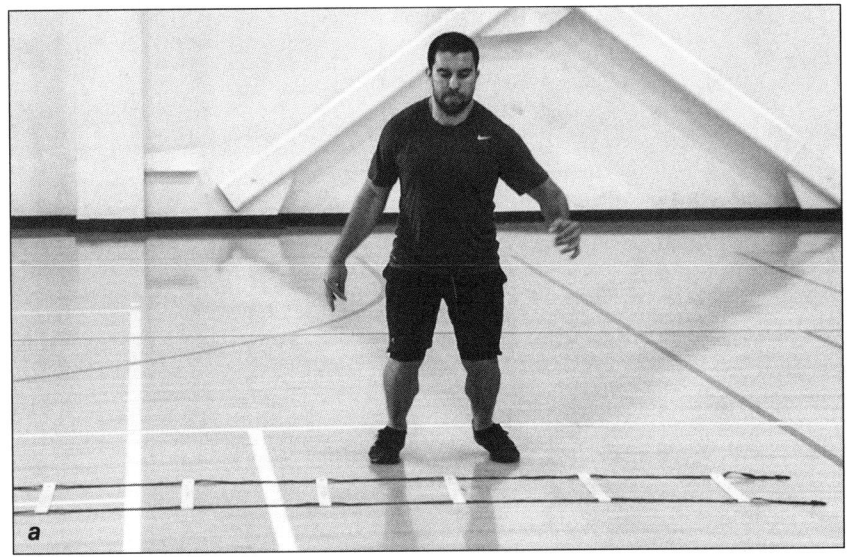

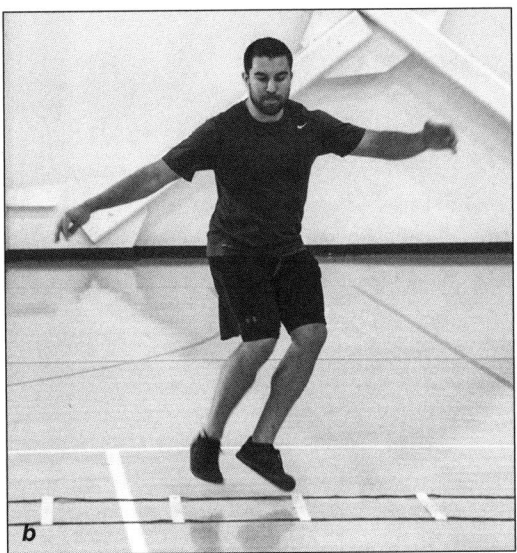

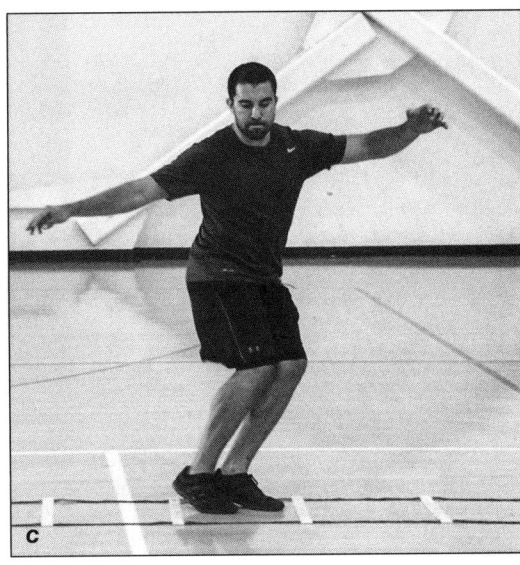

133
Double In–Out Shuffle

Purpose

To develop agility, balance, coordination, and quickness.

Procedure

- Start in a two-point stance.
- Begin standing sideways to the ladder.
- Step with the left foot straight ahead into the first square.
- Follow with the right foot into the first square.
- Step back with the left foot to in front of the first square.
- Follow with the right foot to in front of the first square.
- Step with the left foot straight ahead into the first square again.
- Follow with the right foot into the first square.
- Step back and shuffle with the left foot into the second square.
- Follow with the right foot to in front of the second square.
- Repeat this sequence throughout the ladder.

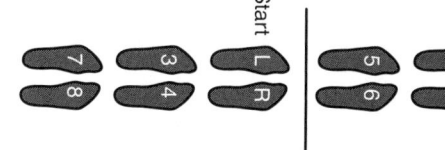

134
Side Left In

Purpose

To develop agility, balance, coordination, and quickness.

Procedure

- Start in a two-point stance.
- Begin standing sideways to the ladder.
- Step with the left foot into the first square.
- Step forward with the right foot over the first square to the other side of the ladder.
- Step laterally with the left foot to the second square.
- Step backward with the right foot in front of the second square.
- Step laterally with the right foot to the third square.
- Repeat this sequence throughout the ladder.

135
Side Right In

Purpose

To develop agility, balance, coordination, and quickness.

Procedure
- Start in a two-point stance standing sideways to the ladder.
- Step with the right foot into the first square.
- Step forward with the left foot over the first square to the other side of the ladder.
- Step laterally with the right foot to the second square.
- Step backward with the left foot to in front of the second square.
- Step laterally with the right foot to the third square.
- Repeat this sequence throughout the ladder.

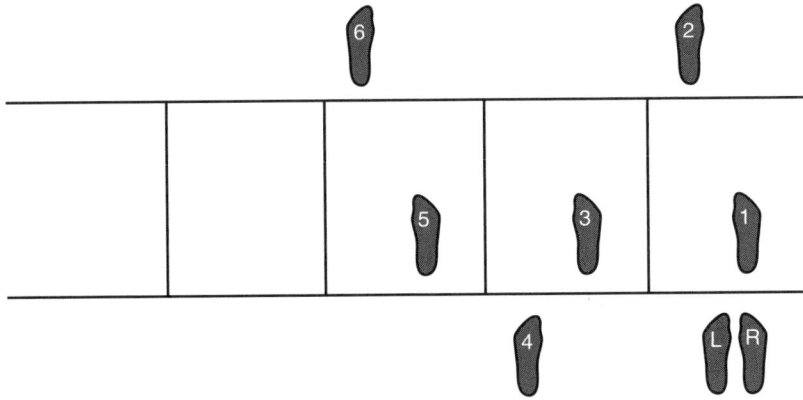

136

 Backward Slalom Jump

Purpose
To develop agility, balance, coordination, and quickness.

Procedure
- Start in a two-point stance with your back to the ladder.
- Straddle the side strap with left foot in the box and right foot out.
- Jump backward across the ladder to straddle the opposite side strap with right foot in the box and left foot out.
- Continue down the ladder in this sequence (see figure).

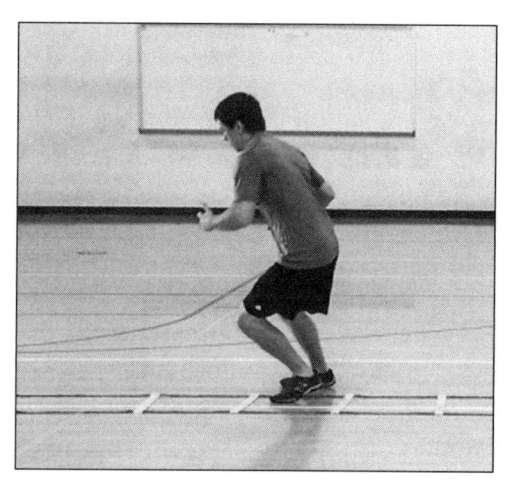

Variation
Perform the drill on one leg as you become more experienced.

137

 Backward Twist Jump

Purpose
To develop agility, balance, coordination, and quickness.

Procedure
- Start in a two-point stance.
- Begin facing the ladder at one end.
- Keeping both feet together, perform a series of quarter-turn jumps (see figure).
- The direction of the feet for each jump is as follows: backward, right, backward, left, and so on.
- This drill enhances the ability to rotate the hips with each jump while moving backward.

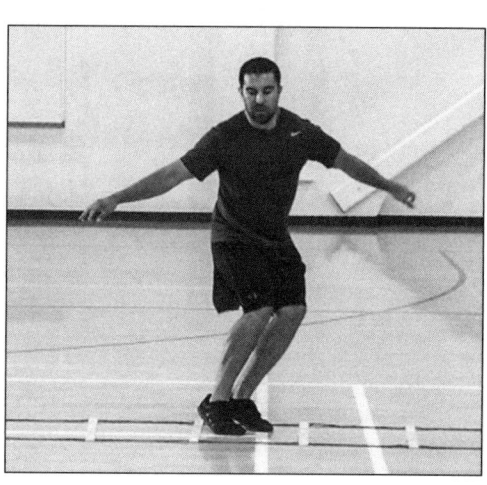

138 Backward Icky Shuffle

Purpose
To develop agility, balance, coordination, and quickness.

Procedure
- Stand in a two-point stance.
- Begin standing sideways to the ladder with your back to the ladder.
- Backpedal with the left foot into the first square (see figure *a*).
- Follow with the right foot into the first square (see figure *b*).
- Step backward and shuffle with the left foot until you are in front of the second square.
- Follow with the right foot until you are in front of the second square.
- Repeat this sequence throughout the ladder.

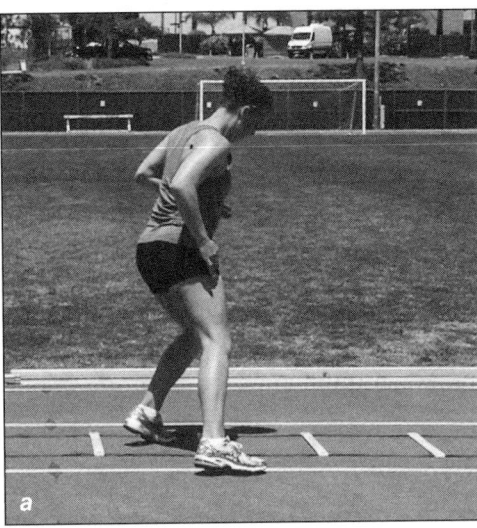
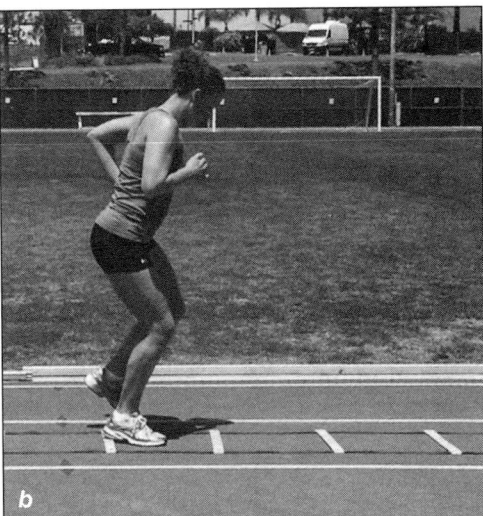

139

Forward Ladder Zigzag

Purpose

To develop foot coordination and flexibility in the abductors and adductors.

Procedure

- Start in a two-point stance on one side of the agility ladder.
- Laterally step into the first square with the outside foot across the front of the inside foot to land alone in the square (see figure *a* and *b*).
- Move laterally across and down the ladder, with the outside foot always crossing the front of the inside foot to land alone in the square (see figure *c* and *d*).

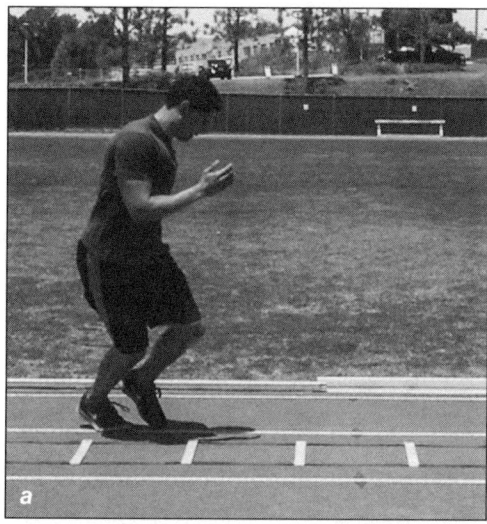
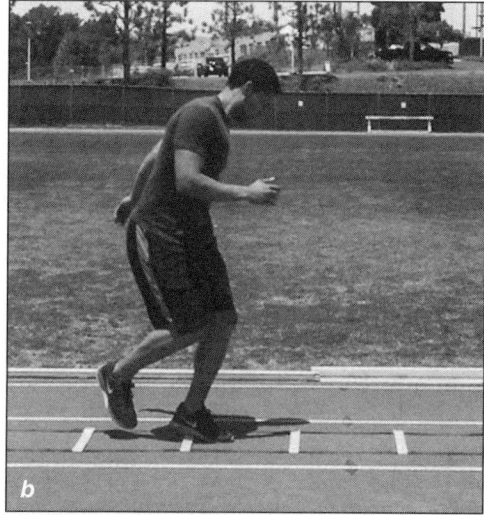
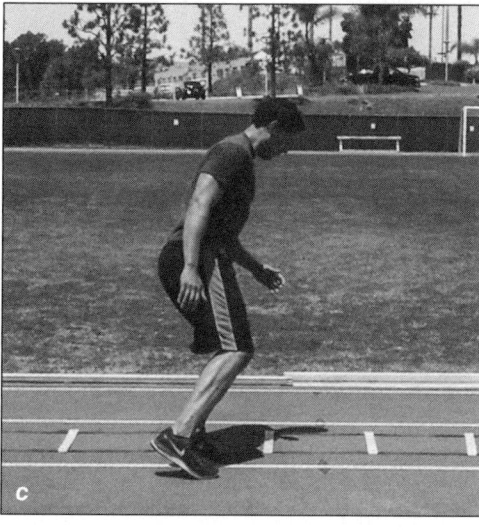
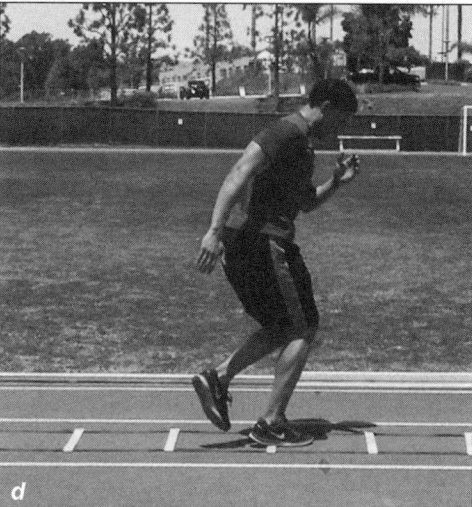

140

Backward Ladder Zigzag

Purpose
To develop foot coordination and flexibility in the abductors and adductors.

Procedure
- Start in a two-point stance.
- Begin standing at one side of the agility ladder with your back to the ladder.
- Backpedal laterally into the first square with the outside foot across the front of the inside foot to land alone in the square.
- Backpedal laterally across and down the ladder, with the outside foot always crossing the front of the inside foot to land alone in the square.

141

Forward Zigzag Same In

Purpose
To develop flexibility in the abductors and adductors and foot coordination.

Procedure
- Start in a two-point stance.
- Standing at the right side of the agility ladder, step with the right foot laterally across the left foot to inside the first square.
- Bring the left foot laterally behind the right foot to the left side of the ladder.
- Bring the right foot to the inside of the left foot.
- Step forward and laterally with the right foot to inside the second square.
- Step across the right foot with the left foot to the right side of the agility ladder.
- Bring the right foot laterally behind to the outside of the left foot.
- Continue down the agility ladder in this pattern.

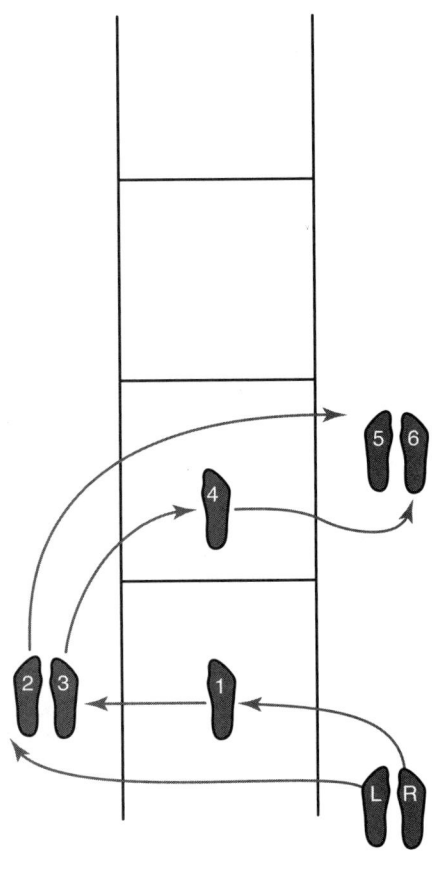

142
Backward Zigzag Same In

Purpose
To develop foot coordination and flexibility in the hip abductors and adductors.

Procedure
- Start in a two-point stance.
- Stand at the left side of the ladder with your back to the ladder.
- Step laterally backward to the left with the left foot into the first square.
- Bring the right foot laterally backward behind the left foot to the right side of the second square in the ladder.
- Step back with the left foot into the second square.
- Bring the right foot laterally backward behind the left foot to the left side of the third square in the ladder.
- Continue down the agility ladder in this pattern.

143

Backward Shuffle Bound

Purpose
To develop flexibility, footwork, strength in the groin area, and change of direction.

Procedure
- Start in a two-point stance on the left side of the ladder, facing backward.
- Shuffle across the ladder by putting the right foot in the first square and then the left foot in the square as the right foot goes to the left of the square.
- Step backward with both feet to the second square, with the left foot in the second square and the right foot to the left of the second square.
- Shuffle across, putting the right foot in the second square and the left foot to the right of the second square.
- Continue this format to the end of the agility ladder.

144 Forward Shuffle Bound

Purpose

To develop flexibility, footwork, and strength in the groin area.

Procedure

- Start in a two-point stance on the left side of the ladder.
- Shuffle across the ladder by putting the right foot in the first square and the left foot in the square as the right foot goes to the right side of the square (see figure *a* and *b*).
- Step forward with both feet to the second square, with the left foot in the second square and the right foot to the right of the second square (see figure *c* and *d*).
- Shuffle across, putting the right foot in the second square and the left foot to the left of the second square.
- Continue this format to the end of the agility ladder.

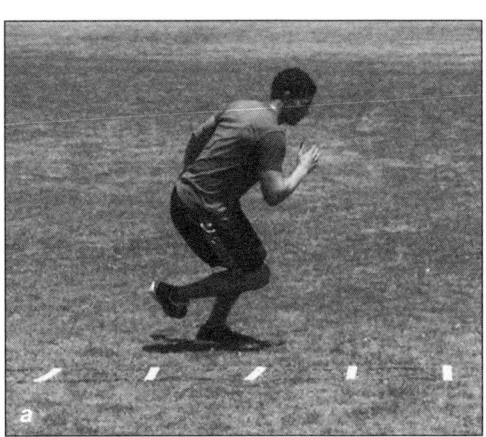
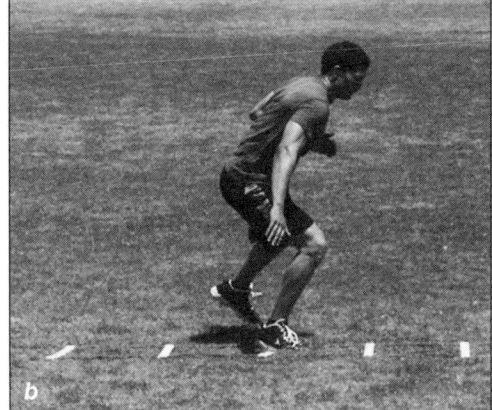
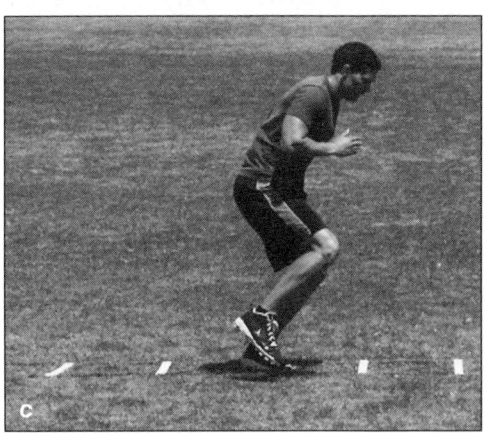
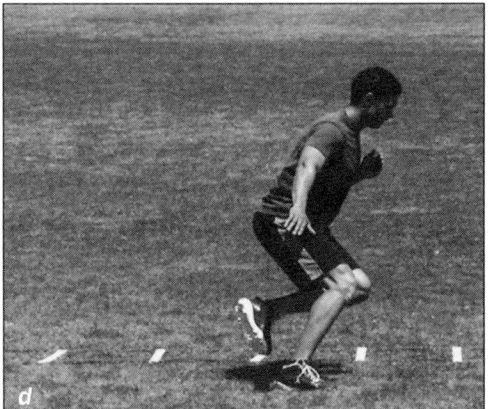

Forward Cross-Step Bound

Purpose
To develop foot coordination, flexibility in the abductors and adductors, and change of direction.

Procedure
- Start in a two-point stance.
- Starting at the left side of the agility ladder, perform a crossover step with the left foot in front of the right foot into the first square (see figure *a*).
- Bring the right leg behind the left leg to the right side of the first square (see figure *b*).
- Laterally step with the left leg to slightly outside the right side of the first square.
- Cross over with the right leg in front of the left leg to inside the second square (see figure *c*).
- Bring the left leg behind the right leg to the left side of the second square (see figure *d*).
- Laterally step with the right leg to slightly outside the left side of the second square.
- Continue down the agility ladder in this pattern.

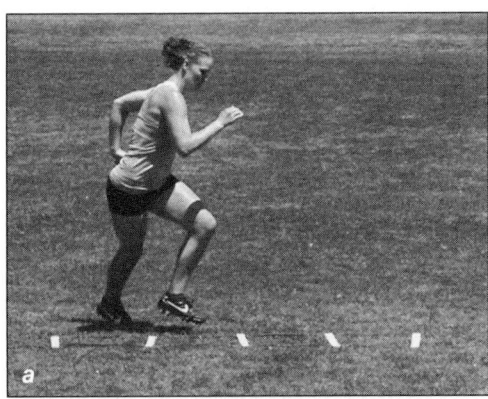
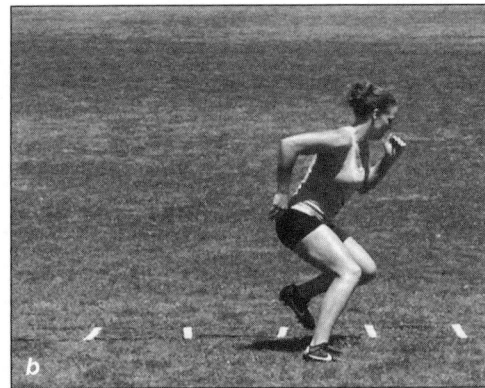
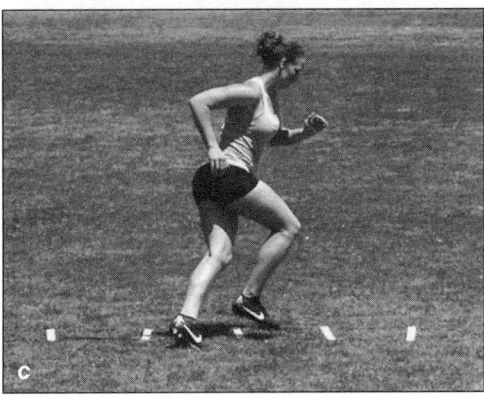
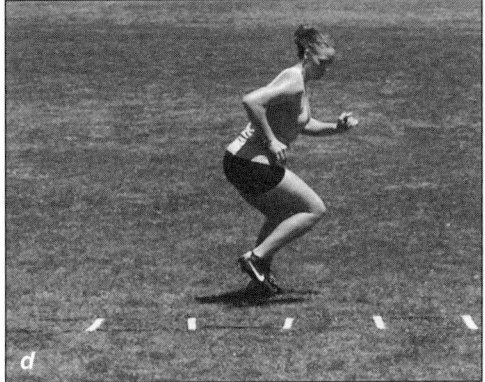

146

▶ Backward Cross-Step Bound

Purpose

To develop foot coordination, flexibility in the abductors and adductors, and change of direction.

Procedure

- Start in a two-point stance on the left side of the ladder, facing backward.
- Perform a crossover step with the right foot in front of the left foot into the first square.
- Bring the left leg behind the right leg to the right side of the first square.
- Laterally step with the right leg in front of the left leg to slightly outside the right side of the first square.
- Cross over with the left leg behind the right leg to inside the second square.
- Bring the right leg in front of the left leg to the left side of the second square.
- Laterally step with the left leg to slightly outside the left side.
- Continue down the agility ladder in this pattern.

147

Crossover Shuffle

Purpose

To increase flexibility and power in the hips; to improve ability to change direction.

Procedure

- Stand with the ladder to your right.
- Cross over with the left foot to the first square of the ladder.
- Laterally step with the right foot to the right side of the ladder. Only one foot is in the ladder at any one time.
- Immediately cross over with the right foot to the second square of the ladder.
- Laterally step with the left foot to the left side of the ladder.
- Repeat.

148

Zigzag Crossover Shuffle

Purpose

To improve footwork, flexibility in abductors and adductors, and ability to change direction.

Procedure

- Start in a two-point stance.
- Begin on the left side of an agility ladder and perform a crossover step with the left foot in front of the right foot into the first square.
- Bring the right leg behind the left leg to the right side of the first square.
- Laterally step with the left leg to slightly outside the right side of the first square.
- Crossover with the right leg in front of the left to inside the second square.
- Bring the left leg behind the right leg to the left side of the second square.
- Laterally step with the right leg to slightly outside the left side of the second square.
- Continue down the agility ladder in this pattern.

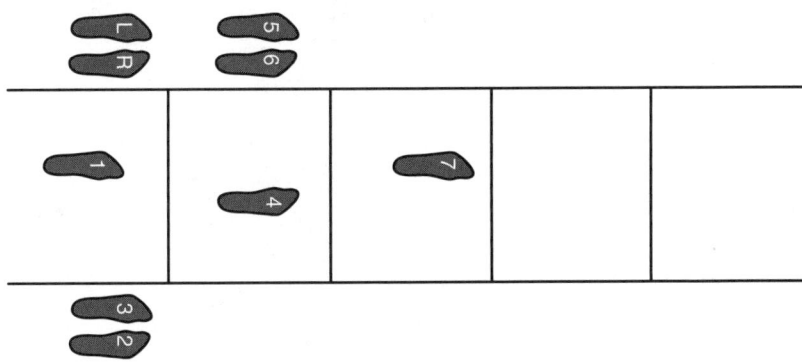

149
Ladder Quick Run With Sprint

Purpose
To develop agility, balance, coordination, quickness, and transitions between skills.

Procedure
- Moving forward through the length of the ladder, step one foot after the other into each space created by the rungs of the ladder.
- Start with the left foot first, and on subsequent runs lead with the left foot (see figure *a*).
- Once through the ladder, sprint 15 yards or meters straight ahead or to the right or left (see figure *b*).
- To add to the drill, have a coach or instructor dictate the direction at the end of the ladder.

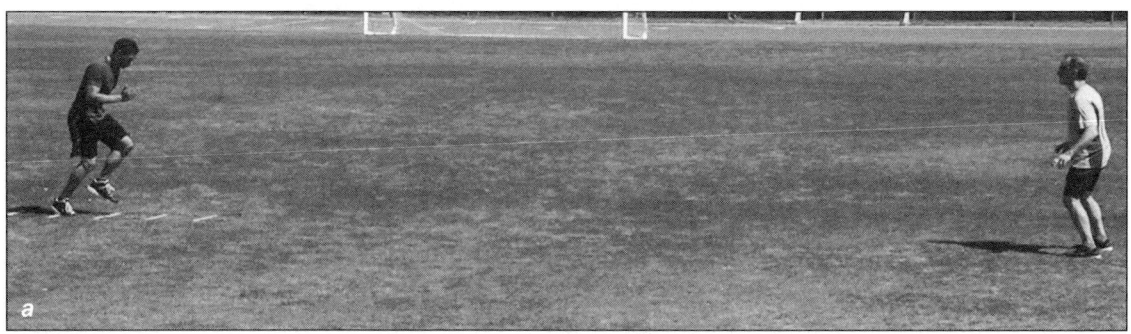

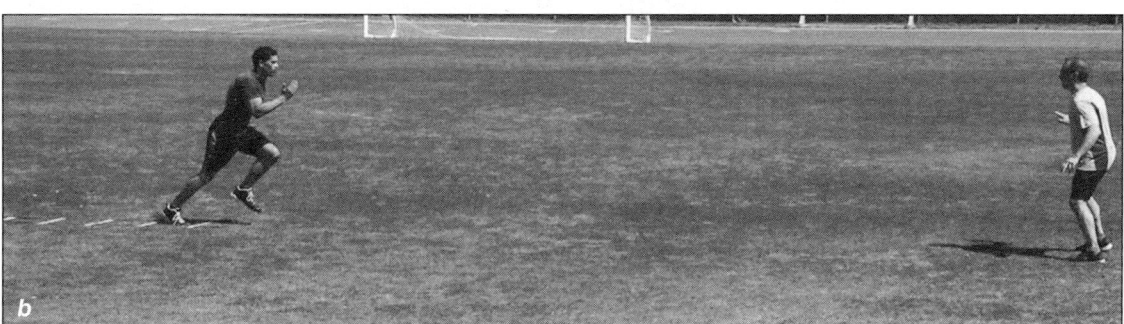

BAG DRILLS

150
Change of Direction

Purpose

To develop change of direction and quick foot action.

Procedure

- Start in a two-point stance.
- Begin at one end of the bags on the right side, and sprint forward toward the left side of the next bag.
- Planting the outside foot at the end of the bag, use a side step to explosively propel forward toward the opposite end of the next bag.
- Complete the sprint through all the bags.

Variations

- Change the distance between bags as well as their orientation.
- Perform various biomotor skill combinations during the drill.

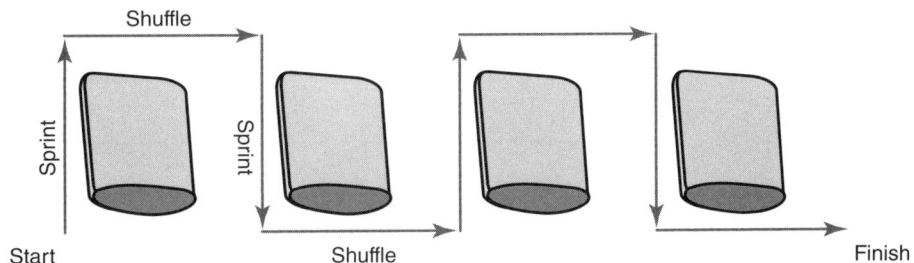

151

Bag Weave

Purpose
To develop flexibility, high knee action, and quick foot action.

Procedure
- Start in a two-point stance.
- Starting on the outside of the first of four bags, sprint forward until you are in front of the bag.
- Shuffle the feet to the right until you reach a space between the bags, but do not cross the feet when moving sideways.
- Backpedal quickly until you are one step past the bag.
- Shuffle the feet again until you reach the outside of the last bag. Remember to always keep your shoulders square and to stay in a two-point stance while keeping your head up; use good running form while moving as fast as possible.

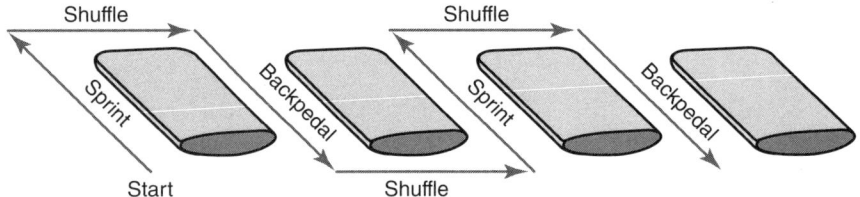

152

Lateral Weave

Purpose
To develop quick foot action and reaction.

Procedure
- Start in a two-point stance with your hands and arms away from the body.
- Laterally sidestep over three or four bags quickly to the right or left.
- After crossing the last bag, immediately reverse directions.
- Once you cross the last bag, sprint forward 5 yards or meters.

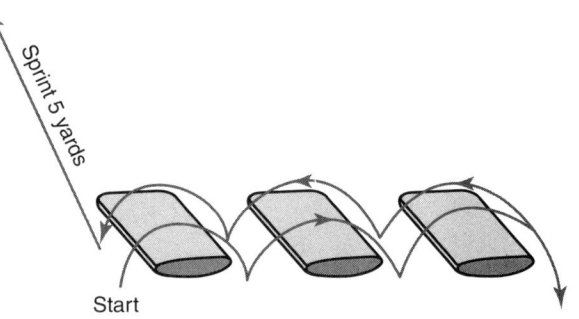

Variation
Add a ball catch.

153

Bag Zigzag

Purpose
To develop foot coordination, flexibility in the abductors and adductors, quickness, and strength.

Procedure
- Start in a two-point stance.
- Start at one end of the first bag on either the right or left side, facing the row of five bags.
- Shuffle diagonally beyond the first bag.
- Switch directions and shuffle diagonally to the end of second bag; continue shuffling through the bags.

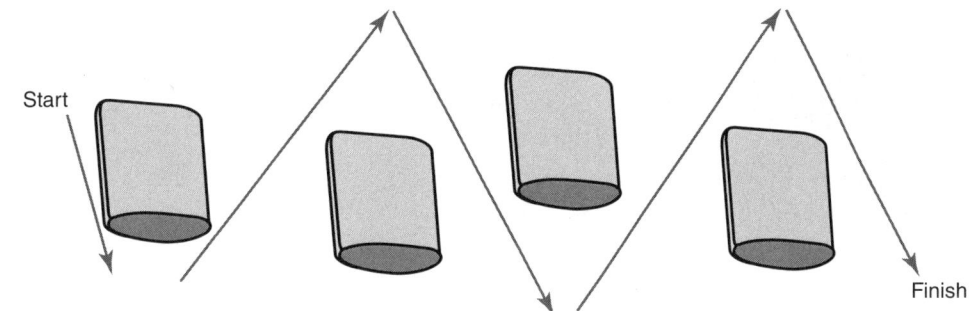

154

Wheel

Purpose
To develop balance and quick foot action.

Procedure
- Arrange four bags in formation as shown.
- With both hands on the ground in the middle area, stand between two of the bags.
- Start by sidestepping over each bag, rotating around all four bags while keeping your hands in contact with the ground until you are back at the original starting position.
- Quickly reverse directions and rotate back, sidestepping quickly over all four bags.
- Finish the drill by quickly sprinting 5 yards or meters straight ahead out of the bags.

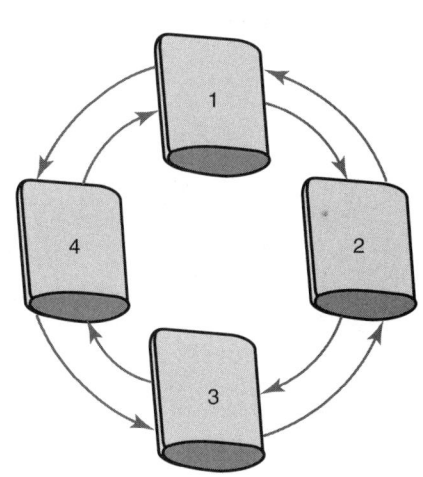

155

Strides

Purpose
To develop flexibility, high knee action, and quick foot action.

Procedure
- Start in a two-point stance.
- Sprint forward over bags using high knee action with a slight forward lean (see figure).

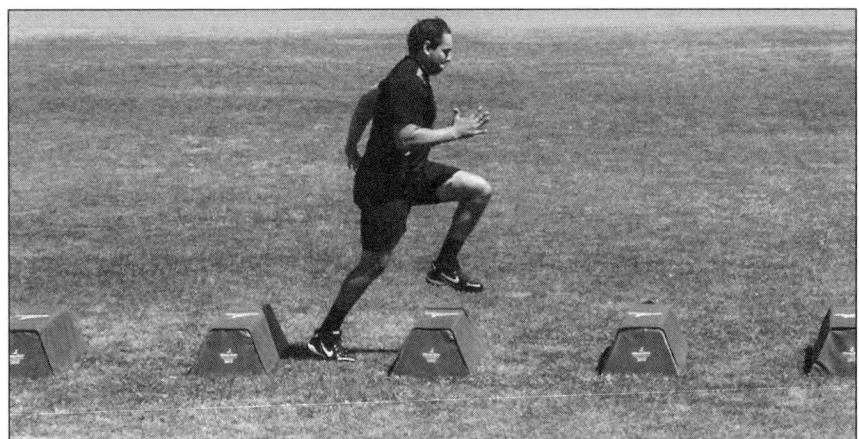

156

Strides With Double Step

Purpose
To develop flexibility, high knee action, and quick foot action.

Procedure
- Start in a two-point stance.
- Sprint forward over bags using high knee action with a slight forward lean.
- Double-step between each bag.

157
Bag Side Step

Purpose
To develop flexibility, high knee action, and quick foot action.

Procedure
- Start in a two-point stance.
- Sprint laterally one direction over bags using high knee action.
- Start with the leg closest to the bag.
- Go over the bags leading with the right foot (see figure), and then lead with the left foot when you reverse directions and go the opposite way.

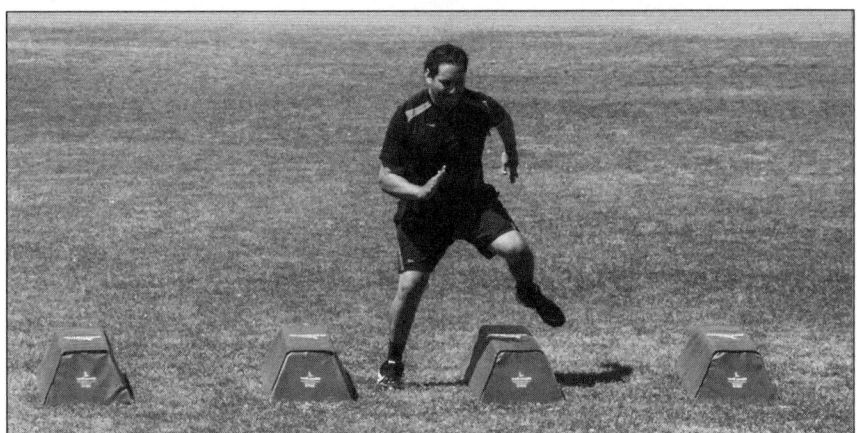

158
Bag Side Step, High Knee Combo

Purpose
To develop lateral movement and high knee action.

Procedure
- Set up four bags going in a forward diagonal line 2 yards or meters apart, then set up four bags in a straight horizontal line 2 yards or meters apart such that the last bag in the diagonal line is 5 yards or meters directly behind the first bag in the straight horizontal line.
- Start in a two-point stance with the arms and hands away from the body.
- Take a quick lateral step diagonally through the first four bags in succession.
- At the completion of the diagonal bags, sprint in a circular pattern to the first of the horizontal bags.
- Turn and run straight through the next series of bags, using high knee action.

159

▶ Bag Side Step With Double Step

Purpose

To develop flexibility, high knee action, and quick foot action.

Procedure

- Start in a two-point stance.
- Sprint laterally using high knee action (see figure *a*).
- Double-step between each bag (see figure *b* and *c*).

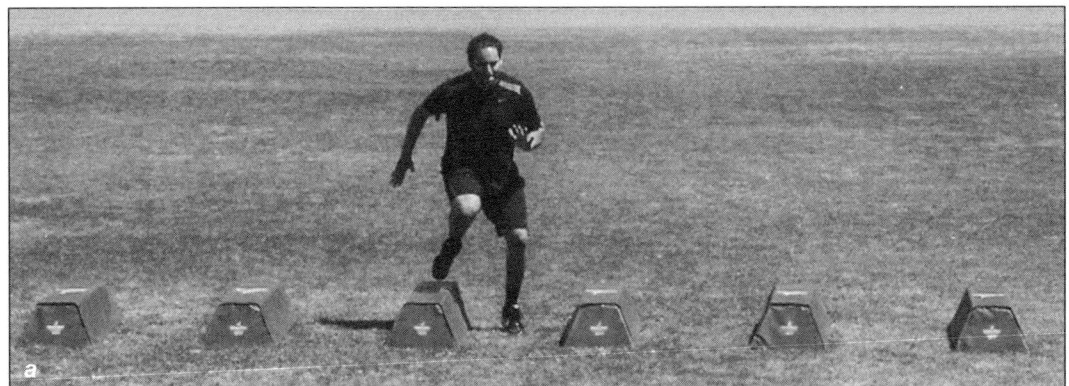

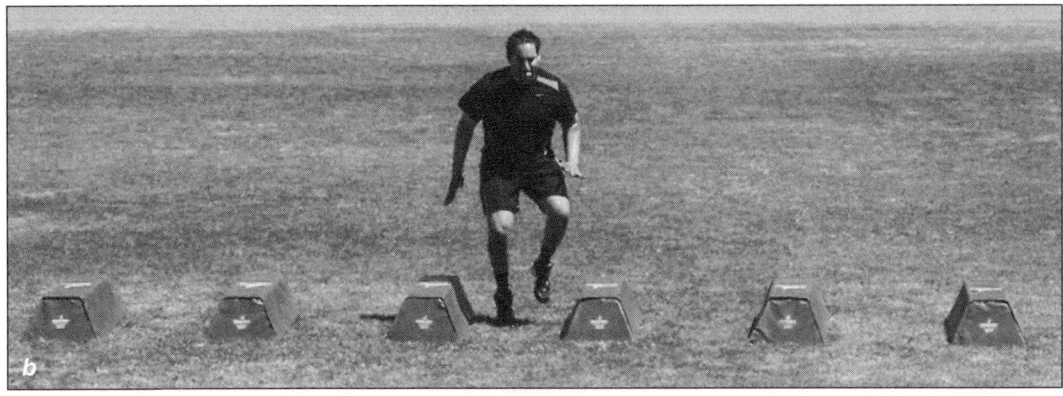

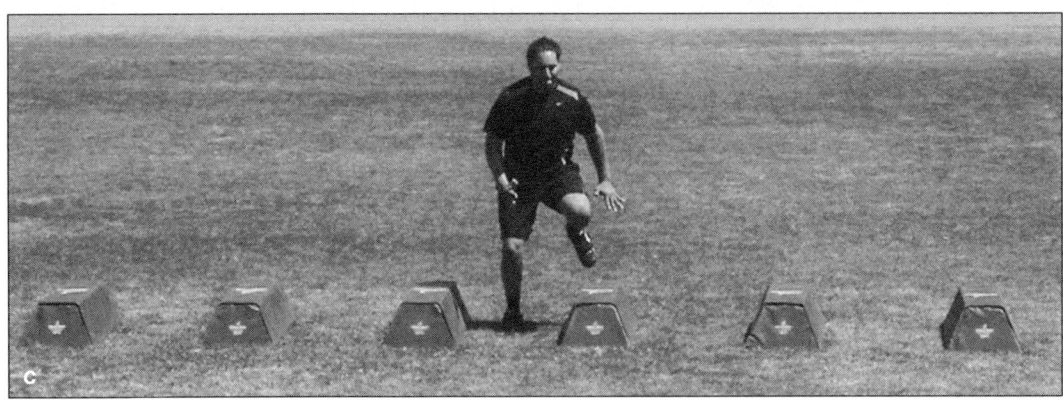

160

Bag Side Step With Two-Hand Touch

Purpose

To keep a low center of gravity with quick foot action.

Procedure

- Start in a two-point stance with hands and arms away from the body.
- Sidestep over the bags, tapping each bag with both hands (see figure *a* and *b*).
- Upon completion of the last bag, sprint forward for 5 yards or meters.

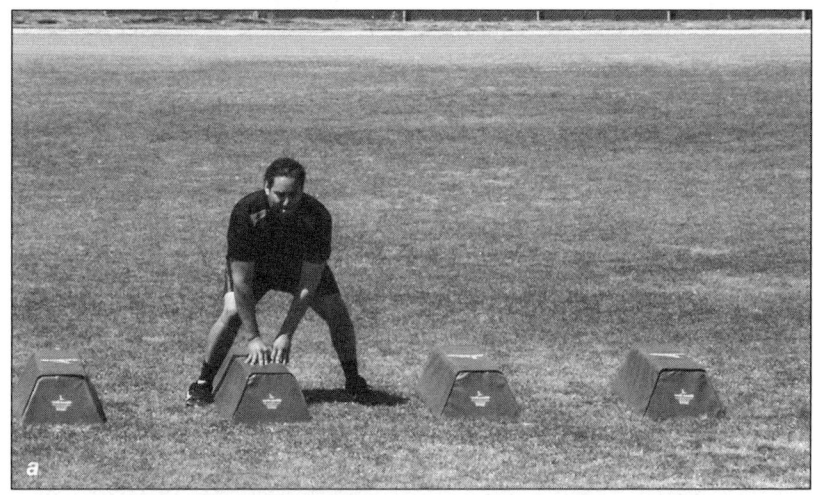

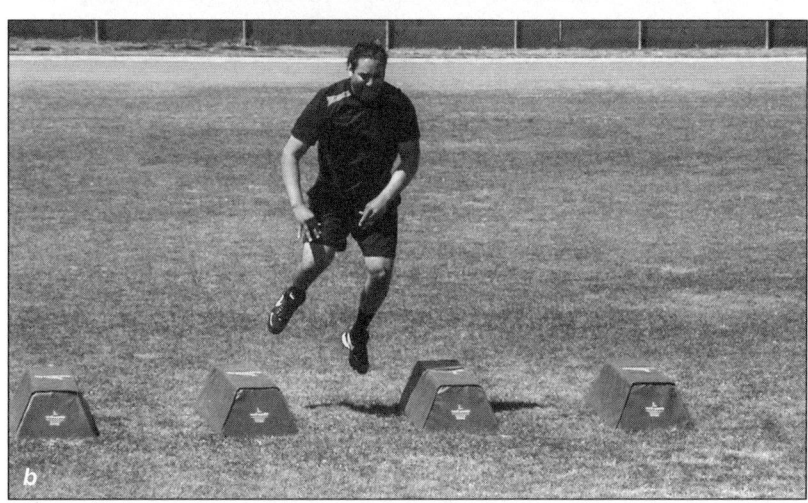

161

 Bag Side Step With Sprint

Purpose
To develop acceleration, change of direction, and reaction.

Procedure
- Start in a two-point stance.
- Sprint forward to the side of the first bag, and take a quick side step over the bag by pushing off with the outside foot.
- Once over the bag, push off the outside foot and sprint to the next bag; take a quick side step over the bag by pushing off the outside foot.
- Repeat for four more bags.

162

Bag Side Step, Forward, and Back Combo

Purpose
To develop change of direction, flexibility, high knee action, and quick foot action.

Procedure
- Start in a two-point stance with hands and arms away from the body.
- Sprint laterally over the first two bags.
- Sprint 5 yards or meters to the front of the third bag and shuffle.
- Backpedal 5 yards or meters and laterally step over bags four and five.
- Sprint 5 yards or meters to the front of the sixth bag and shuffle.
- Backpedal 5 yards or meters and laterally step over bag seven.

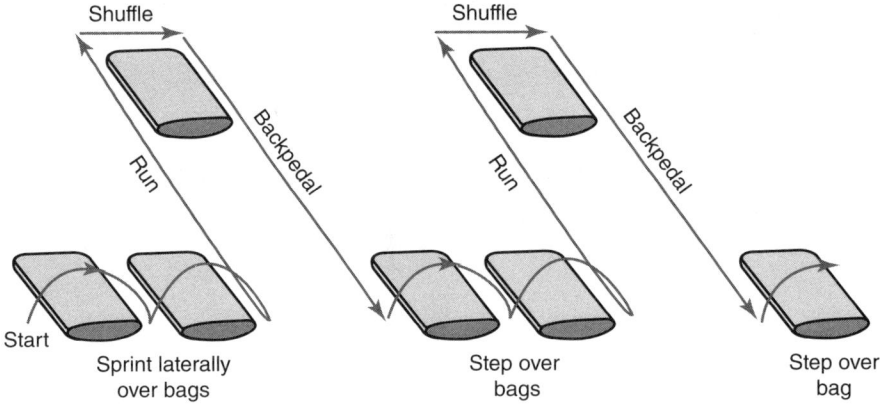

163

Bag Jumps With 180-Degree Turn

Purpose

To develop foot quickness and hip flexibility while providing plyometric training.

Procedure

- Start in a two-point stance.
- Laterally hop over the first bag, rotating 180 degrees while in the air (see figure *a*).
- Land between two bags (see figure *b*) and immediately hop over the second bag, rotating 180 degrees in the opposite direction (see figure *c*).
- Hop and rotate over four to six bags.

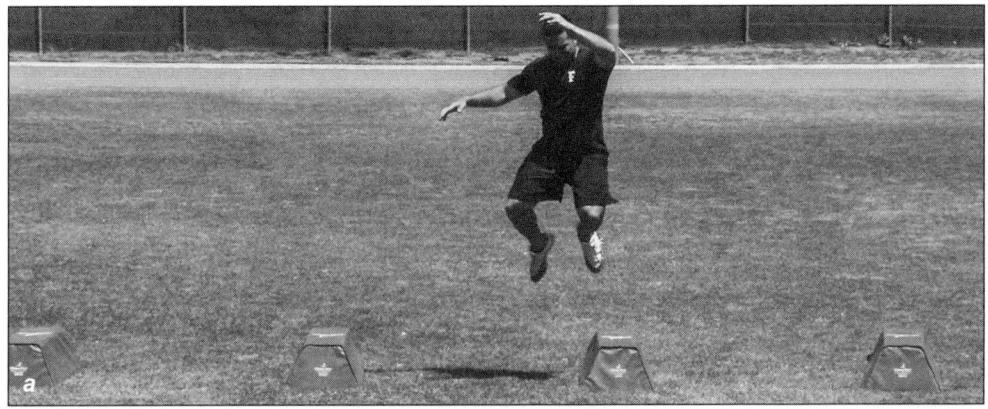

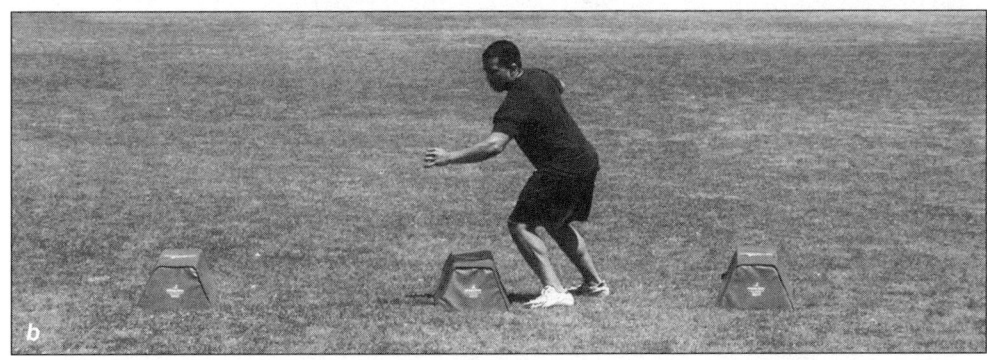

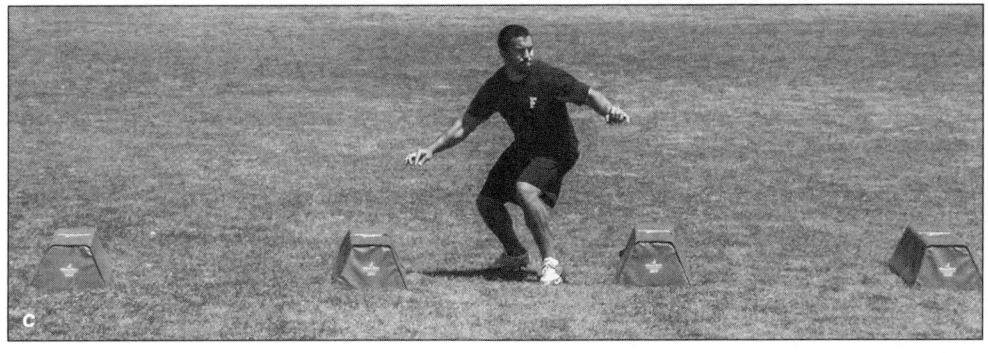

BACKPEDAL DRILLS

164

Backward Run

Purpose

To mobilize hips and thighs by having them move through an exaggerated range of motion and propelling you backward.

Procedure

- Set up as performing a forward run.
- Push off backward bringing your heel up as close to your butt as possible.
- Perform movement in a fluid manner.

165

Backpedal–Sprint on Line

Purpose

To develop hip rotation.

Procedure

- Start in a two-point stance with your back toward the line.
- Backpedal for 5 yards or meters, pivot your hips to the right, and run for 5 yards or meters, staying on the line with eyes on the start.
- Pivot back to the left and backpedal for 5 yards or meters, pivot your hips to the left, and run for 5 yards or meters, staying on the line with eyes on the start.

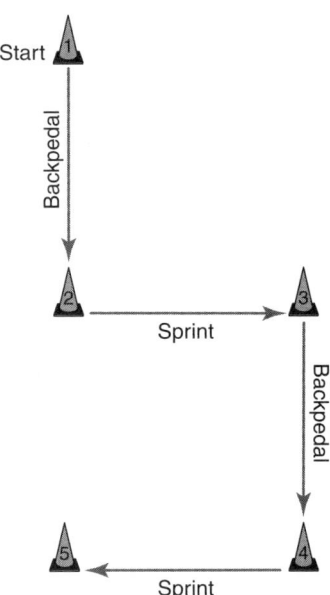

W Backpedal Break

Purpose
To develop change of direction.

Procedure
- Start in a two-point stance.
- Backpedal for 10 yards or meters at a 45-degree angle.
- Plant the outside foot and sprint forward for 10 yards or meters at a 45-degree angle.
- Repeat twice.

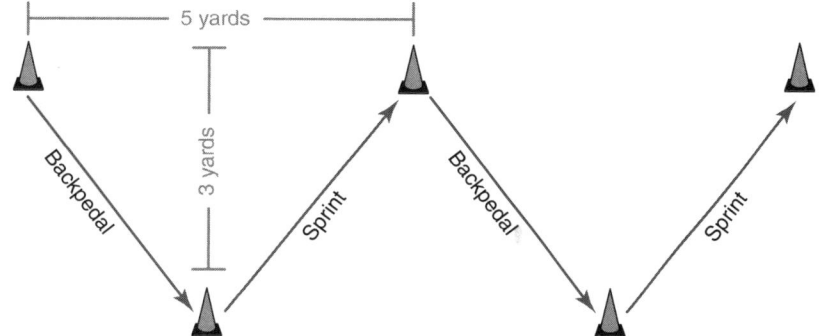

167

Backpedal–High Knees–Sprint

Purpose
To develop change of direction and quick feet.

Procedure
- Start in a two-point stance.
- Backpedal 15 yards or meters quickly.
- At 15 yards or meters, plant the feet and come forward 5 yards or meters with quick steps and high knees before sprinting 10 yards or meters.
- Repeat three times.

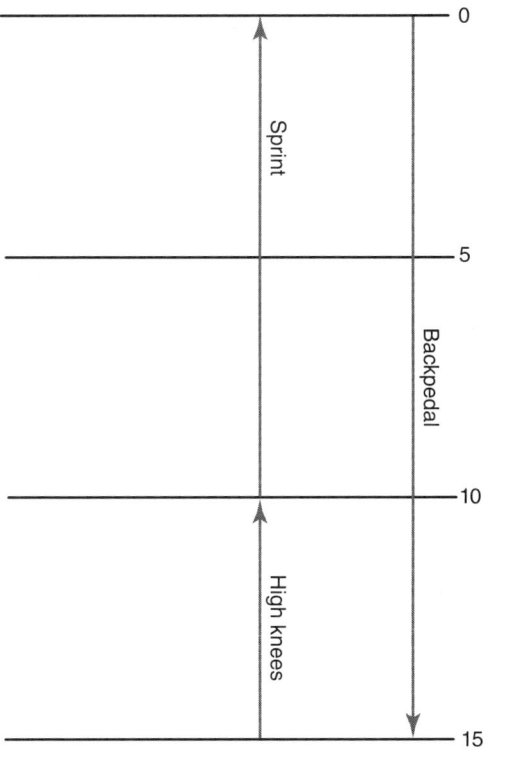

168

Backpedal Weave

Purpose
To develop backpedal technique.

Procedure
- Start in a two-point stance.
- Backpedal in a weaving motion for 15 yards or meters, changing direction every 3 to 4 yards or meters.

MINI-HURDLE DRILLS

169
Side High Knees

Purpose

To develop lateral explosive change of direction.

Procedure

- Start in a two-point stance.
- Sprint laterally in a running motion across mini-hurdles (see figure).
- Focus on lifting your knees and pumping your arms quickly and explosively.
- Reverse directions at the end, and return in the same format.

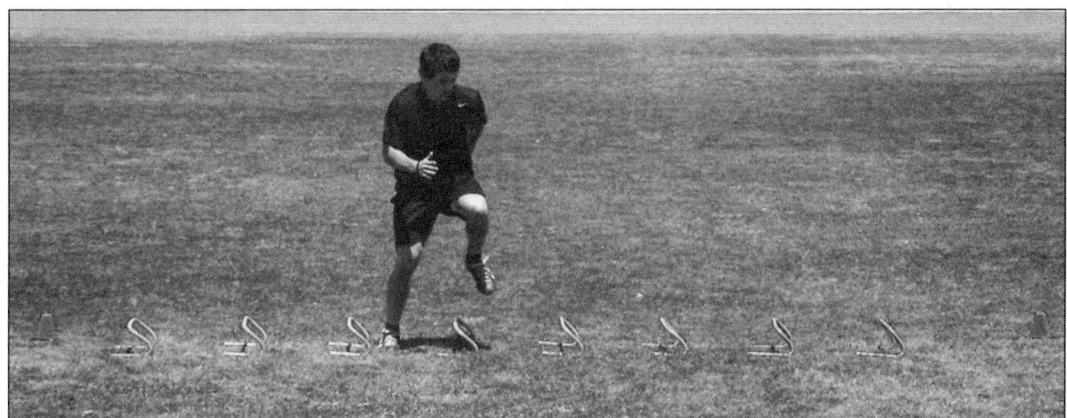

170

Resisted Side High Knees

Purpose

To develop resisted and overspeed lateral explosive change of direction.

Procedure

- Start in a two-point stance.
- While wearing a sport cord attached to a fixed object or held stationary by a coach or athlete, sprint laterally in a running motion across the hurdles (see figure).
- Focus on lifting your knees and pumping your arms quickly and explosively.
- Reverse directions at the end, and return in the same format.

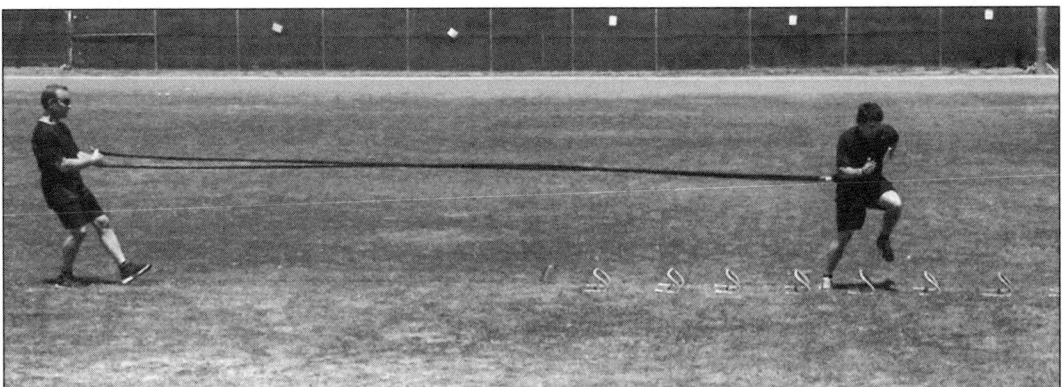

TOTAL-BODY AGILITY

171

Forward Roll Over Shoulder

Purpose

To develop total-body agility and kinesthetic awareness.

Procedure

- Start in a two-point stance (see figure *a*) with the left foot forward.
- Bend over and start to fall forward (see figure *b*).
- As you are about to make contact with the ground, roll over the left shoulder (see figure *c*).
- Roll and come back to your feet (see figure *d* and *e*).
- Perform forward rolls over both shoulders and with either foot forward.

Variations

- Add a sprint in any direction before or after the roll.
- React to any stimuli after the roll (for example, a visual cue to run to a cone).
- Add a sport-specific skill after the roll.

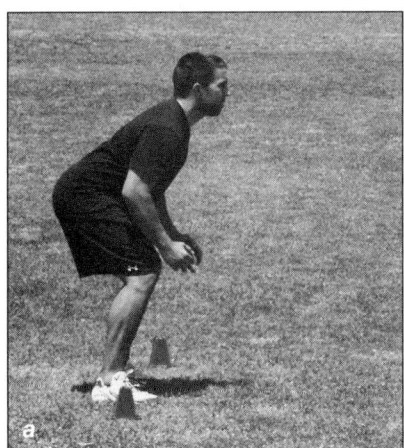 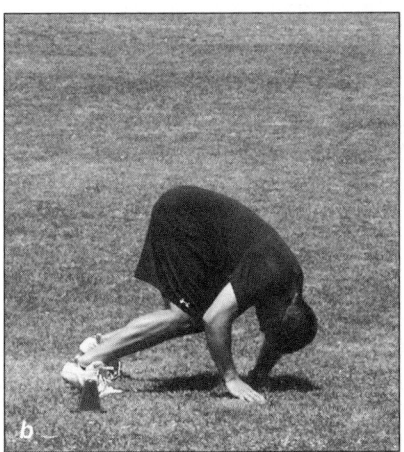 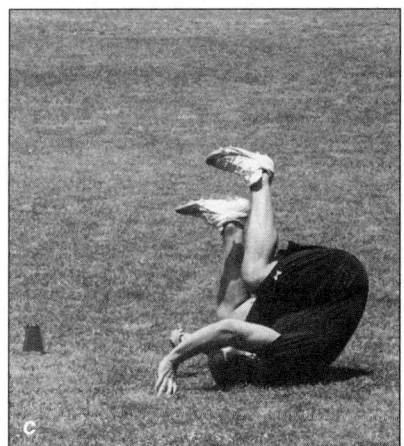

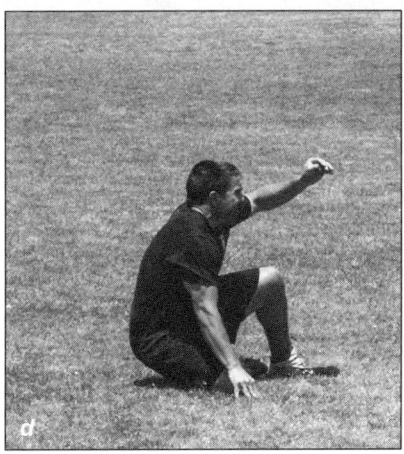 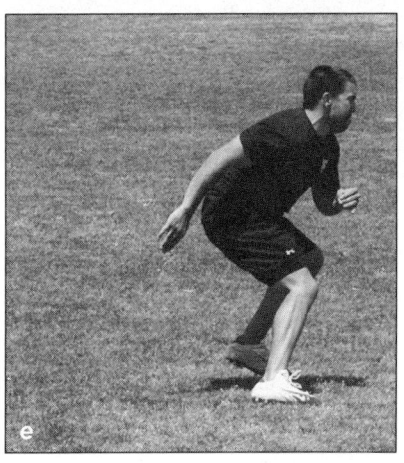

172

Backward Roll Over Shoulder

Purpose
To develop total-body agility and kinesthetic awareness.

Procedure
- Start in a two-point stance.
- Bend the legs and start to sit on the ground behind you (see figure *a*).
- As you are about to make contact with the ground, roll back over the left shoulder (see figure *b*).
- Continue to roll and come back up to your feet (see figure *c* and *d*).
- Perform backward rolls over both shoulders.

Variations
- Add a sprint in any direction before or after the roll.
- React to any stimuli after the roll (for example, a visual cue to run to a cone).
- Add a sport-specific skill after the roll.

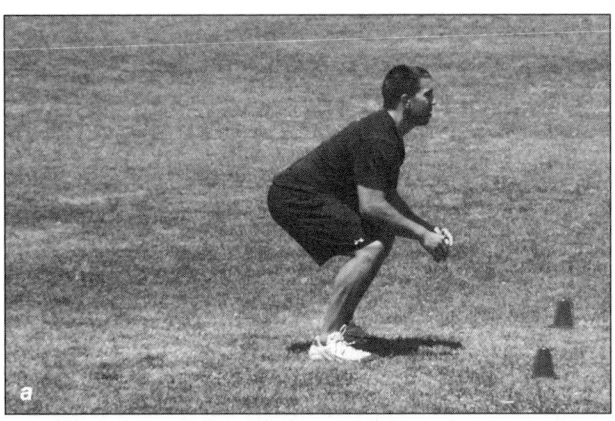
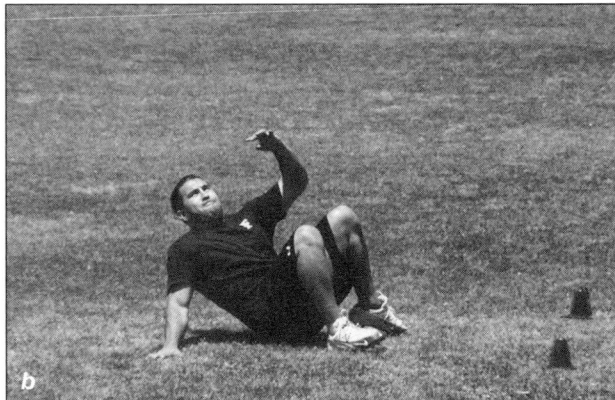
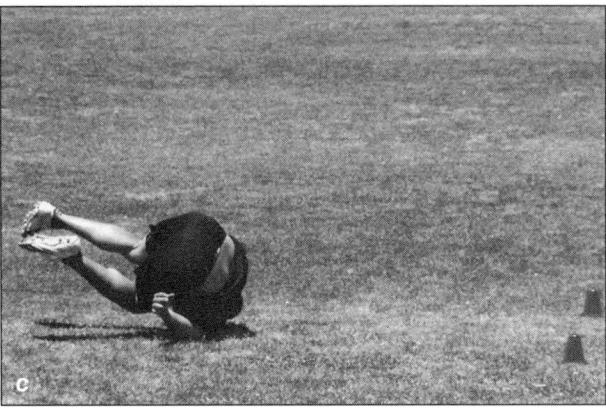
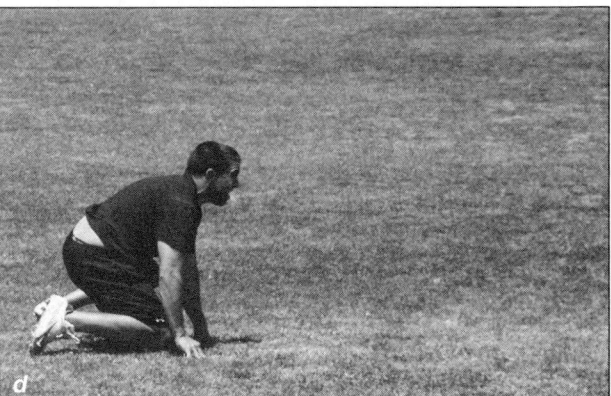

173

Forward Roll–Backward Roll Combination

Purpose
To develop total-body agility and kinesthetic awareness

Procedure
- Start in a two-point stance.
- Perform a forward roll to your feet.
- Immediately go into a backward roll with a hands push-off.
- You may start and end this drill on your knees to reduce amplitude and difficulty.

Variations
- Add a sprint in any direction before or after the roll.
- React to any stimuli after the roll (for example, a visual cue to run to a cone).
- Add a sport-specific skill after the roll.

Outside of sport-specific training, agility training may be the primary determining factor to predict success in a sport. Sports are not straight ahead; they require changes of direction in which lateral movements are used in several planes of movement simultaneously. Because movements in sport are initiated from various body positions, athletes need to be able to react with strength, explosiveness, and quickness from these different positions. Unfortunately, because of the focus placed on physical attributes in sports, the focus on off-season programs often revolves around strength training and conditioning exclusively. Often agility and speed development at sport-specific speeds are neglected or focused on only during small blocks of time in the preseason. Agility is a neural ability that is developed over time with many repetitions (Halberg 2001). Researchers found that an increase in speed and strength was not as effective in developing agility as participation in activities specifically designed to develop agility (Barnes and Attaway 1996; Cissik and Barnes 2011).

The performances of athletes in sports today have dramatically elevated the level of agility necessary for performance success. There is a direct correlation between improved agility and the development of athletic timing, rhythm, and movement (Costello and Kreis 1993). Agility training provides the athlete with performance benefits: neuromuscular adaptation, improved athleticism, injury prevention, and decreased rehabilitation time. A comprehensive agility program will address components of agility such as strength, power, acceleration, deceleration, coordination, balance, and dynamic flexibility. When instructing athletes on the execution of agility exercises, it is critical to stress technique as a priority and then speed of movement only after technique has been mastered. When designing an agility training program for athletes, many variables should be considered: training factors, sequence of drills, repetitions, sets, duration of exercise and drills, intensity, recovery, volume load, frequency, drill selection, and equipment.

Chapter 6

Quickness and Reaction-Time Training

Diane Vives

Successful performance by an athlete depends heavily on her ability to react quickly. In sports performance, this usually requires the athlete to quickly decelerate and just as quickly accelerate. Whether it involves reacting to a starter's pistol at the beginning of a running race, outjumping an opponent for a rebound on the basketball court, or being able to juke an opponent on the football field, the athlete with greater quickness and better reaction time (RT) usually maintains a competitive advantage.

Speed, *rapidity*, and *instancy* are all words that are used in defining quickness. These terms refer to the rate of movement of an object, or the measurement of the distance it has traveled in a certain amount of time. When an athlete performs a task or a movement in a relatively brief time, he is described as being *quick*.

When discussing quickness, such factors as speed, acceleration, and agility are not always clearly distinguished: "Did you see how *quickly* he accelerated?" "It's amazing how *quickly* she made those cuts!" "Notice the *quick* leg turnover in that sprinter." All these factors are, of course, to some degree interconnected with quickness. But are they merely components of quickness, or is quickness instead something that can be trained and improved separately to promote successful athletic performance?

RT, which is predicated on one's ability to react quickly to a stimulus, also plays a major role in many sports. How quickly a hockey player can react to the drop of a puck will determine what percentage of face-offs she can win. Can we improve our RT? The answer is yes. In this chapter, we discuss how sport-specific quickness and RT can be improved. We present exercises and drills, from simple to complex, that can be employed specifically for this purpose and that apply to a wide variety of sport-related movements.

Developing Quickness Skills

Athletes perform certain biomotor skills with an end result or purpose in mind. These experienced skills are recorded as memories of the varying patterns of movements, primarily in the sensory, sensory association, and motor control areas of the brain. These memories are referred to as sensory *engrams* of the movement patterns. Success with learning these skills is probably achieved through successive performance of the same skill activity until an engram for the movement is created (Guyton 1991).

New movements will always take a bit longer to improve while their patterns are burned into an engram. If performed slowly, even highly complex motor skills can be accomplished the first time through. The movement must be slow enough at first for sensory feedback to occur. This allows proper adjustments to be made that serve as guides for improvement. However, when faced with having to learn quick athletic movements, one must always perform quickly the biomotor patterns associated with the movements. In any case, movements that have been repeatedly performed before can be recalled from memory. Without needing to focus on learning the patterns associated with these movements, the athlete can place particular emphasis on performing them at speed.

Training for Quickness

In considering training progression, coaches can employ simple drills to help athletes improve their ability to be aware of the intricacies involved in movement generally, as well as to help them enhance their level of skill with stopping and maintaining correct body position, optimal body angles, plant-foot position, and control of their center of mass. Coaches can also emphasize improving their athletes' ability to stop with good body position and control, decrease the time it takes for them to begin accelerating (i.e., the amortization phase), and then immediately accelerate. By making an athlete *conscious* of successful movement strategies, over time and through numerous successful attempts he will begin to feel these movement patterns becoming more *unconscious*, or "second nature" (Young and Farrow 2013). The focus here should be on progression, precision, and repetition.

After an athlete masters the more basic patterns of movement, the coach can focus on the true nature of sport-specific quickness, which involves the athlete performing skills with multiple or chaotic stimuli intended to increase reactive demands. More advanced drills with more complex decision-making requirements (such as open drills that include an increase in chaotic patterns) mimic the more unpredictable environment found in the sporting arena. By performing these drills, the athlete can continue to progressively respond to increased reactive and physical demands.

When training for quickness, keep in mind that the movements athletes perform when doing drills should always progress from

- slow to fast,
- simple to complex,

- active to reactive,
- predictable to unpredictable (in terms of reactive demands), and
- low-level to high-level plyometrics.

Reaction-Time Training

RT can be considered the precursor of quickness. In other words, the athlete must first see and recognize the need to react to an opposing player, for example, and then she must move at a high speed to accomplish the task at hand. Considering most decisions in the athletic arena occur in 200 milliseconds or less, enhancing mental processing time should be viewed as equal in importance to the training program that is implemented (Prentice and Voight 1999; Schmidt and Lee 1998). In fact, it is arguable that mental processing speed is the sole defining feature of athletic greatness. Think about it. At the upper level of athletics, everyone is gifted physically. Take professional football players, for example. Relative to each position, most of them possess similar physical gifts: similar speed, strength, and jumping ability. Yet, there is a distinct separation between the 98 percent who are merely great and the 2 percent who are truly exceptional. How is this possible? Why do athletes who possess similar physical gifts vary so widely in performance? Current research suggests that focusing on mental processing speed, or RT, gets us closer to answering this question; it suggests that mind speed is the new frontier in athletic development.

It is important to differentiate some key variables that make up what is often mistakenly referred to as RT. RT is defined as the length of time it takes to initiate a movement. It includes the sensation and perception of a stimulus, as noted already, and the selection of an appropriate response to the stimulus. But it does *not* include the movement itself. This movement is instead called movement time. Movement time describes the time in which an action is taken, whether it is successful or not, relative to the stimulus or signal. Consequently, when describing athletic movement, it is more accurate to describe an athlete's reaction to a signal in terms of total response time. Total response time takes into account the mental processing time as well as the actual movement selected and performed. The sections that follow describe these two components and the various stages associated with each. Practical examples are provided to help you understand each component better.

Mental Processing Speed

Mental processing speed is composed of three stages: sensation, perception, and response selection.

Sensation During the sensation stage, an environmental stimulus acts on the athlete's body. As a result, an electrical impulse is sent to the brain for extensive processing. The interval of time that elapses while the athlete detects the sensory input (light, sound, touch, and so on) from an object or the environment is referred to as sensation time. Let's consider the example of a volleyball serve-receive to put sensation time into a practical context. During a serve-receive, all six athletes on the receiving team must prepare to receive the ball. Each athlete must detect not only if the ball is coming toward him but also at what speed and with what characteristics. In this case, the visual amalgamation of colors and borders of the ball and the environment begins to reveal such characteristics of the ball as its direction, velocity, and disposition (Schmidt and Wrisberg 2000). Discerning these initial stimuli in the sensation stage begins to give meaning to the situation presented to the athlete and ushers in the second stage of mental processing speed, perception.

Perception During the perception stage, the results of the sensation stage are further processed, resulting in usable patterns of object movement that bring fuller meaning to the athlete's situation. The length of time needed to acknowledge and correlate the array of sensations discovered in stage one is defined as perception time. Continuing with our volleyball serve-receive example, all six athletes combine the visual amalgamation (which is gradually gaining meaning) with the audible cues given by the defensive specialist to detect the serve as a deep, right-corner floater (note that audible cues register faster than visual stimuli) (Schmidt and Wrisberg 2000). At this point, each athlete must decide if a response is necessary. The information gathered in the perception stage is then passed on to the third stage of mental processing speed, response selection.

Response Selection During the response selection stage, the athlete decides whether or not a response is necessary to address the stimulus. In the volleyball example, all six players have detected that the serve is a deep, right-corner floater. As a result, five players will decide no response is necessary, while one player must respond in a manner that results in proper body position for a successful pass. The total time required to organize a response, or to decide not to respond, to the environmental stimuli is called response selection time. Please note, for the sake of simplicity, that the serve-receive example describes the decision process involved in assessing whether or not to receive the serve. It does not consider off-ball movements that are required of the other five players on the court.

Movement Time

The second component of total response time, as noted already, is movement time. Movement time is the time required to initiate and complete a specific movement or task. It involves the mechanisms in the brain stem and spinal cord that control neuromuscular organization as well as the actual orchestration of the muscles required for adequate force production, force reduction, force stabilization, and timing (Clark 2001; Schmidt and Wrisberg 2000). It is important to understand that movement time describes the time to initiate and complete a specific movement. It does not describe whether or not that movement achieves the desired objective, such as making contact with the ball during a serve-receive.

Factors Affecting Total Response Time

Although psychologists use the stages of processing model just described to simplify the explanation of motor activity, in reality this process is a continuous cycle of stimulus action and reaction and a resulting evaluation performed by the central nervous system. This cycle occurs to improve neuromuscular efficiency. Because of the interrelated properties that make up total response time, any improvement in the operation of one or more of the stages will enhance total response time. Likewise, any weakening of the operation of one or more of the stages will be detrimental. Following are the three most influential factors directly affecting RT and thus total response time. It becomes easy to see that achieving good mental processing speed is not only preferable in sports but absolutely essential, and it can be improved through appropriate training.

Stimulus Choices

One of the most important factors influencing the time it takes to initiate an action is the number of possible stimulus choices presented at a given time. In this section, we discuss the three different types of response selections—simple, choice, and recognition—and provide practical examples of each.

A simple reaction is the fastest of the three types of reactions. In this situation, there is only one impending signal with one corresponding response. An example of this sort of reaction is the response athletes make when hearing the starter's gun at a swim meet. Because of the simplicity of the reaction, athletes often try to anticipate when the signal will occur to decrease their processing time and thus their RT. As a result, most competitions employ fore periods or catch trials, in conjunction with predetermined typical RT standards (100 milliseconds is the Olympic standard), to determine whether or not an athlete anticipated or reacted to the signal. In this example, if a swimmer has a better simple response time off the block, she could gain a 1-meter lead while the other swimmers are just coming off the blocks. In other sports such as soccer, the faster the athlete responds to a single stimulus in the open field the more time he may have to shoot the ball or apply the subsequent sports skill. This gives the athlete that first layer of fundamental reactive ability to improve over all response time and quickness.

When an athlete is confronted with a choice reaction, two essential components must be processed that are not required during a simple reaction: signal distinction and response selection. The former term refers to determining which signal occurred and the latter to selecting an appropriate response based on signal specificity. Choice reaction time is determined by the interval of time that elapses from the presentation of one of several possible unanticipated signals to the beginning of one of several possible responses (Schmidt and Lee 1998; Schmidt and Wrisberg 2000). As a result, perception time is longer, and by consequence, RT is slower. American football provides an example when a running back in possession of the ball in the open field is confronted by a defender and responds by choosing to cut left or right because both options are available. A faster choice reaction gives the runner a better possibility to get a lead on the defender and gain yardage.

Recognition reaction comes into play in situations where there are various impending signals but only one correct response. In this situation, the athlete initiates a reaction when one signal occurs but declines to react when others are presented. Hence, RT is substantially slower than with simple reactions and even with choice reactions. Take a basketball player who is in possession of the ball and is dribbling down the court. She assesses the layout of teammates and opponents in front of her, hears a teammate calling for the ball behind her, and is distinguishing which opponents closing in are the biggest threat. She then chooses among throwing an overhead pass to a faraway teammate, sending a bounce pass to a closer teammate, or juking the opponent in front of her and continuing to dribble toward the basket. In this scenario, the athlete distinguishes the signals present, chooses which signal to respond to, and then chooses among several possible responses to the chosen signal. The complexity inherently creates more demands on overall response time.

Anticipation

At this point, one might think that athletes will be plagued by prolonged RTs. But in reality there is an abundance of information readily available to the vigilant athlete that can be used to plan and process future movements. Two essential means of combating potentially long RTs are to anticipate *what* and *when* particular events are likely to occur. Psychologists use the terms spatial and temporal anticipation, respectively, to describe these two strategies.

Spatial anticipation, also referred to as event anticipation, is defined as the capacity of an athlete to predict what is going to occur in a given situation (Schmidt and Lee 1998; Schmidt and Wrisberg 2000). This strategy allows the athlete to preplan his future movements with respect to a signal and therefore to eliminate stages two and three of mental processing speed. When successfully accomplished, spatial anticipation provides the athlete with a tremendous advantage, reducing RT by as much as 40 to 80 milliseconds. However, when executed erroneously, this strategy results in devastating consequences, often costing the athlete as much as 200 to 300 milliseconds of RT (Prentice and Voight 1999). An example of spatial anticipation is seen on the soccer field during a penalty kick. In this event, for instance, the goalie anticipates the kicker's placing the ball in the upper right side of the goal.

Temporal anticipation is defined as the capacity of an athlete to predict when an event is going to occur during a given situation (Schmidt and Lee 1998; Schmidt and Wrisberg 2000). The tactical interplay that occurs in football between the quarterback and the defensive linemen during the snap is a good example of this strategy. During the snap, the quarterback uses a well-orchestrated presentation of visual and audible cues to attempt to draw his opponents offside while communicating to his offense when to move.

As one can see, the combination of both spatial and temporal anticipation allows the seasoned athlete to initiate her movements faster or at a time that is more relevant with respect to the demands of the environment (Schmidt and Lee 1998). For the sake of simplicity, the practical applications of these strategies just described were presented as isolated events. But in reality, the athlete's playing environment is a continual flow of audible, visual, and tactile signals from which she must readily detect and process those cues that can gain her the competitive edge over the opponent. It is this ability to efficiently interpret the continual flow of signals stemming from the environment that allows the best athletes to complete one action while processing the next, and quite possibly the one after that (Jeeves 1961; Leonard 1953; Prentice and Voight 1999; Schmidt and Lee 1998; Schmidt and Wrisberg 2000).

Skill-Specific Practice

The law of specificity states that the degree of performance adaptation that occurs during training is strongly related to the mechanical, neuromuscular, and metabolic similarity of the training program to competition itself (Clark 2001). In other words, the more similar the practice is to the actual activity for which the athlete is training in terms of movement mechanics, movement velocity, energy metabolism, and cardiorespiratory function, the greater the transfer of the training effect (Clark 2001). Therefore, if a baseball player needs to improve his ability to hit a baseball, the best activity to prescribe is typically batting practice.

With respect to total response time, the amount of skill-specific practice and the relativity of the practice to functional application are the two primary elements that govern choice response time. Simply stated, greater amounts of skill-specific practice produce shorter processing times and faster choice reaction times. The implementation of repetitive functional training will stimulate the conversion of conscious programming to unconscious programming (Prentice and Voight 1999). As a result, the response to a given stimulus is stored as a triggered response and is ultimately performed without continuous reference to conscious processes (Clark 2001; Prentice and Voight 1999). Triggered responses offer the trained athlete a tremendous advantage because there is the added benefit of negligible effect on the athlete's speed.

Quickness and Reaction-Time Training Drills

As described already, skills developed to enhance quickness and game-performance RT are most successful when they are task specific. The added experience of position-specific practice increases the athlete's ability to extract relevant information from her environment, resulting in quick and highly accurate response selections during different game situations. Practice of this sort also allows the trained athlete to cancel out false signals; eliminate distracting audible, visual, and mental "noise" from her environment; and reduce perception and response selection time. All this can be accomplished while increasing the accuracy of movement selection for various environmental signals. This, in turn, will lead to quicker movements by the athlete through enhanced rapidity of activity.

Having said this, and understanding that skills developed to enhance quickness and game-performance RT must be ingrained on the microlevel, there are still a number of ways to incorporate the factors discussed in this chapter into the macrolevel to improve general RT and enhance overall athleticism through body quickness and increased speed. Coaches should keep in mind the law of specificity in their exercise prescription and tailor the exercises to the athlete's specific needs.

BALL REACTION DRILLS

174
Medicine Ball Bull in a Ring

Purpose

To improve quickness and elastic strength.

Procedure

- Stand facing a partner.
- Chest-pass a medicine ball while moving in a circle (see figure).

Variation

- One of you leads and is free to change direction at will. The other athlete reacts and follows.
- Perform the drill using a carioca step.

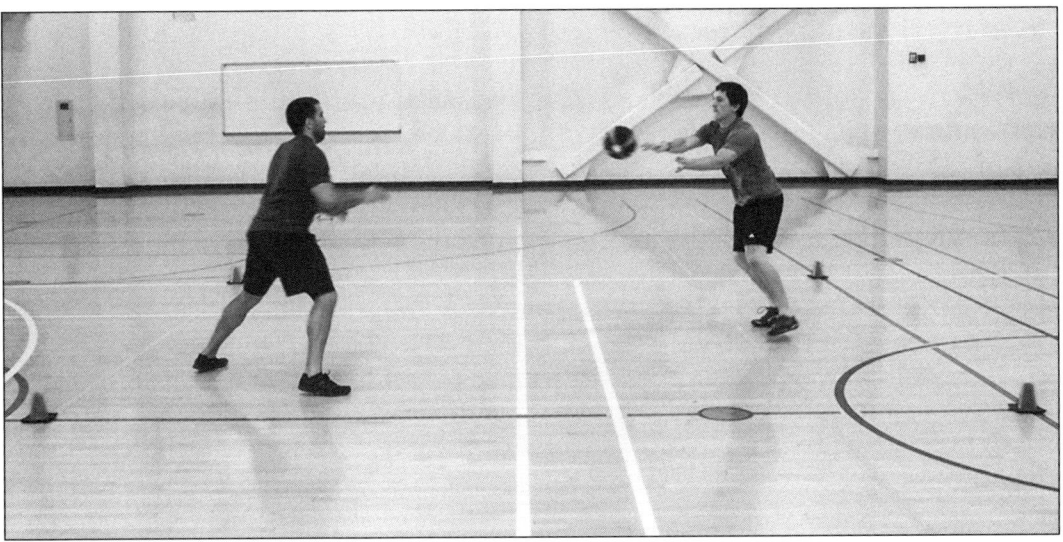

175

 # Medicine Ball Lateral Shuffle With Pass

Purpose
To improve quickness and elastic strength.

Procedure
- Stand facing a partner. The distance you travel depends on the weight of the medicine ball: The lighter the ball, the farther you will travel.
- Shuffle laterally while performing a chest pass back and forth along the predetermined route (see figure).
- Upon reaching the target distance, return in the opposite direction while continuing to pass the ball.

Variation
- One of you leads and is free to change direction at will. The other athlete reacts and follows.
- Perform the drill using a carioca step.

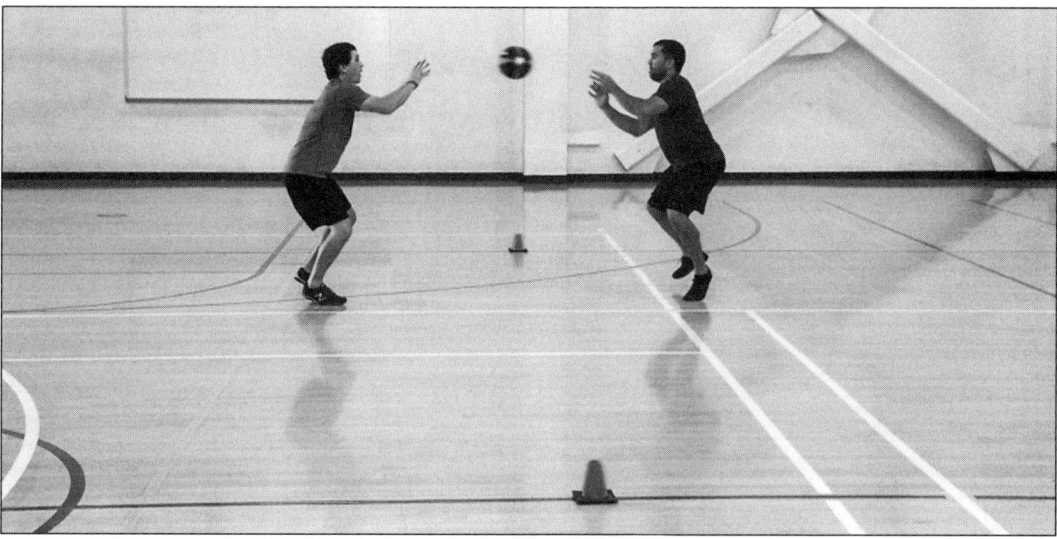

176

Medicine Ball Squat, Push Toss, Bounce, and Catch

Purpose

To improve reactive and elastic strength and total body power.

Procedure

- Begin by holding a rubber medicine ball (one that can bounce) chest high while squatting down, and then throw the ball for height and distance (see figure *a* and *b*).
- You must be quick enough to chase after the ball and catch it before it bounces twice.

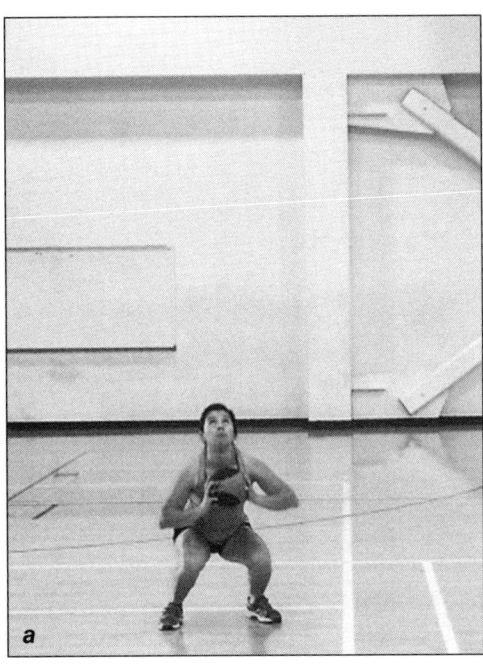
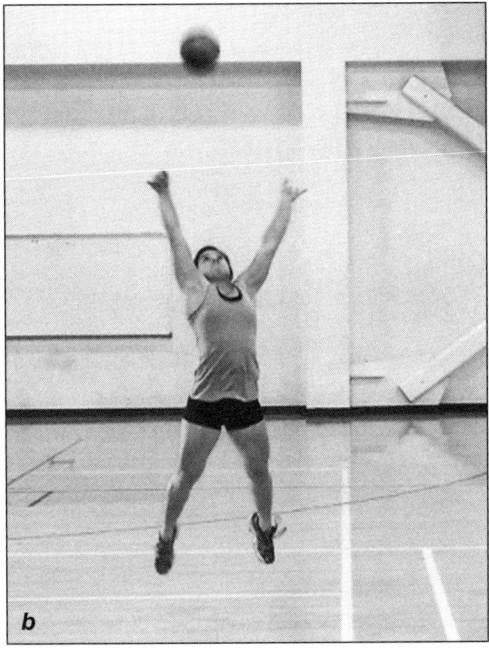

177

Medicine Ball Forward Scoop Toss, Bounce, and Catch

Purpose
To improve total body power and reactive strength.

Procedure
- Swing the medicine ball between your legs as you squat down, and then throw it up and forward, releasing the ball at about shoulder height (see figure *a* and *b*).
- Sprint forward toward the ball and try to catch it before it bounces twice.

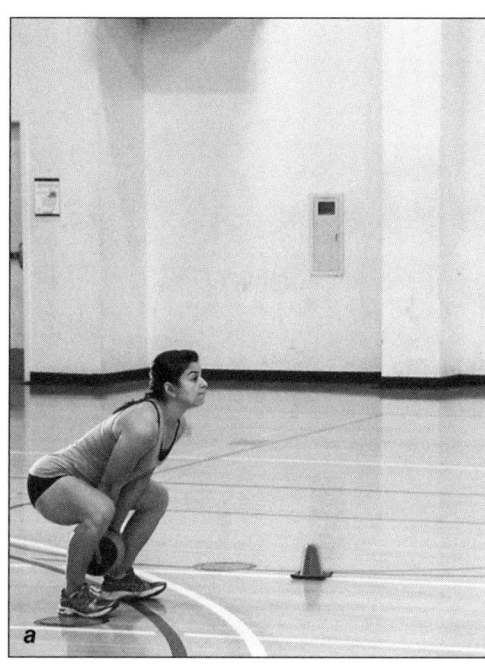
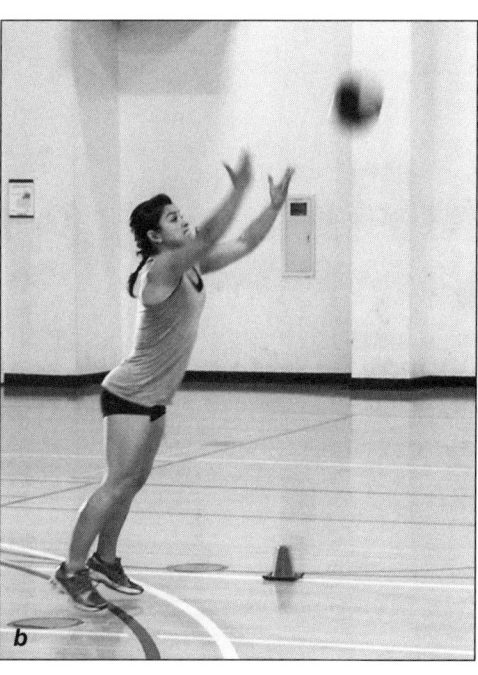

178
Partner Ball Drops

Purpose
To improve visual stimulus response and first-step quickness.

Procedure
- A partner stationed 5 to 10 yards or meters away from you drops a ball from shoulder height (the ball can be specific to the target sport) (see figure *a*).
- You must catch the ball after the first bounce but before a second bounce (see figure *b*).

Variations
- The height of the drop, or distance between partners, can be changed to accommodate skill level.
- Use a ball in each hand in order to increase the difficulty of responding.

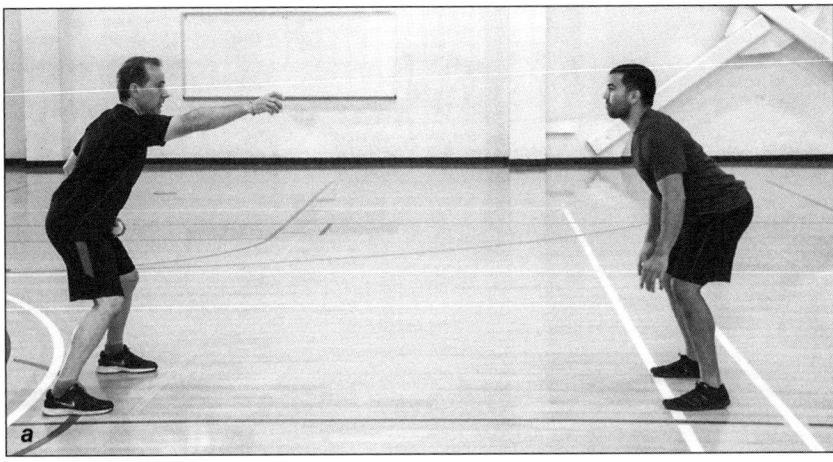

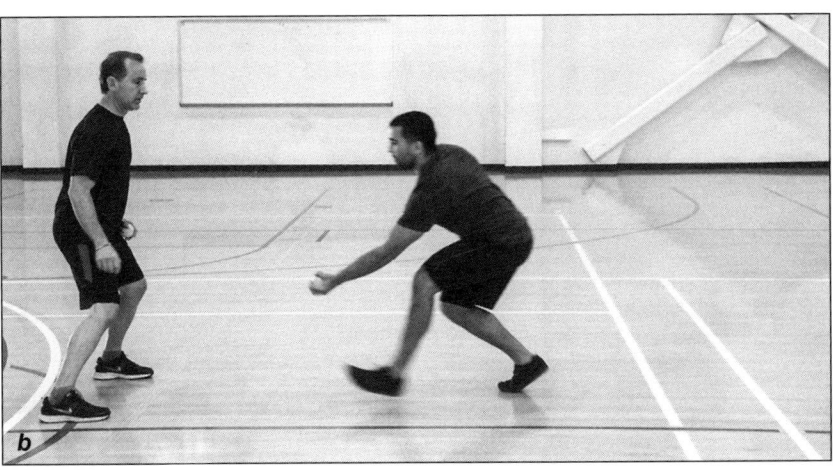

179

Goalie Drill

Purpose
To improve quickness in the upper body.

Procedure
- You are the goalie, and a partner is the shooter.
- Your partner passes the ball high or low toward the goal, which is defined by a line and cones (see figure *a*).
- Try to stop the ball from crossing the line using the hands (see figure *b*).
- Switch roles and repeat.

Variation
You have a bungee attached from your waist to each wrist.

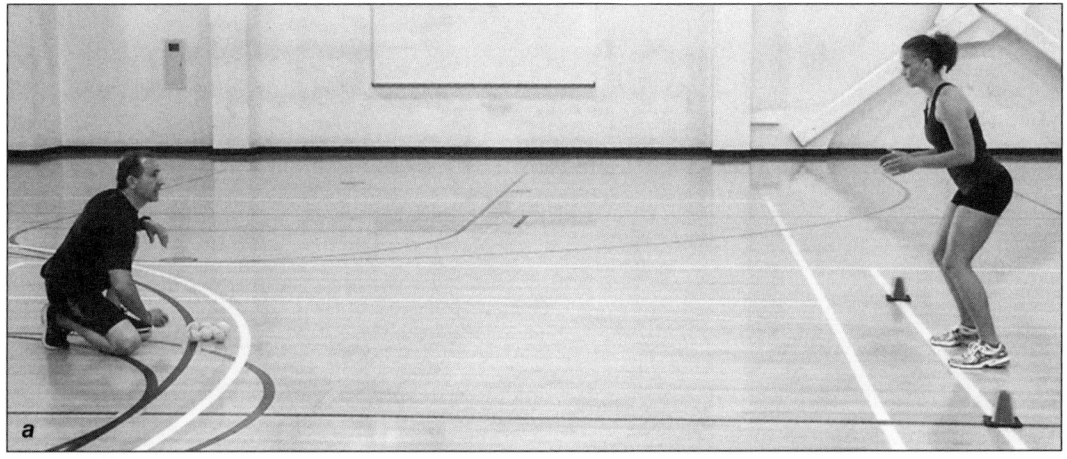

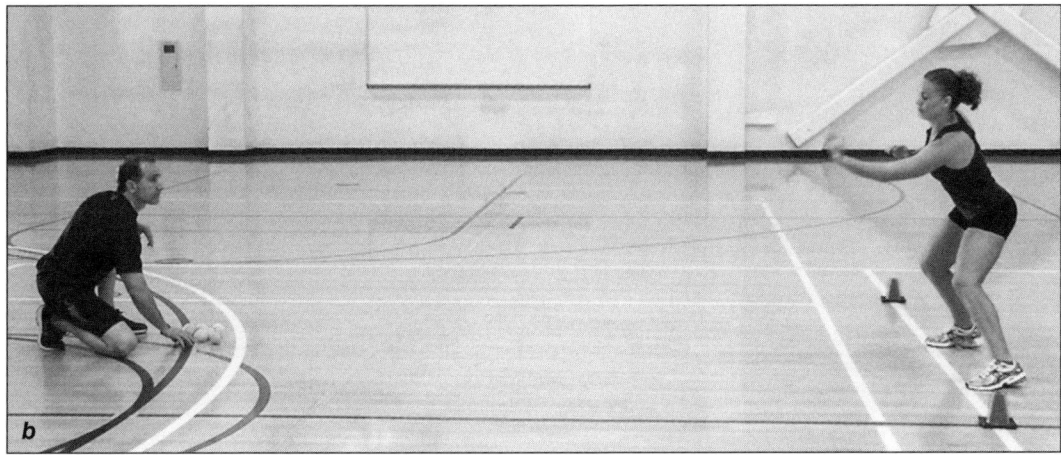

180

Partner Blind Tosses

Purpose

To improve upper and lower body quickness and reaction time.

Procedure

- Stand in a ready position.
- A partner stands behind you and tosses a tennis ball or Z-ball over one of your shoulders (see figure *a*).
- Reacting as you see the ball, sprint and catch it before it bounces twice (see figure *b*).

Variation

Perform this drill with a reaction ball.

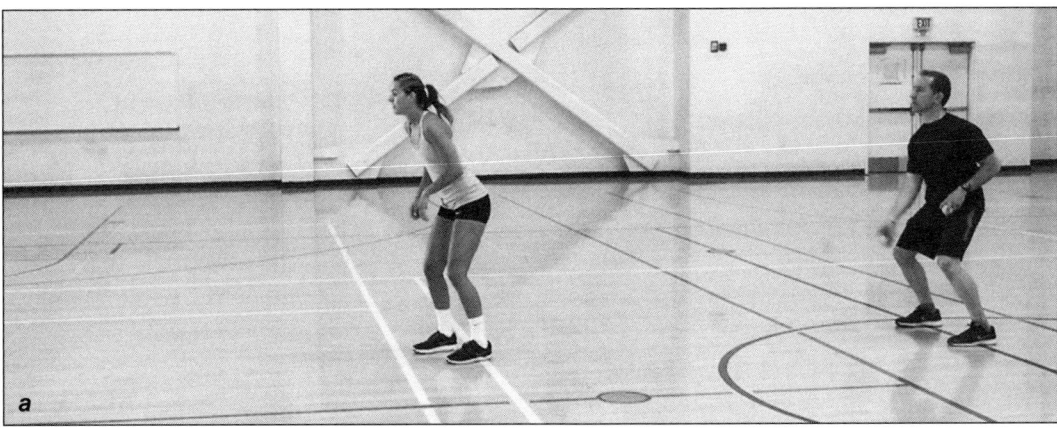

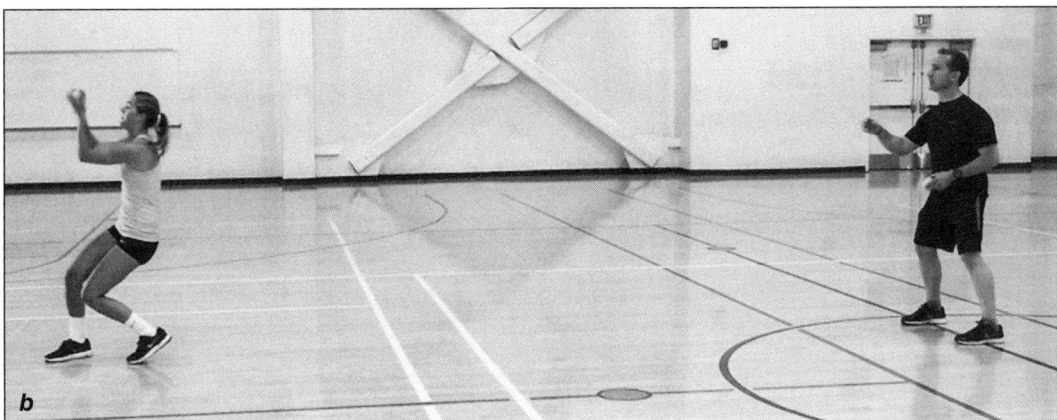

PLYOMETRIC DRILLS

181
Stability Ball Impact Lockouts

Purpose
To strengthen the core and improve the body's ability to absorb impact.

Procedure
- Assume a hand-on-ball push-up position, keeping the core (abdominal muscles, lower back, and hips) tight (see figure *a*).
- Release the ball, allowing yourself to fall on the ball, making impact on the upper abdominals (see figure *b*).
- As you bounce off the ball, secure it with the hands and lock out the arms.

Variations
- Reach out and touch a target while bouncing.
- Clap your hands behind your body while bouncing.

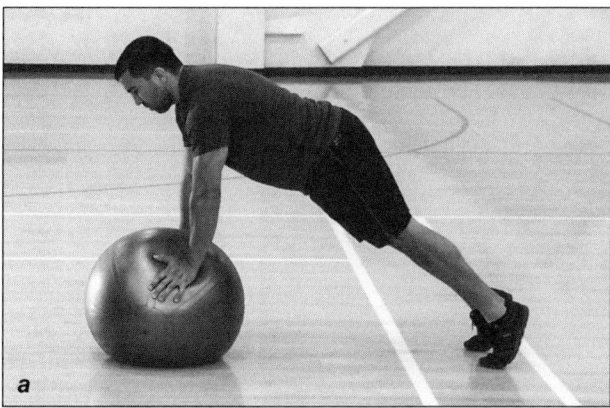

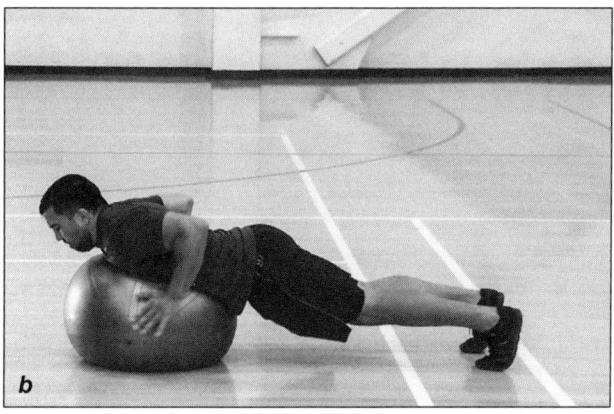

182
Stability Ball Hops

Purpose
To improve quickness in the pushing musculature in the upper body.

Procedure
- Place your feet on the stability ball and hands on the floor (push-up position).
- Hop backward and forward and from side to side, maintaining your balance on the ball with your feet (see figure *a-c*).
- Do not allow the abdominals and hips to sag. Maintain a firm body position.

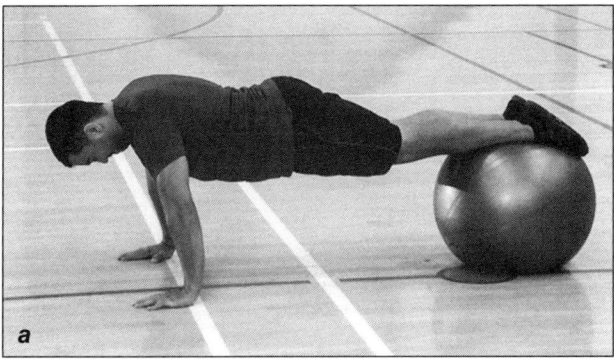

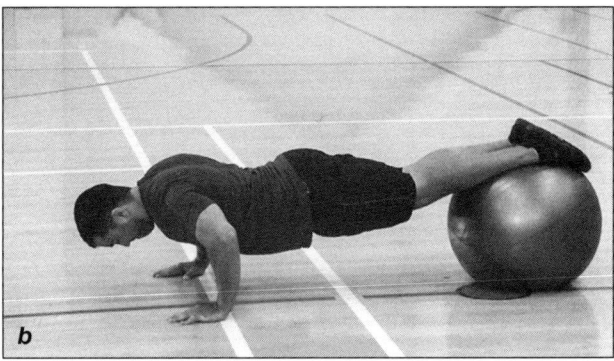

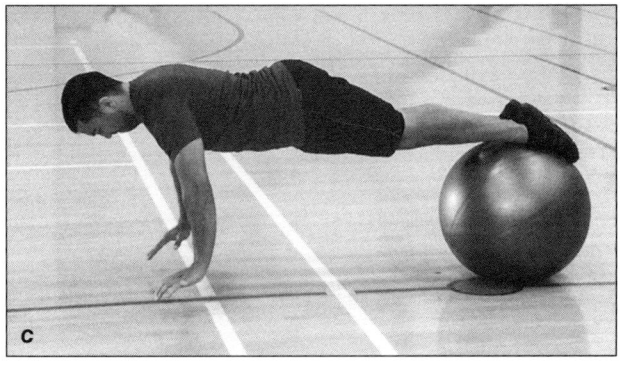

183 Wheelbarrow Drill

Purpose
To improve power in the upper body and core.

Procedure
- A partner holds your feet while your hands perform a predetermined pattern or task (see figure *a* and *b*).
- This should be done as quickly as possible while maintaining a straight body.

Variations
- Perform jumps instead of hand runs.
- Perform lateral shuffles or circular walks with the hands.
- Time the drill to judge improvements.
- Use visual cues, such as ladders, mini-hurdles, or dot patterns.

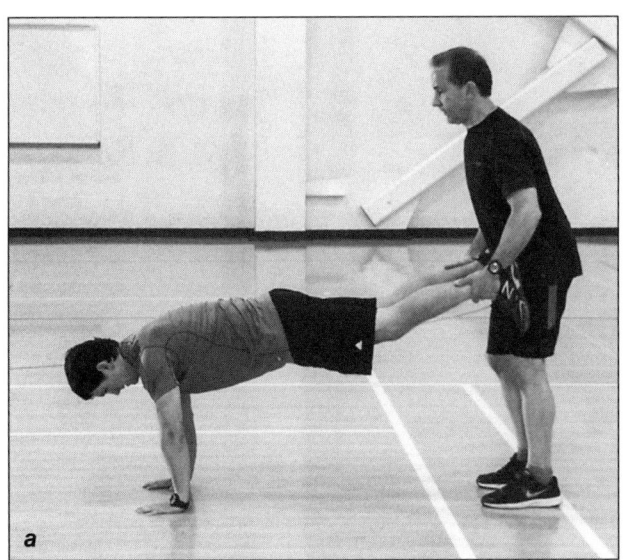
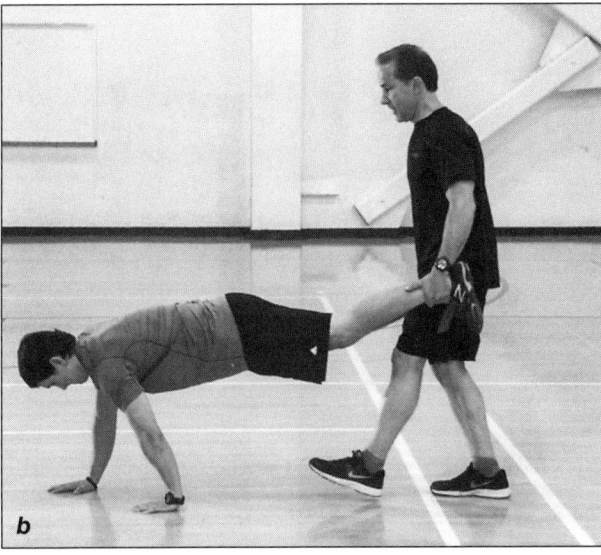

184

Plyo Push-Ups

Purpose

To improve quickness in the pushing musculature in the upper body.

Procedure

- Beginning in the up position, perform an explosive push-up (see figure *a-c*).
- The hands should leave the ground, achieving as much space between the hands and the ground as possible. Finish with the arms extended.
- When landing, keep your arms stiff but not locked. Spend as little time on the ground as possible, and explode back up.

Variation

You and a partner are both in push-up position with your heads facing the same direction; you are positioned 1 yard or meter apart. Perform a push-up with a clap. Your partner reacts to your movement, performing a push-up and attempting to clap at the same time you do.

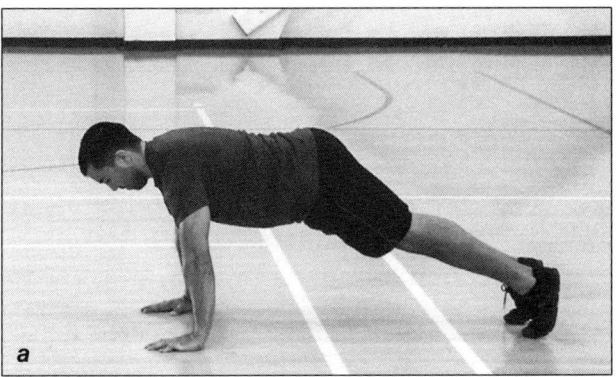
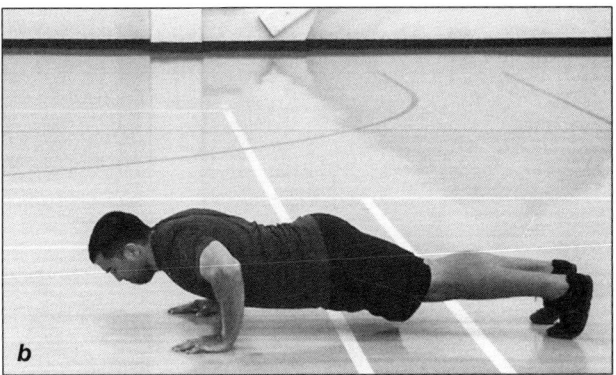
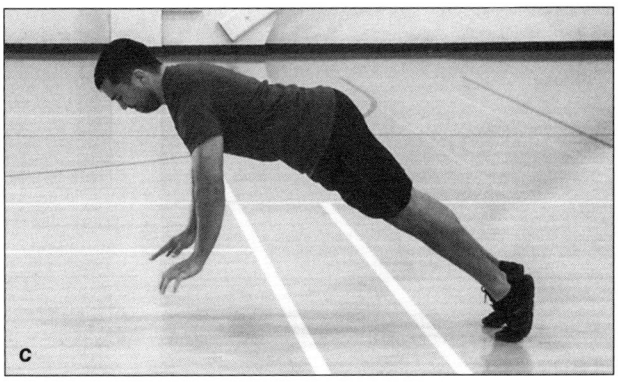

185
Medicine Ball Wall Chest Pass

Purpose
To improve total body transmission of power.

Procedure
- Perform chest passes to a wall (see figure).
- Receive the ball with your arms extended before performing the next pass.
- This can be done for any number of repetitions, for time, or for distance.

Variations
- Perform the drill with one arm.
- Perform the drill while moving laterally up and down the wall.

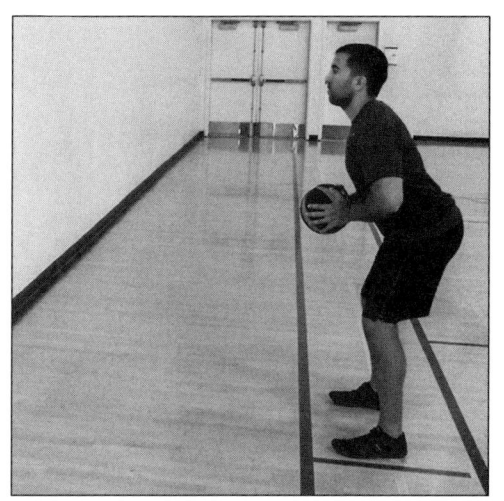

186
Medicine Ball Release Push-Ups With Partner

Purpose
To improve quickness in the pushing musculature in the upper body.

Procedure
- Starting in a kneeling position, throw the medicine ball to a partner and then fall into a push-up (see figure).
- Push up back into the start position while the partner returns the medicine ball.
- Repeat the exercise as quickly as possible.

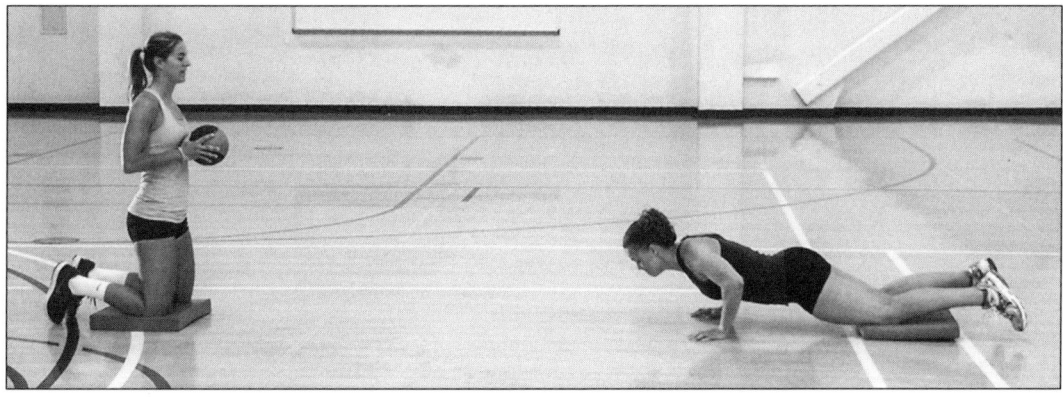

187
Medicine Ball Wall Side Toss

Purpose

To enhance explosive rotational mechanics and changes in direction.

Procedure
- Begin by facing the wall in an athletic position, with a medicine ball held at your side (see figure).
- Throw the ball, striking the wall directly in front of you.
- Catch the rebound, using the momentum to load the body and immediately reverse the throw to perform the next repetition.

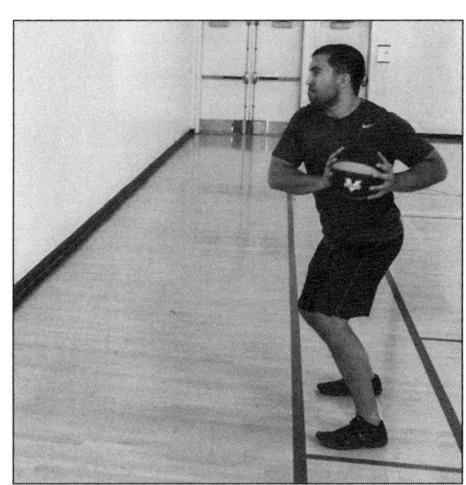

Variations
- Use different stances, such as perpendicular to the wall.
- Use a parallel stance, and toss the ball so that it rebounds to the other side of your body.

188
Medicine Ball Wall Scoop Toss

Purpose

To enhance total body extension, quickness, and power.

Procedure
- Face a wall in an upright athletic stance with a medicine ball.
- Quickly squat and extend your entire body (see figure).
- Toss the ball against the wall as fast as possible while maintaining a tight-backed, low-squat stance.
- Perform this drill for time or for a predetermined number of repetitions.

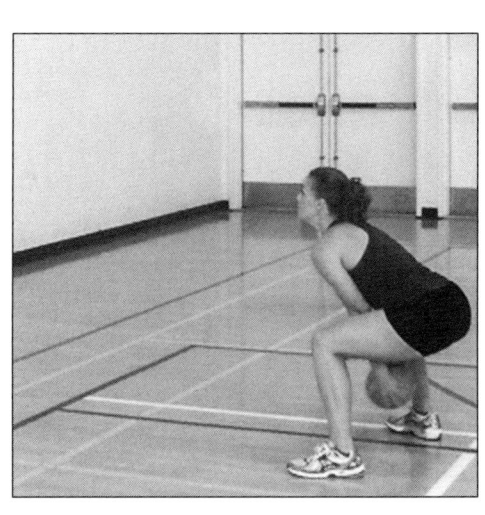

Variations
- Perform a reverse scoop toss backward.
- Perform a long jump and then a scoop toss.

Medicine Ball Wall Overhead Throw

Purpose

To improve explosive power in throwing and overhead activities.

Procedure

- Load the ball over and behind the head with both hands, extending the entire body (see figure).
- Throw the ball at a wall with both hands, and catch it with both hands.
- Keep a parallel stance and feet flat during the loading, or cocking, phase.

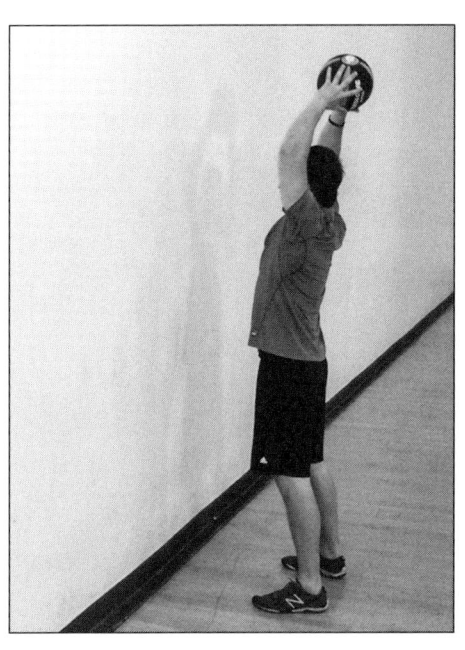

Variations

- Step forward while throwing (alternate legs).
- Throw from a kneeling position.
- Throw with one arm from a two-leg stance.
- Throw with both arms from a single-leg stance.
- Balance on one leg and throw on the same side, with one arm, or opposite-side arm.
- Throw with both arms and incorporate multidirectional hops.

190

Medicine Ball One-Arm Push-Off

Purpose
To improve power and quickness in the pushing musculature in the upper body.

Procedure
- Begin in a push-up position; your body should be straight, with one hand on the medicine ball.
- Drop down into a push-up, and explosively push off with the hand that is on the ground (see figure *a* and *b*).
- The hand on the ball stays on it throughout the exercise. The hand pushing off the ground leaves the ground until it is at the same height or just above the height of the medicine ball.
- Be sure to lower the hand back to the ground in a controlled manner, and then repeat the explosive push-off again once that hand makes contact with the ground.
- Your goal is to spend the least amount of time possible in contact with the ground by delivering an explosive push with the hand that is on the ground.

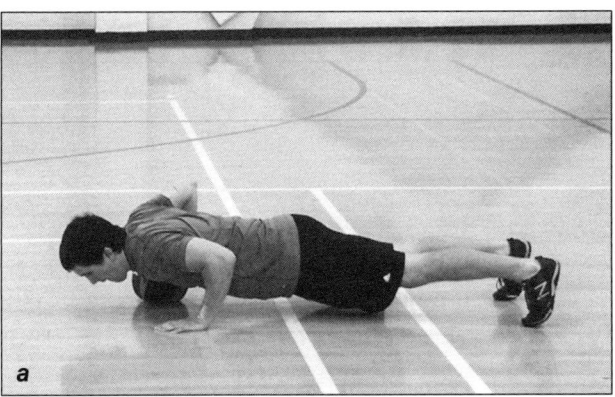
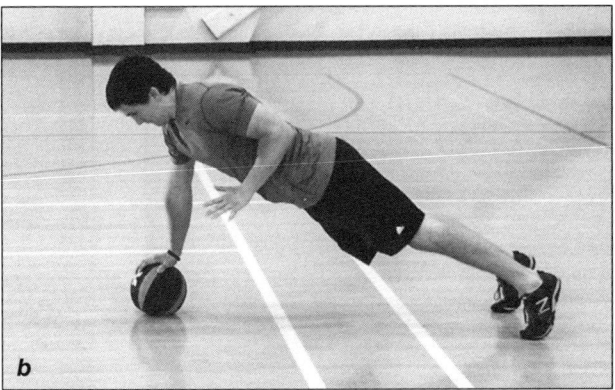

191

Medicine Ball Upper Body Shuffles

Purpose
To improve power and quickness in the pushing musculature in the upper body.

Procedure
- Begin in a push-up position; your body should be straight, with one hand on the medicine ball and your shoulders parallel to the floor.
- Drop down into a push-up, and explosively push off laterally with the hands so that your body passes over the ball and the opposite hand lands on the ball (see figure *a-c*).
- Your feet should remain about hip-width apart, and your core should remain tight throughout the movement.

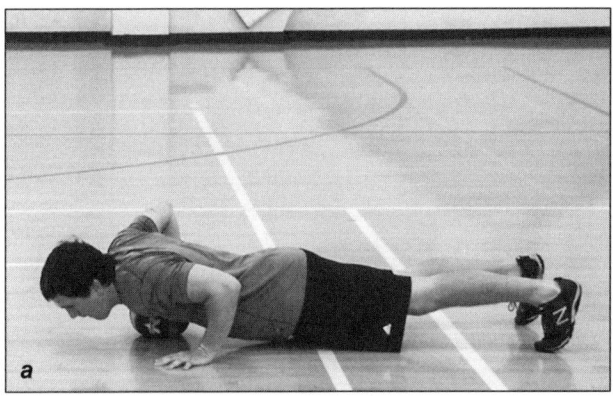
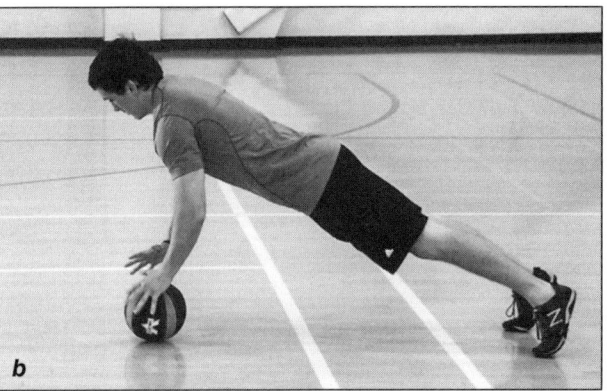
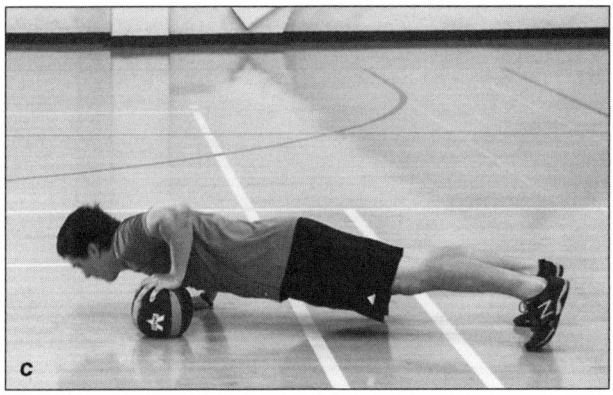

192
Upper Body Shuffles

Purpose
To improve quickness in the upper body pushing musculature.

Procedure
- Begin in a down push-up position, with your hands placed underneath each shoulder (see figure *a*).
- Explosively push yourself up into the air (see figure *b*).
- Land in the down push-up position and repeat (see figure *c*).

Variations
- Start in the up position with your hands shoulder-width apart.
- Shuffle the hands out wider than the shoulders as you drop into a push-up.
- Explosively push up and shuffle the hands back underneath the shoulders while in the air.

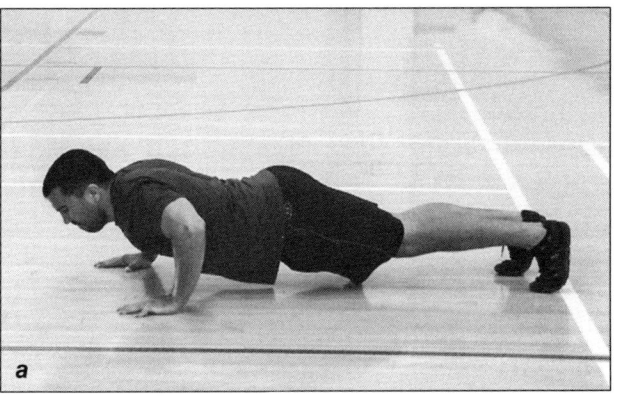

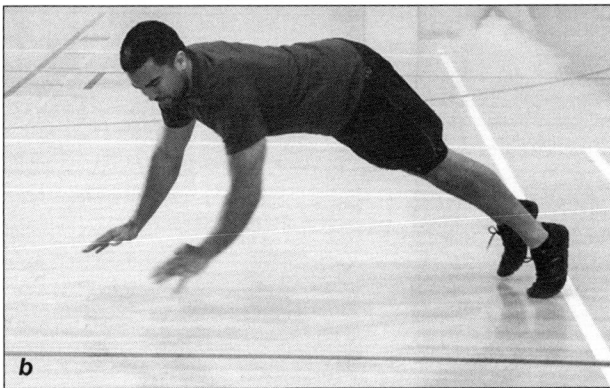

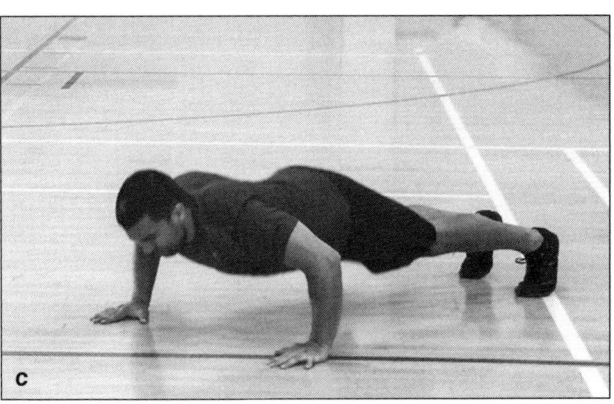

193
Upper Body Box Shuffles

Purpose
To improve power and quickness in the pushing musculature in the upper body.

Procedure
- Start in the push-up position, with one hand on a box or step and one hand on the ground.
- Drop to the floor (see figure *a*).
- Explosively push up into the air and return with the opposite hand on the box or step and the opposite hand on the ground (see figure *b* and *c*).
- Try to get off the ground as quickly as possible.

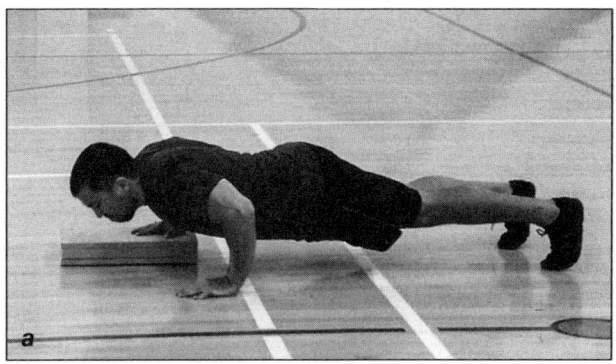

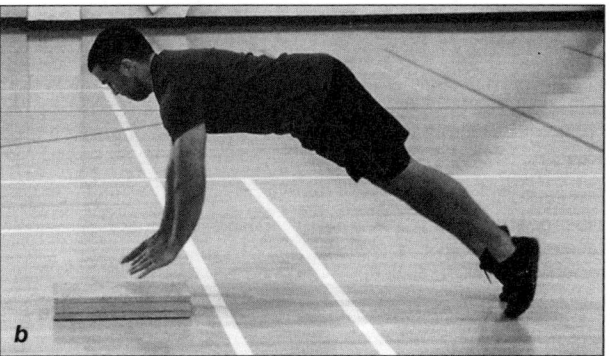

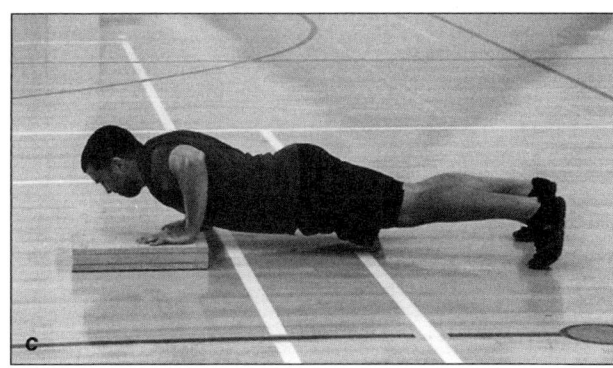

194

Explosive Reclined Pulls

Purpose

To improve power and quickness in the pulling musculature in the upper body.

Procedure

- Begin with a rope—at least 2 inches (5 cm) in diameter with a nonslippery surface—draped over a secured bar or through a secured hook.
- Hold onto the rope with the arm extended, your body reclined to 45 degrees and straight with a tight core (see figure *a*).
- Explosively pull on the rope to quickly elevate your body (see figure *b* and *c*).
- Regrip the rope and repeat.

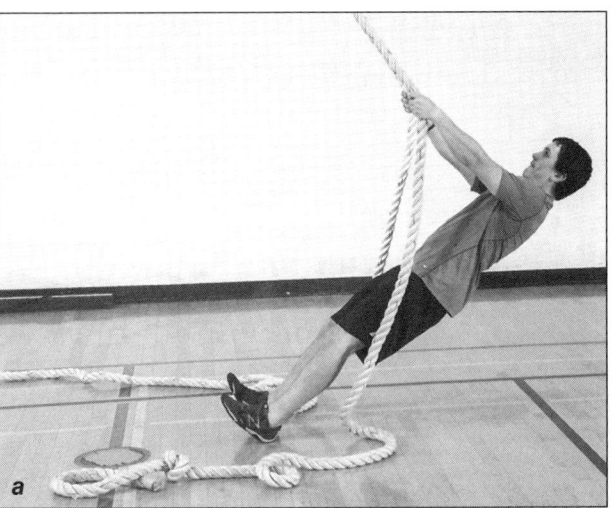

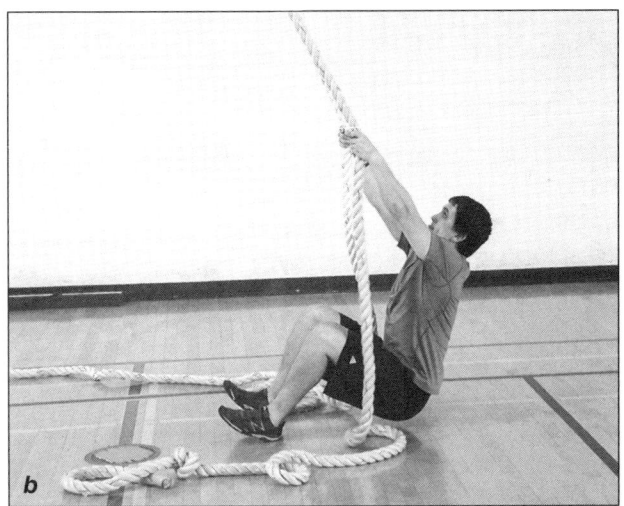

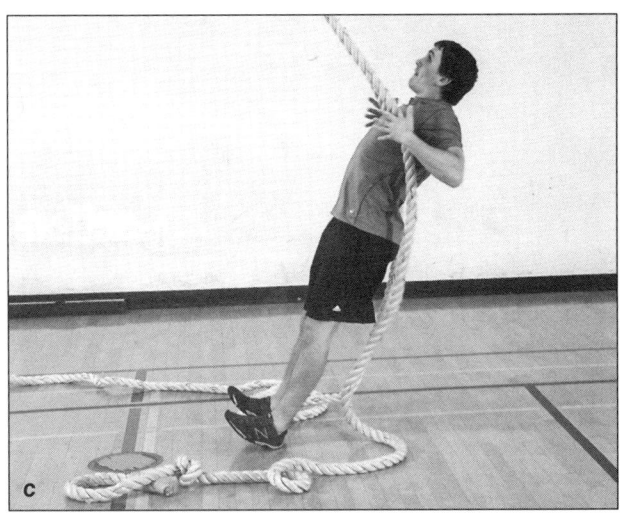

195

Rope Skipping

Purpose
To improve quickness and elastic strength in the lower body.

Procedure
- Skip rope while jumping to designated spots on the ground.
- This drill may be performed with both legs or a single leg.

Variations
- Variable patterns: Skip rope while changing patterns in response to commands. This variation may be performed with both legs or a single leg.
- Weighted rope skipping: Perform the drill with a weighted rope.
- Side skipping: Perform the drill to the left or right. The arm and knee sequence should remain the same throughout. This drill can be the most challenging of all the skips.

196

Ankle Jumps

Purpose
To improve elastic strength and quickness in the lower body.

Procedure
- Perform jumps using just the ankle (see figure *a* and *b*).
- Spend a minimum amount of time on the ground.

Variations
- Jump over a line on the ground, back and forth or sideways.
- Use varied stances and foot positions with feet together, staggered, toes-in, or toes-out.

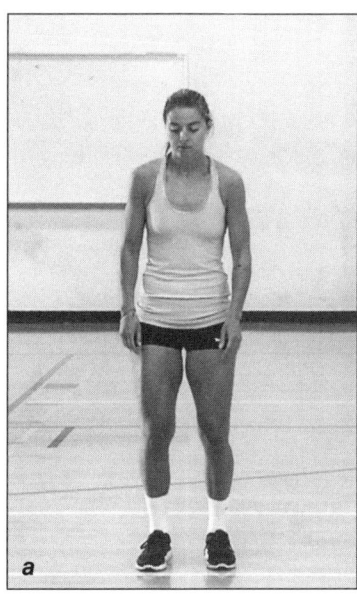
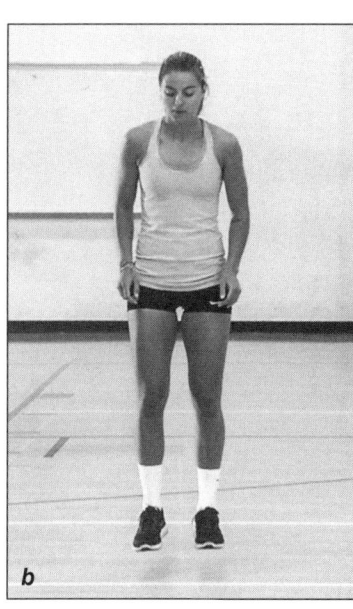

197 Scissor Jumps

Purpose
To improve quickness in the hips and enhance balance.

Procedure
- Begin in a staggered stance with the knees and hips slightly flexed (see figure *a*), then jump off the ground.
- While in the air, switch feet and land in a staggered stance with the opposite foot forward (see figure *b* and *c*).
- Keep your torso upright and avoid leaning the torso forward.
- Repeat as quickly as possible for a predetermined number of reps or for time.

Variations
- For increased intensity, use a split jump with a longer, staggered stance and lowered center of gravity.
- Move forward or backward on each jump.

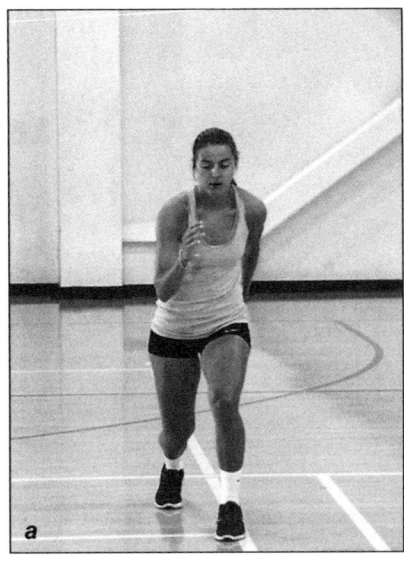
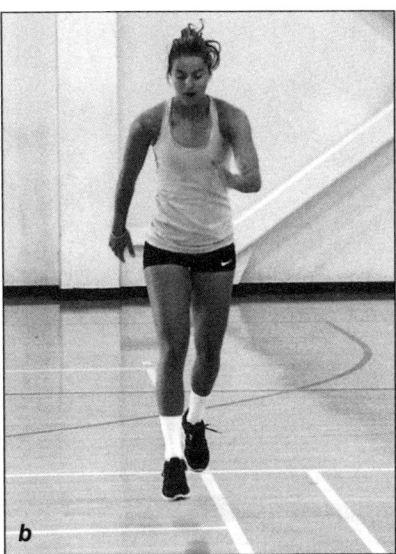
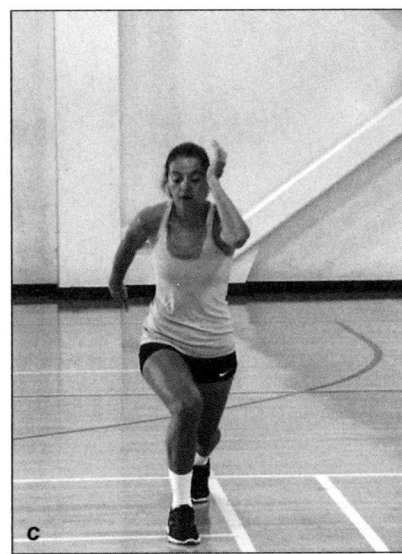

198

Lateral Skaters

Purpose
To improve cutting ability and first-step lateral quickness.

Procedure
- Begin with both feet together, and push off laterally with one leg (see figure *a* and *b*).
- Upon landing, immediately push off in the opposite direction, and continue the drill for either reps or time (see figure *c*).
- To develop quickness, perform as many reps as possible for time (10 seconds or less).

Variation
Jump diagonally so as to move laterally and forward.

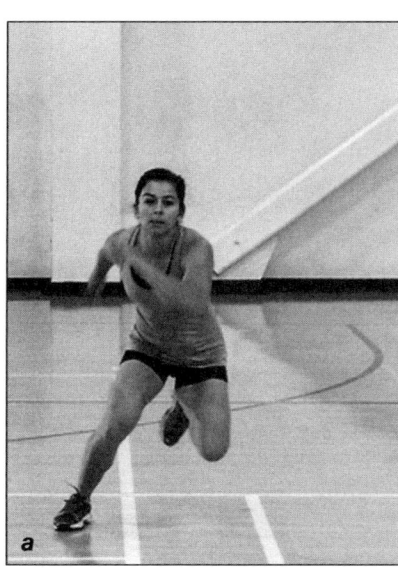
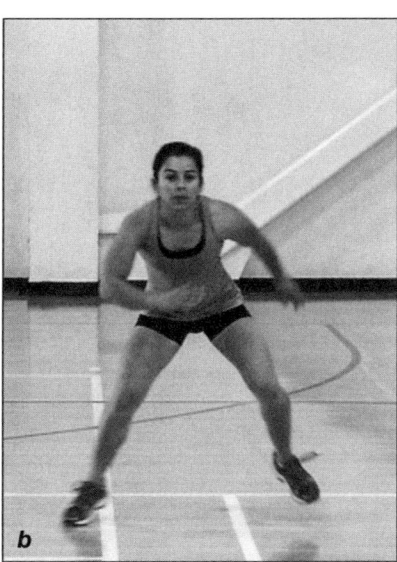
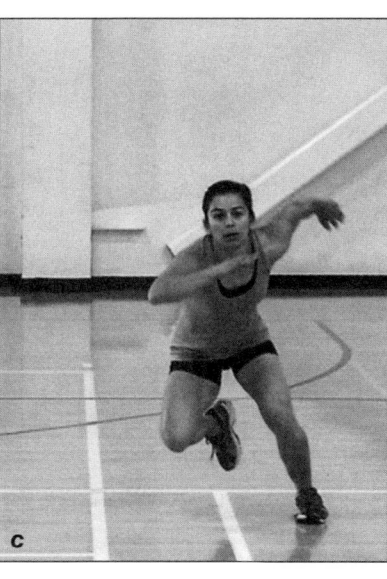

199

Tuck Jumps

Purpose

To improve power in the lower body.

Procedure

- Standing in the power position, load the lower body by swinging both arms back while flexing the hips and knees (see figure *a*).
- Begin the extension of the hips, knees, and finally ankles as the arms swing forward but close to the body.
- Jump straight in the air, tucking both knees to the chest (see figure *b*).
- Upon landing, repeat immediately with the same technique.
- For quickness, perform as rapidly as possible for time while counting reps, or for a fixed number of reps as rapidly as possible.

Variations

- Perform the jump and land a short distance to the side or add rotation and land 90 degrees from each start position.
- Perform this drill with a single leg.
- Perform a pike jump, keeping your legs straight while tucking.
- Perform this drill while moving forward, backward, or side-to-side.

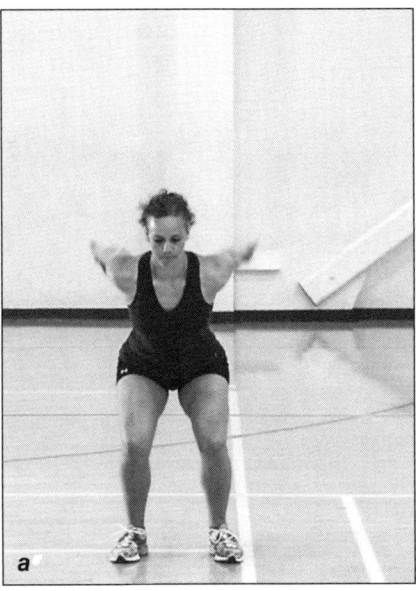
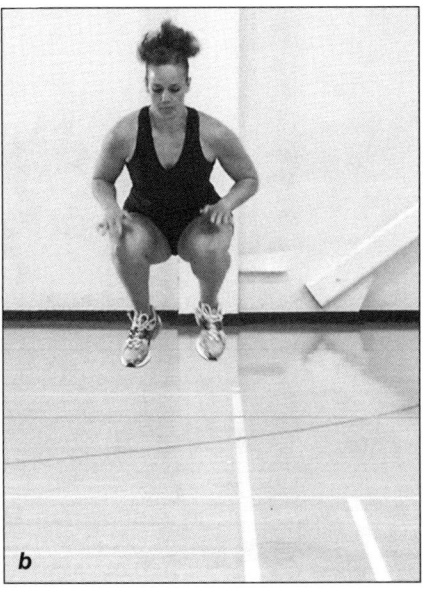

200
Vertical Jump

Purpose
To improve quickness and explosive power in the lower body.

Procedure
- Stand with the feet shoulder-width apart (with the knees and hips flexed in a prestretched position and with the arms back and shoulders over the toes), and quickly dip into the power position.
- Perform a vertical jump by sequentially extending the ankles, knees, and hips, followed by reaching the arms straight up into the air (see figure).

Variation
Upon landing, immediately reload the legs and perform another vertical jump sequence, spending as little time as possible on the ground.

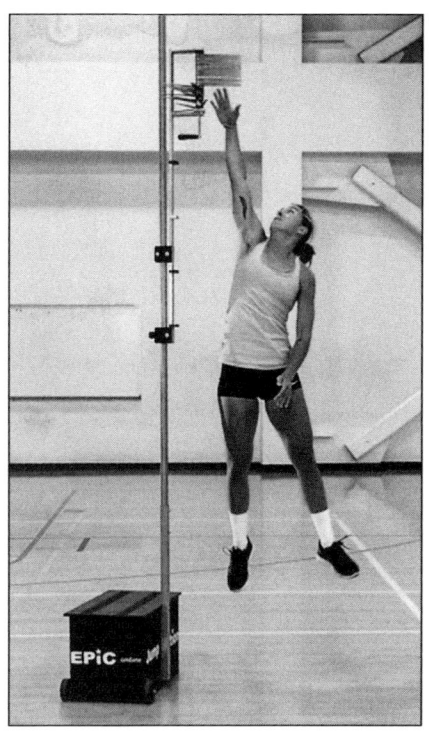

201
Standing Long Jump

Purpose
To improve power in the lower body.

Procedure
- Stand with both feet about shoulder-width apart or slightly narrower.
- Load the legs by flexing the knees and hips and cocking the arms backward.
- Propel your body up and out for distance by extending the legs and using the arms to help thrust the body forward.

202

Barrier Jumps

Purpose
To improve power and quickness in the lower body.

Procedure
- Using something for a barrier (a hurdle, cones, boxes), propel your body over the barrier by jumping forward using the extension of your hips, knees, and ankles (see figure *a* and *b*).
- Maintaining a vertical body posture, tuck your knees to your chest while clearing the obstacle.
- Use a double-arm swing to maintain balance and assist in achieving vertical height.

Variations
- Perform a cut and sprint after the jump.
- *Lateral barrier jumps*: This variation is the same as barrier jumps except the barrier is conquered laterally. Begin by standing parallel to the barrier. Use the same loading action as previously described, but now propel your body over the obstacle laterally. Upon landing, load the legs and arms once again and immediately jump laterally back over the barrier. Continue as quickly as possible for a set amount of jumps or for time.
- *Single-leg barrier jumps*: This variation is the same as barrier jumps but is performed with one leg at a time. This adds a high degree of difficulty to the jump and should be performed over shorter obstacles at first, with gradual increases in height.

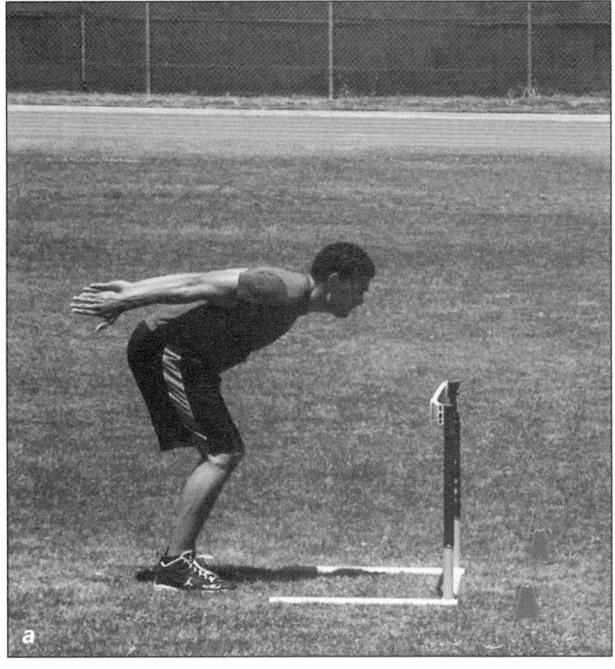 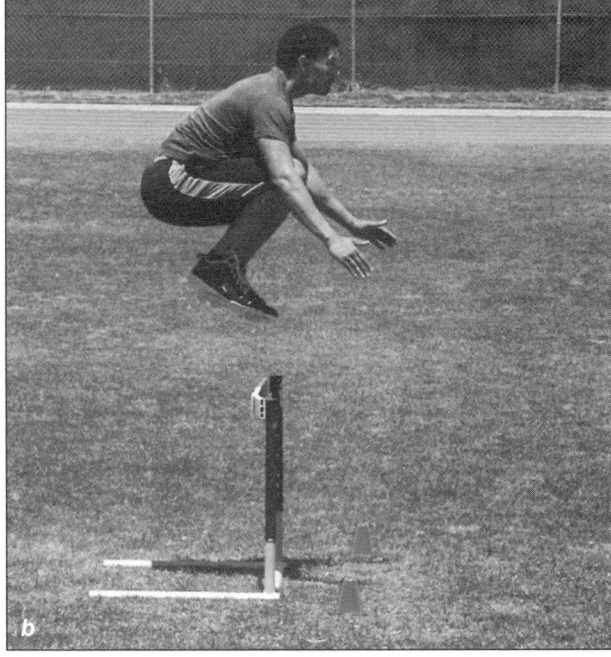

203

Barrier Jump With Cut and Sprint

Purpose

To improve power and quickness in the lower body.

Procedure

- Set up a barrier (such as a hurdle, cone, or bag), and place two cones at 45-degree angles from the barrier and about 10 yards or meters forward; your coach stands between the cones, facing you.
- Jump over the barrier using the extension of your hips, knees, and ankles (see figure *a*).
- While you are in the air, your coach gives either a visual or auditory signal to sprint to the left or right.
- As soon as your feet hit the ground, open your hip position and drive with your first step to sprint in the signaled direction (see figure *b*).

Variation

After jumping the barrier, use a crossover step and sprint in the intended direction.

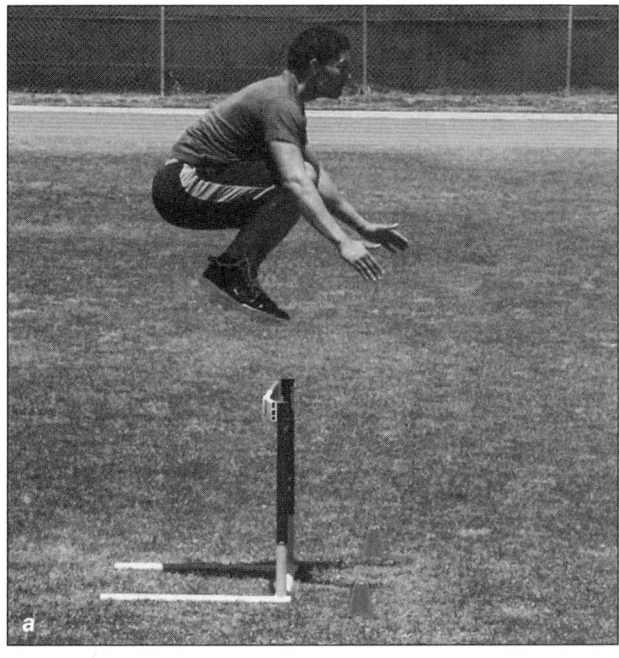 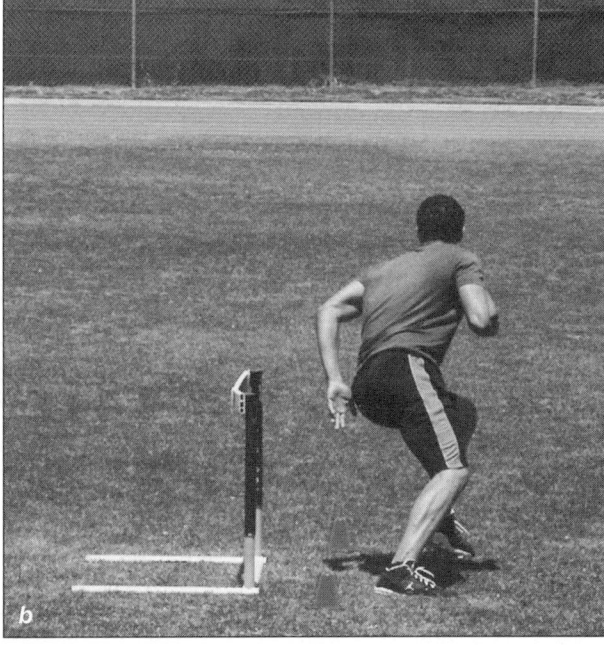

204

Speed Skips

Purpose

To improve power and quickness in the lower body.

Procedure

- Skip with quick lower-body turnover.
- The goal is to achieve fast skipping movement without excessive vertical displacement.
- Spend the least amount of time in contact with the ground.
- Shoulders move forward on the same horizontal plane.

205

Lunge With Power-Up Jump

Purpose

To improve power and quickness in the lower body.

Procedure

- Step into a lunge position and shift your weight toward your front leg (see figure *a*).
- Drive off of the front leg into a forward motion and then land on two feet (see figure *b* and *c*).
- Step out with the other leg and repeat.

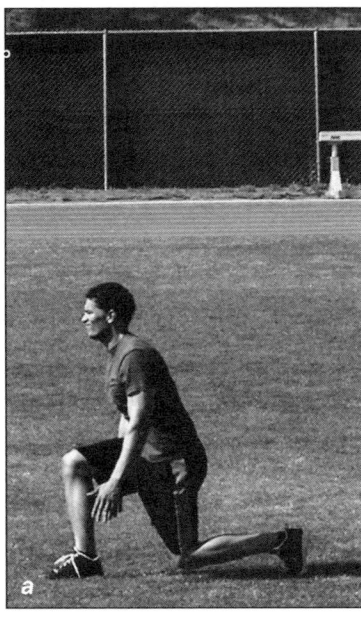 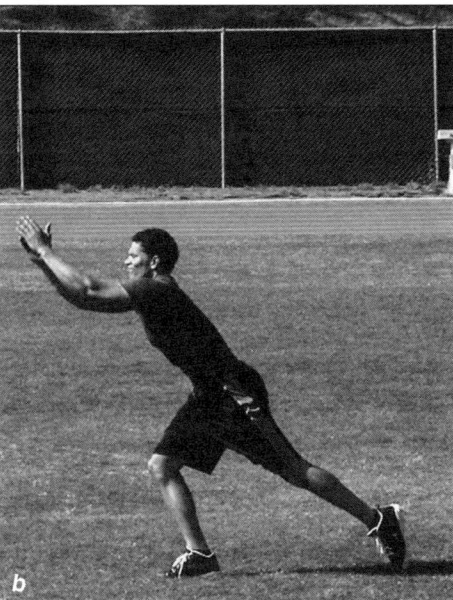 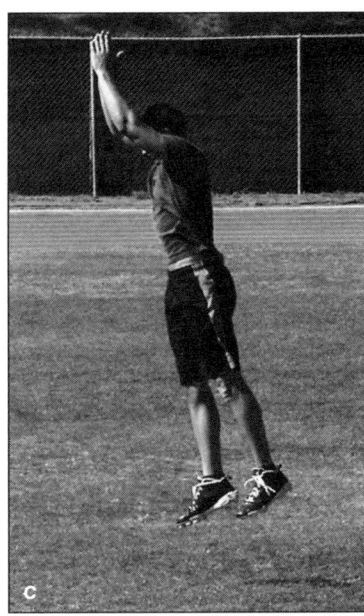

206
Push-Off Box Shuffle

Purpose
To improve power and quickness in the lower body.

Procedure
- Use a box (or step) that rises no higher than halfway up your shin.
- Place one foot completely on the box, and slightly lean forward so your shoulders are over the edge of the box (see figure *a*).
- Quickly push off the box with the foot that is on it, and exchange feet in the air (see figure *b*).
- The back foot should land with stiffness in the ankle to encourage an immediate rebound, or elastic response (see figure *c*).
- The goal is to spend more time in the air and less time in contact with the box or the ground.

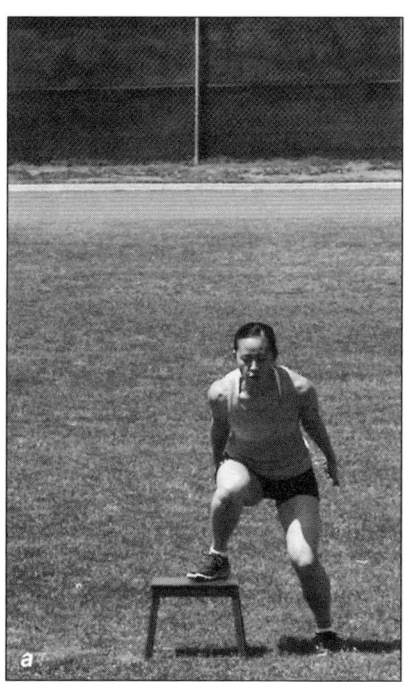
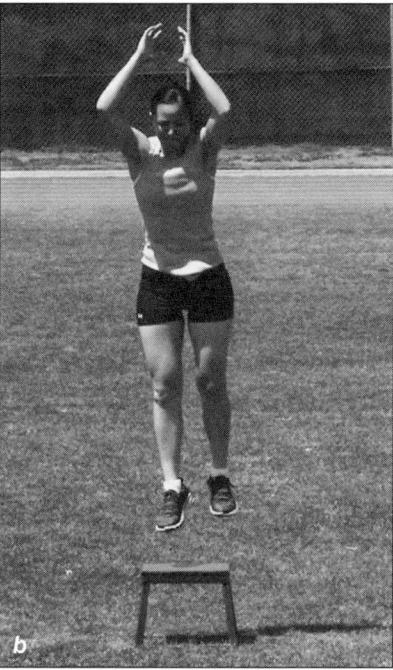
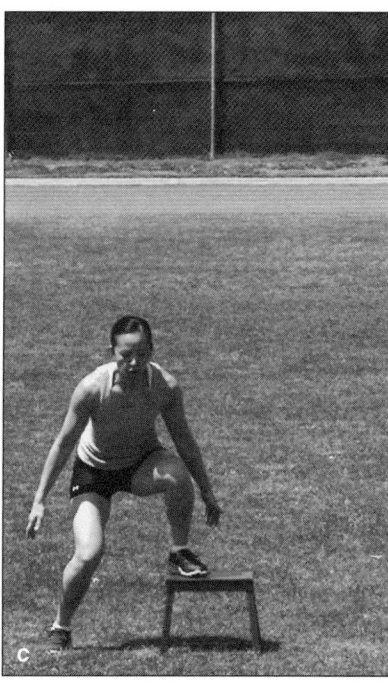

207

Jump Rope With Multidirectional Jumps

Purpose

To improve power and quickness in the lower body.

Procedure

- Jump rope while alternating between two foot positions.
- Start in a split-foot position with one foot up and one foot back and then switch to a straddle position with the feet hip-width apart.
- Continue to repeat this sequence as fast as you can and alternate the lead foot in the staggered position (see figure *a* and *b*).
- Repeat for a designated number of repetitions and then use other jumps, such as bilateral, where the feet move narrow to wide, and rotational, where one foot opens 90 degrees.

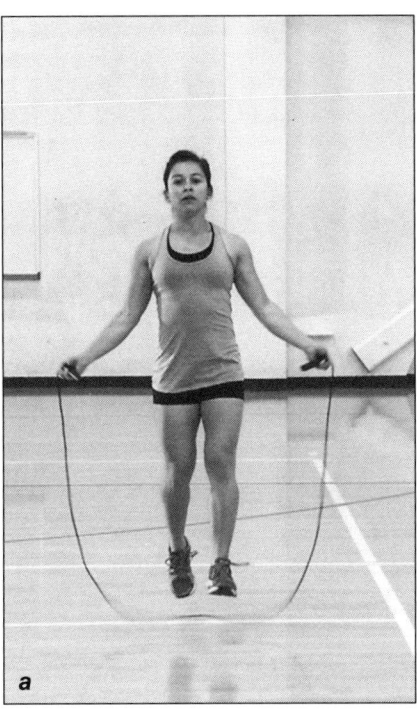
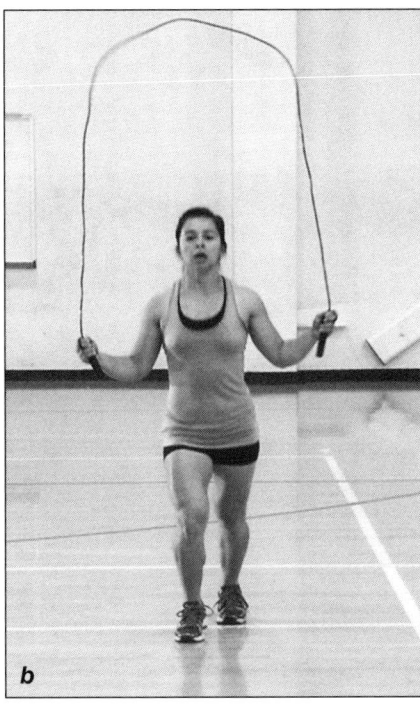

208

Jumping Jacks

Purpose

To improve power and quickness in the lower body.

Procedure

- Perform jumping jacks, mixing a variety of arm and leg motions.
- Start with your feet hip-width apart and perform a jumping jack.
- Follow this by doing a jumping jack with the feet split forward and back while alternating the lead foot each time you split (see figure *a* and *b*).
- Return to the start position and repeat.

Variations

- Add a jump in which you land in a crossover foot position.
- Perform the jumping jack while moving the body forward, backward, laterally, or while rotating your body position.

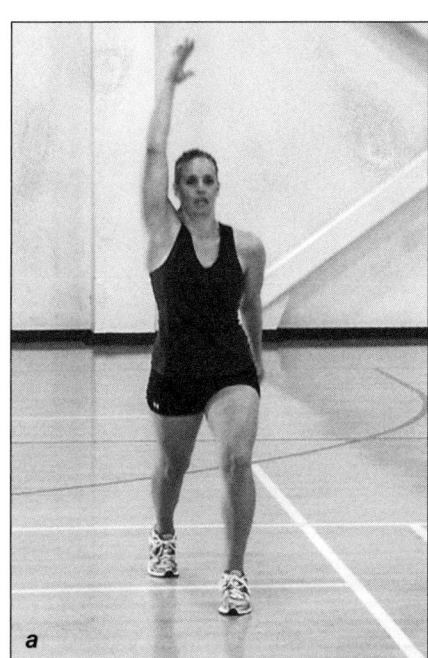
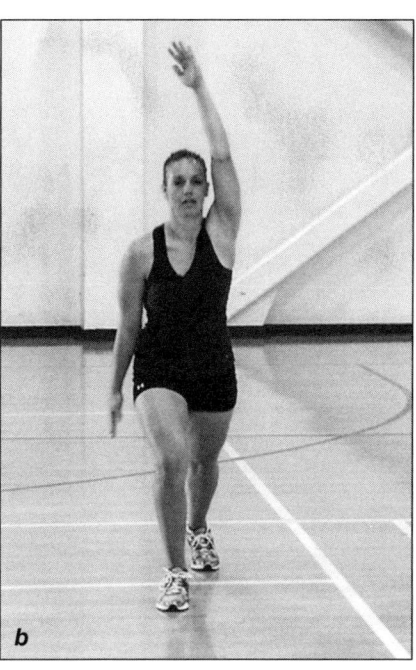

HALF AGILITY LADDER REACTION DRILLS

Note: To avoid duplication, we have split the agility ladder drills between this chapter and chapter 5. The drills in this chapter emphasize short, first-step quickness. They employ half a standard agility ladder to make the drill quicker and prevent neural fatigue from becoming a significant factor. Additionally, a reaction command will add the reaction–response component emphasized in this chapter.

The coach can designate predetermined cones—for example, one cone on each side of the ladder, 5 to 10 yards or meters from the ladder—for you to run to on receiving an audible or visual command. Every drill can be performed laterally or backward for increased difficulty.

209

Quick Feet

Purpose

To enhance stride frequency on the first step.

Procedure

- Run through an agility ladder using the pattern of one foot down between each run (see figure *a* and *b*).
- Concentrate on foot speed, not linear running speed.

Variation

React to a command and run to a designated target.

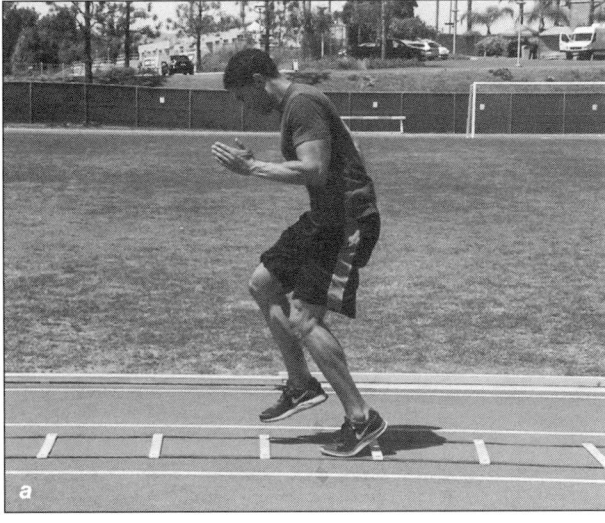
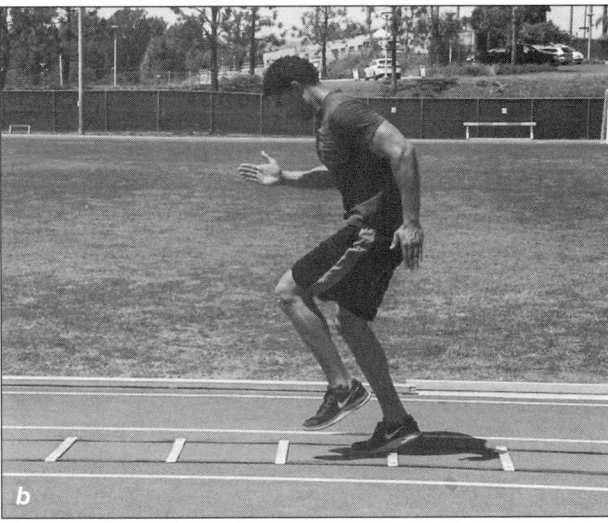

210
Bunny Jumps

Purpose
To enhance elastic strength in the ankle complex.

Procedure
- Perform fast multiple jumps into every square of the ladder (see figure *a-c*).
- Use a quick ankling motion, and minimize ground contact.
- Look straight ahead, not at the ground.

Variation
Add a skill to the drill.

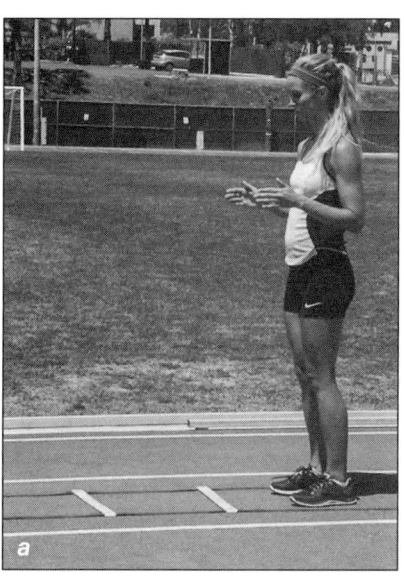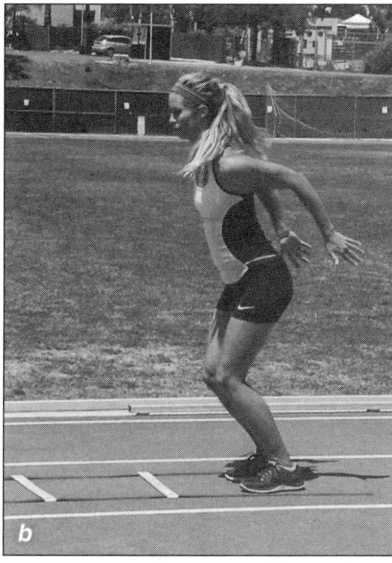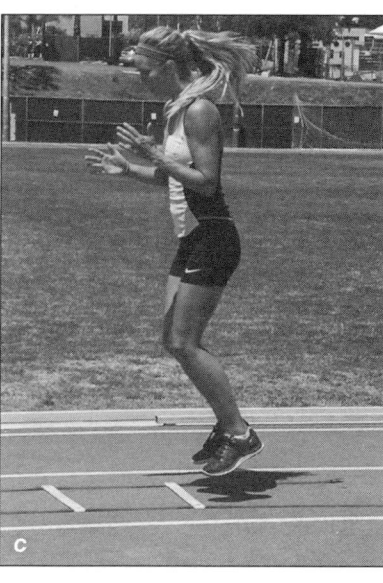

211

Hopscotch Drill

Purpose
To enhance elastic strength in the ankle complex.

Procedure
- Start with one foot on each side of the ladder.
- Jump with both feet into the first space (see figure *a*), then to the next space with feet spread apart so that each one lands on the outside of the ladder (see figure *b*).
- Jump with both feet into the next square of the ladder (see figure *c*), and continue to repeat.
- Look straight ahead, not at the ground.

Variations
- Land on one foot inside the ladder squares.
- Add a skill to the drill.

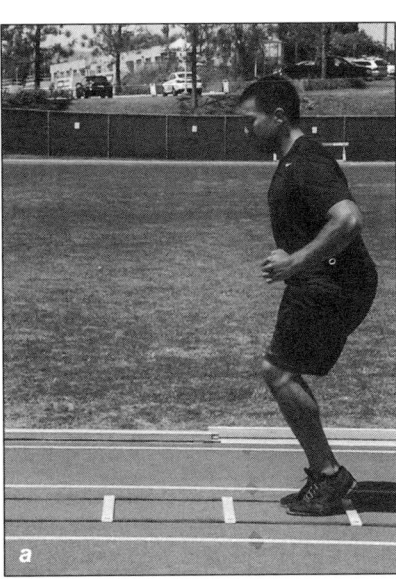
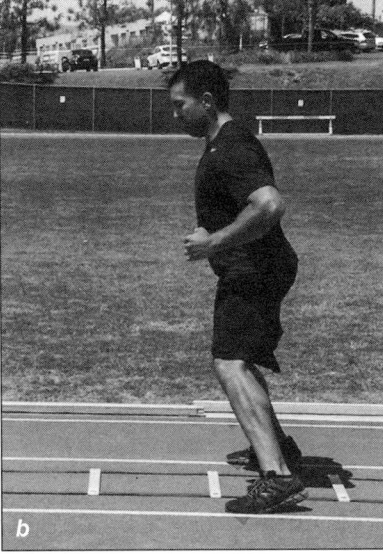
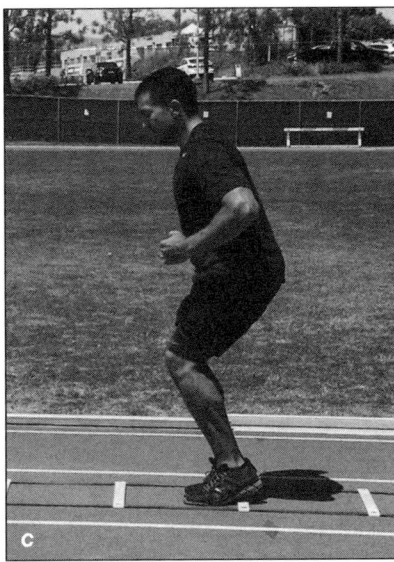

212
Single-Leg Hop

Purpose
To improve quickness in the lower body.

Procedure
- Hop in every square of a ladder, using only one leg (see figure *a* and *b*).
- Emphasize minimizing ground contact.
- Look straight ahead, not at the ground.

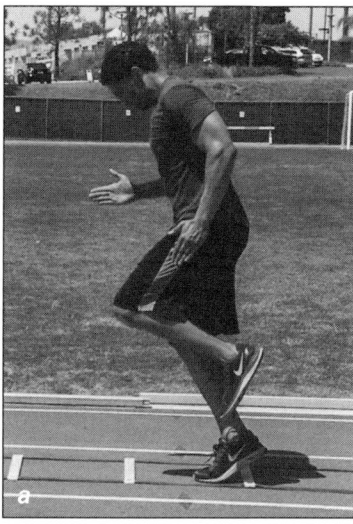
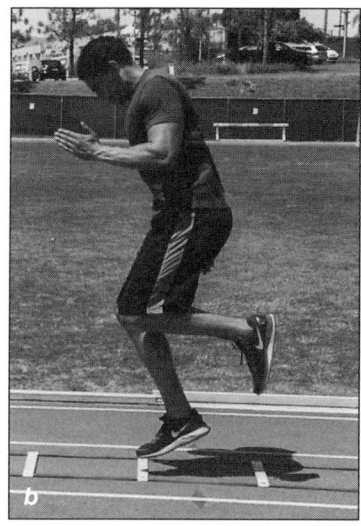

Variations
- Move forward, backward, or laterally.
- Add a skill to the drill.

213
Half Ladder Skill to Sport-Specific Skill

Purpose
To improve quickness in the lower body.

Procedure
- You can perform any of the agility ladder drills while looking at your coach, who is positioned on the opposite side of the ladder.
- React as your coach throws a sport-specific ball to either side of the ladder.
- React in midrun to the side to which the ball is thrown, and catch or hit the ball.

REACTION DRILLS

214

The Bob

Purpose

To improve mental processing speed, upper body reaction time to visual stimuli, and total body quickness.

Procedure
- Stand in a ready position or in a position particular to your sport, with a partner standing in front of you.
- Using a foam bat, focus mitt, or oversized boxing glove, your partner initiates the drill by attempting to lightly contact your head area (see figure *a*).
- The attack is made along the sagittal plane (i.e., straight on).
- Respond by avoiding contact, moving to either side of the attack (see figure *b*).

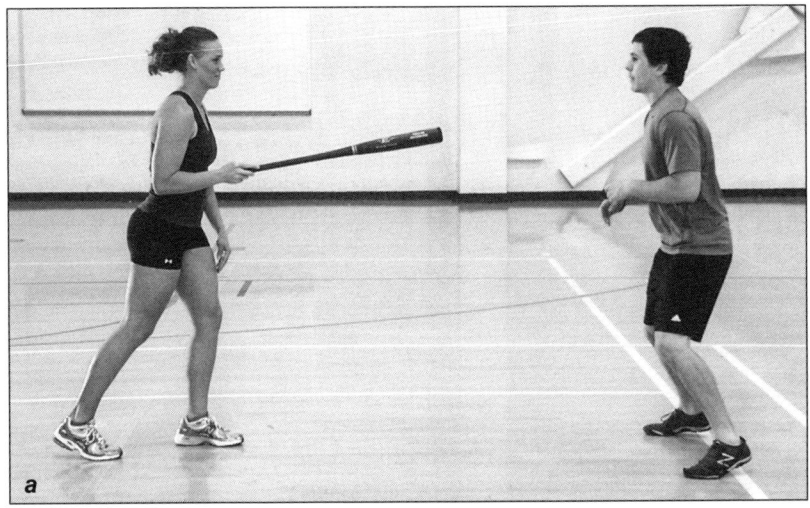

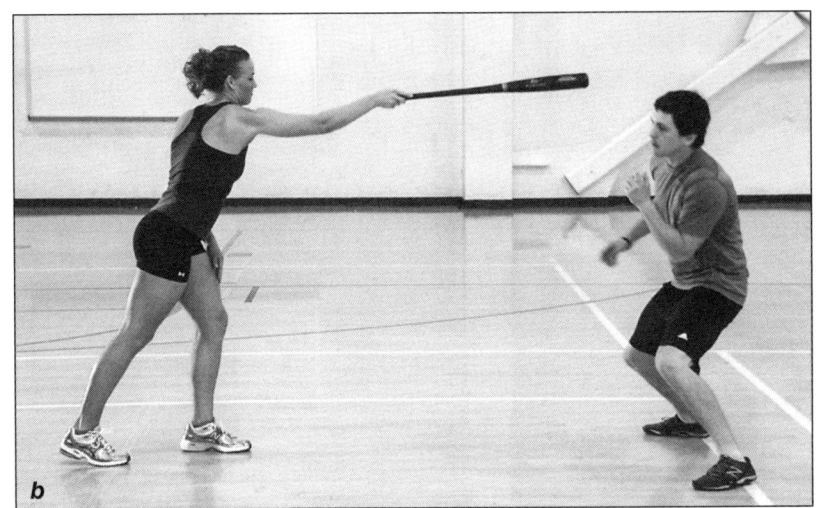

215

The Parry

Purpose

To improve mental processing speed, upper body reaction time to visual stimuli, and total body quickness.

Procedure

- Stand in a ready position or in a position particular to your sport, with a partner standing in front of you.
- Using a foam bat, focus mitt, or oversized boxing glove, your partner initiates the drill by attempting to lightly contact your head area (see figure *a*).
- The attack is made along the sagittal plane (i.e., straight on).
- Respond by using your hands and slapping off the attack just before contact (see figure *b*).

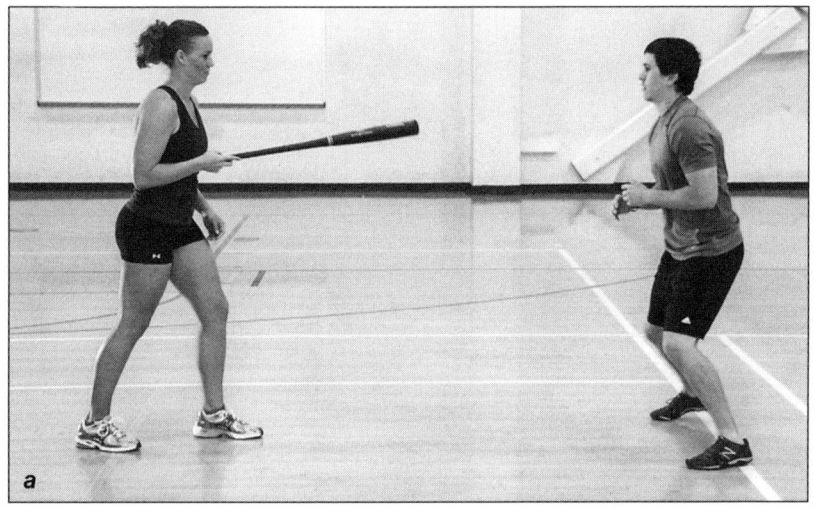

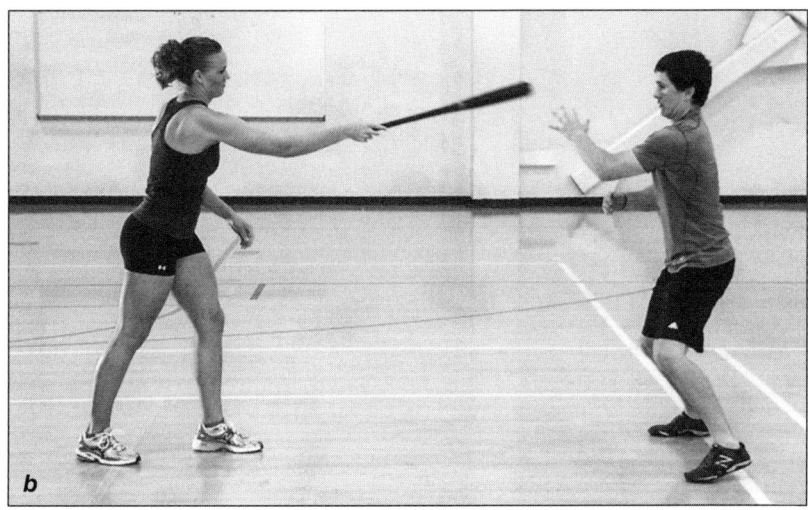

216

The Weave

Purpose

To improve mental processing speed, upper body reaction time to visual stimuli, and total body quickness.

Procedure

- Stand in the ready position or in a position particular to your sport, with a partner standing in front of you.
- Using a foam bat, focus mitt, or oversized boxing glove, your partner initiates the drill by attempting to lightly contact your head area (see figure *a*).
- The attack is made along the sagittal plane or transverse plane (i.e., straight on or via a roundhouse).
- Respond by ducking and weaving under the attack (see figure *b*).

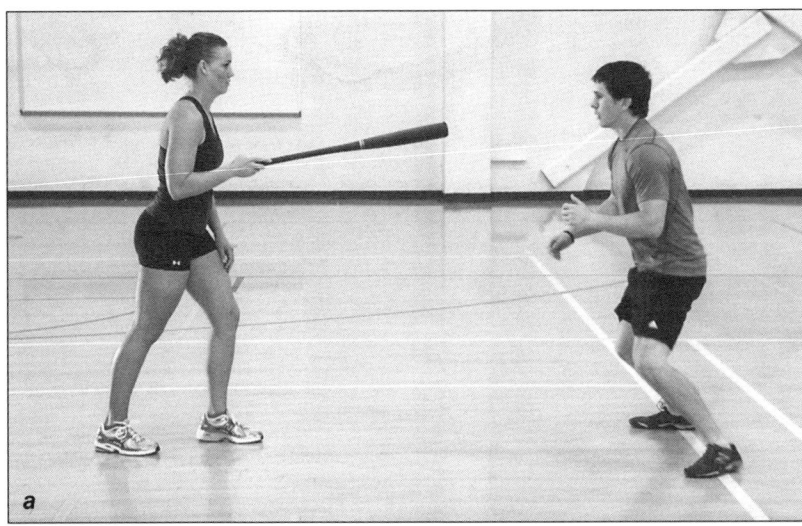

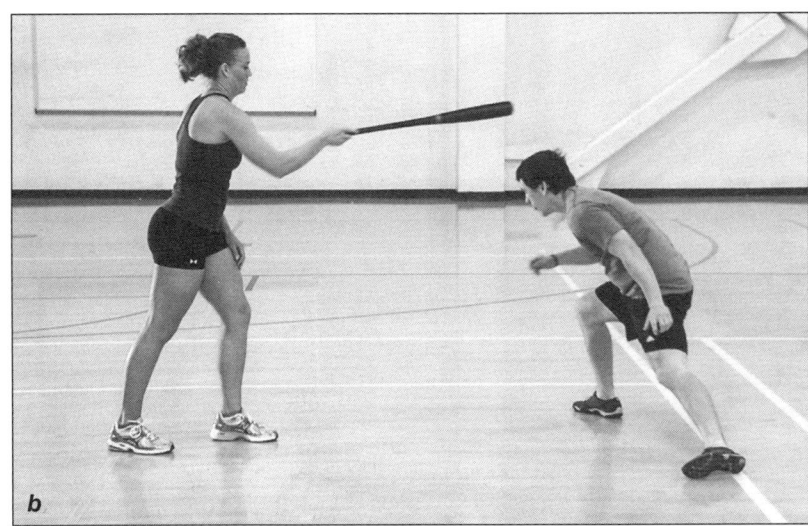

217

Partner-Resisted Lateral Shuffle and Chase

Purpose

To improve lower body quickness and reaction and enhance ability to change direction.

Procedure

- Start by facing a sideline in the athletic position, ready to side shuffle.
- Your partner places a hand on the hip with which you will be leading the side shuffle (see figure *a*).
- On your coach's command, your partner resists your side shuffle; your partner then lets go and sprints in the same direction (see figure *b* and *c*).
- Chase your partner and try to tag her as quickly as possible.

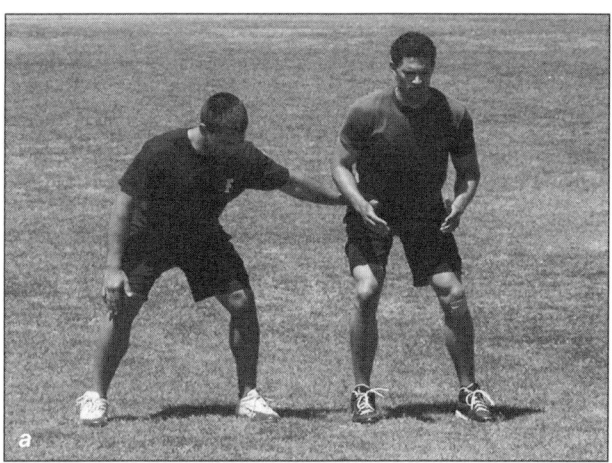

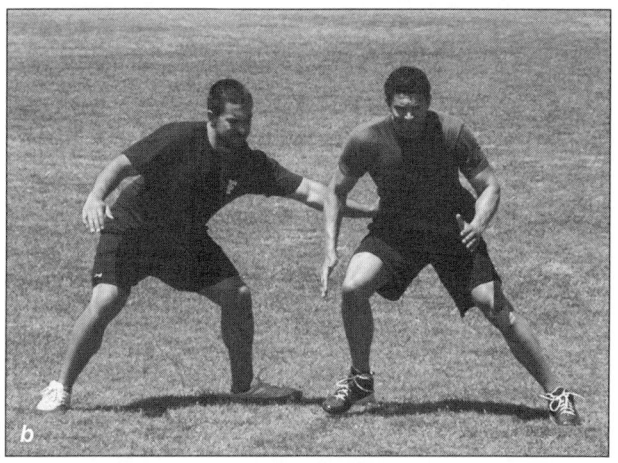

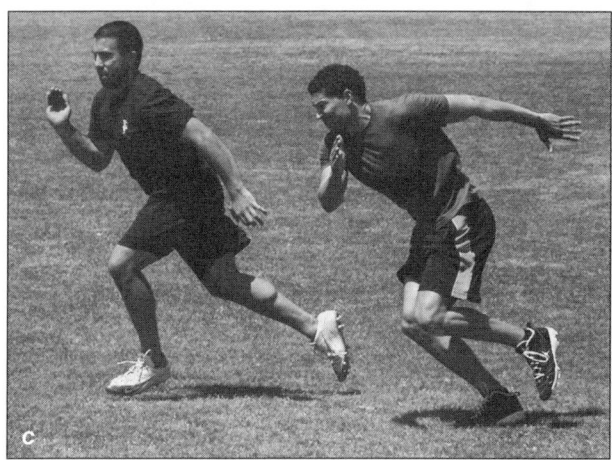

218

Mirror Partner Sprints

Purpose

To improve ability to change direction.

Procedure

- Set up lines or cones over a distance of approximately 20 yards or meters.
- Start on the start line with your partner 5 yards or meters ahead and facing you.
- Sprint forward for 10 yards or meters while your partner backpedals in front of you.
- Stop and backpedal as your partner stops and sprints forward 5 yards or meters; try to always maintain the same distance between you.
- Repeat the sequence until you reach the end of the line.

219

Containing Opponent Drill

Purpose

To improve ability to change direction and react.

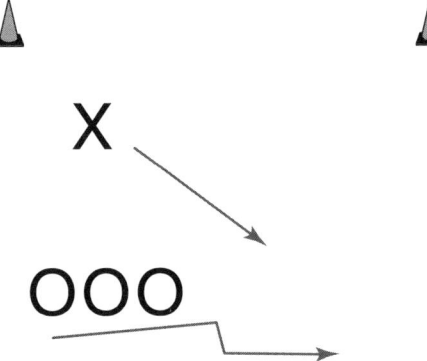

Procedure

- Set up lines and cones over a distance of approximately 20 yards or meters wide by 80 yards or meters long.
- Stand on the end line to start.
- Three or four opponents face you in a line to act as a wall to contain you.
- The opponents backpedal as well as move side to side in order to prevent you from sprinting though their line.

220
Mirror Two-Box Sprint Drill

Purpose
To improve ability to change direction and react.

Procedure
- Mark two boxes with four cones each, with 5 yards or meters between each cone.
- Begin by standing in the middle of one box while a partner stands in the other.
- Sprint to any given cone, touch it, and return to the center of the box.
- Your partner must mirror you, reacting to your movements.

221
Mirror Two-Box Shuffle Drill

Purpose
To improve lower body quickness in a lateral direction and ability to react.

Procedure
- Mark two boxes with four cones each, with 5 yards or meters between each cone.
- You start as commander on the line of one box, and your partner starts on the same line of the other box.
- You can only shuffle on the outside of the box, staying on the lines.
- Your partner must react and mirror you by only shuffling on the same lines of his box.

222
Triangle Drill With Commands

Purpose
To improve quickness of the foot plant and change of direction.

Procedure
- Place three cones in a triangle with sides 5 yards or meters apart.
- Start at the designated cone, sprinting as fast as possible.
- Stay close to the cones.
- Change the direction of the sprint after two to four turns based on the coach's verbal command.

Variation
Triangle chase drill: Stand on the line between two cones. Add a partner who is the chaser and starts at the third cone. Start the chase on the verbal command of the coach, and finish when tagged by the chaser.

223
Three-Step Foot-Tap Drill With Sprint

Purpose
To improve first-step quickness and reaction time.

Procedure
- Start by standing outside of a hoop; quickly tap your foot twice outside the hoop and then tap one foot laterally, touching inside the hoop.
- Tap inside the hoop with the foot closest to it.
- Your coach then gives a visual or auditory command; you must quickly take a step forward and sprint to a cone 5 yards or meters in front of you, touch the cone, return to the beginning position, and continue with the original foot-tapping pattern.

224
Three-Point Fire Drill With Reaction

Purpose
To improve lower body quickness, reaction, and ability to change direction.

Procedure
- Set up a box with hoops in each corner, spaced 10 yards or meters from each other.
- Put two more hoops in the middle of the square about 1 yard or meter apart; you and a partner are in the middle of the box, one assigned to each hoop.
- Both of you start the drill using a fast tap, or "fire feet," while keeping one foot in your hoop.
- Your coach stands at the base of the box and gives visual signals (such as hands up or hands down) to direct both of you to sprint to the back side of the hoop or the front side on your side of the square, to turn, and to sprint back to try to beat your partner to the start position.
- Always maintain a fast tap when returning to the start position.

Variation
Your coach can ask that you use hand touches in all hoops, requiring more total body quickness.

225
Three-Step Foot-Tap Drill With Sprint to Ball Drop

Purpose
To improve first-step quickness and upper body reaction time.

Procedure
- Start by standing outside a hoop; quickly tap your foot twice outside the hoop and then tap your foot once laterally, touching inside the hoop.
- You should tap inside the hoop with the foot closest to the hoop.
- A partner stands 5 yards or meters away and drops a tennis ball from shoulder height.
- You must quickly make a first step forward and sprint to catch the ball before it bounces twice.

226

Four-Box Plus Drill

Purpose

To perform a predictable multidirectional agility movement with multiple reactive agility challenges on command.

Procedure

- Perform a two-foot jump in a box pattern, following the sequence from box 1, 2, 3, 4, and then back to 1 for a continuous pattern.
- Use a hip-width foot jumping stance, and maintain an athletic position throughout the box jump repetitions
- The coach calls out the number of the box you are moving to for the next jump.
- The number called out has an assigned movement at the corresponding numbered cone; you must immediately associate the movement with the number and react to perform that movement.
  - 1: Run to cone 1 and perform upper body shuffles for four repetitions.
  - 2: Run to cone 2 and perform lateral skaters for four repetitions.
  - 3: Run to cone 3 and perform a figure-eight pattern around cones 3 and 4 for four repetitions.
  - 4: Run to cone 4 and perform a bear crawl forward and back between cones 3 and 4.
- After the reactive agility movement, run back to box 1 and wait the for coach's whistle to repeat the drill again.

Variation

Choose more advanced patterns and movements for the reactive movements at each cone.

227
Mirror Two-Box Drill

Purpose
To improve total body quickness and ability to change direction.

Procedure
- Mark two boxes with four cones each, with 5 yards or meters between each cone.
- You start as commander in one box, with your partner in the other box.
- Start by making any move you choose (a squat, a side shuffle, a jump, giant circles, sprinting and touching a cone, and so on).
- Your partner must react and follow your movements.
- At any time, your coach will give an audible signal and your partner will become the commander; now you must react and mirror.

228
Color Dot Drill

Purpose
To train reactive agility and multidirectional movement.

Procedure
- Place multicolored agility dots or cones in rows, mixing the colors throughout the rows. Assuming an athletic position with a hip-width stance, start on a color.
- The coach calls out a color, and you must pogo jump to a correctly colored dot of your choice.
- Always stay facing the same direction, and use lateral jumps to move sideways, forward jumps to move to a dot in front of you, and backward jumps to move to any dot behind you.
- This drill continues for a specific number of called colors in a row or for time.

Variations
- Perform single-leg hops to move forward and laterally to the correctly colored dot that has been called.
- Use 16 dots of mixed colors, and have two athletes responding to the called colors with two-foot jumps or single-leg hops. The athlete that reaches the correctly colored dot first gets to complete the movement on that dot. Therefore the athletes must anticipate the direction the other athlete is going in order to find an open dot of the correct color.

229
▶ Directional Foot Movement

Purpose

To improve mental processing speed and first-step movement time.

Procedure

- Move your foot in the direction of a stimulus (e.g., a hand signal, foot signal, shoulder signal, or ball toss).
- Work only on your first-step reaction.

Variations

- Add a second step, progressing to a full skill movement.
- Preplan a signal to which you respond, but have your coach give multiple signals.

230
▶ Directional Hand Movement

Purpose

To improve mental processing speed and upper body movement time.

Procedure

- Move your hand in the direction of a stimulus (e.g., a hand signal, shoulder signal, or ball pass).
- Work only on your hand reaction.

Variations

- Add footwork to your hand-response work, progressing to a full skill movement.
- Preplan a signal to which you respond, but have your coach give multiple signals.

231
Directional Mirror Drill

Purpose
To improve mental processing speed and quickness of movement time.

Procedure
- This drill is performed with a partner.
- Perform all directional foot movements and variations.
- Initiate the leg or arm movements (or a combination of both); your partner reacts by mirroring the same movement.
- Switch roles and repeat.

Variation
Perform offensive or defensive mirroring with a training tool, such as a basketball.

DIRECTIONAL CHANGE DRILLS

232

Sprint and Backpedal on Command

Purpose

To improve reaction time and ability to change direction.

Procedure
- Start in a two-point stance.
- On command, sprint.
- On the next command, backpedal.
- Repeat.

Variations
- Start from different stances.
- Change biomotor skills throughout the drill or on each command.
- Add a plyometric exercise on each command.
- Vary the distances traveled between commands.

233
Sprint and Cut on Command

Purpose
To improve mental processing speed, quickness of movement time, and ability to change direction.

Procedure
- Start in a two-point stance.
- Sprint on command, cut sharply, and sprint in the instructed direction.

Variations
- Start from different stances.
- Change biomotor skills throughout the drill or on each command.
- Add a plyometric exercise on each command.
- Vary the distances traveled between commands.
- Change the cut angle.

234
Backpedal and Cut on Command

Purpose
To improve mental processing speed, quickness of movement time, and ability to change direction.

Procedure
- Start in a two-point stance.
- Backpedal on command, cut sharply, and sprint in the instructed direction.

Variations
- Start from different stances.
- Change biomotor skills throughout the drill or on each command.
- Add a plyometric exercise on each command.
- Vary the distances traveled between commands.
- Change the cut angle.

235

Circle Reaction Drill

Purpose
To improve mental processing speed and multidirectional quickness.

Procedure
- Stand in a hoop placed in the middle of an eight-hoop circle.
- Assume a ready position and wait for a signal.
- React to the signal and run to each hoop, putting one foot in the hoop.
- Run back until both feet are inside the middle hoop.

Variations
- Start from different stances.
- Use a defensive lateral slide instead of a sprint.
- Add a skill movement on command (e.g., sprawl on the whistle, intercept a passed ball, pass to a target).
- Vary the commands given both audibly and visually.

236

Side Shuffle Reactive Drill

Purpose
To improve mental processing speed, lateral agility, and quickness.

Procedure
- Begin in a ready position—your knees and hips slightly flexed, arms relaxed and to the sides, and shoulders over toes—and wait for a signal.
- Shuffle laterally in the direction of a command from your coach without crossing your feet.
- This should be done by accelerating and then decelerating in order to stop as soon as subsequent commands to change direction are given.

Variations
- Use visual cues instead of audible cues.
- Have your coach move in a semicircle in front of you while you are shuffling to develop court sense.

X Drill

Purpose

To train powerful first-step power for the diagonal step needed in reactive agility.

Procedure

- Place two hurdles side by side lengthwise at 1 yard or meter apart.
- Take one powerful diagonal step, pushing off the inside edge of the right shoe from position 1 to position 2.
- Backpedal and sidestep to position 3.
- Take a powerful diagonal step off the inside edge of the left shoe from position 3 to position 4.
- Backpedal and sidestep to reset at position 1.
- Repeat three times, staying in the athletic position at all times.

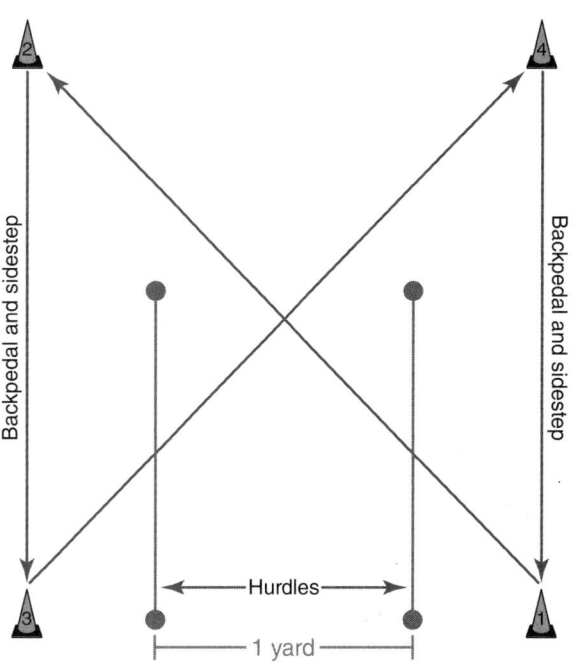

Variations

- Add a ball toss while maintaining the pattern and the rhythm of the movements.
- Use quick fire feet to keep the body in an active ready stance, and perform a reactive diagonal step on the coach's auditory signal or visual signal. After each explosive diagonal step, return to position 1 or 3, and continue quick fire feet until the coach's next signal or the completion of the drill.

GROUND-BASE QUICKNESS DRILLS

238

Four-Point Pop-Up

Purpose

To improve mental processing speed, total body agility, kinesthetic awareness, and quickness.

Procedure

- Start on the ground on your hands and knees and wait for a signal (see figure *a*).
- Explode as fast as possible as you stand up (see figure *b* and *c*).

Variations

- Follow standing up with a skill movement done on command.
- Follow standing up with a tennis ball catch.

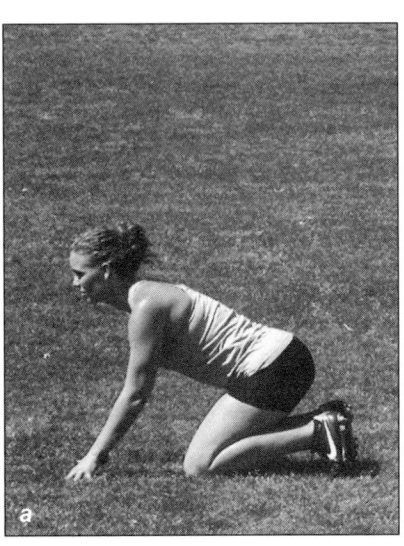 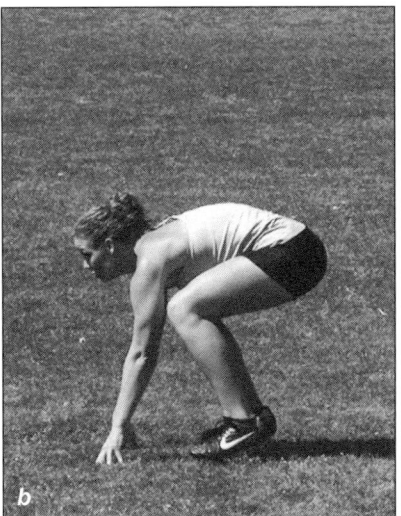 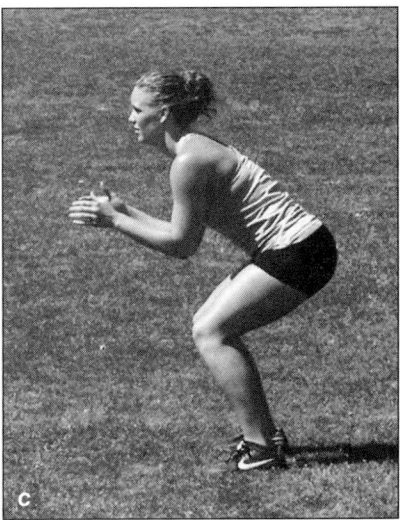

239
Sit-to-Stand Pop-Up

Purpose
To improve mental processing speed, total body agility, kinesthetic awareness, and quickness.

Procedure
- Start from a sitting position on the ground and wait for a signal (see figure *a*).
- Explode as fast as possible as you stand up (see figure *b-e*).

Variations
- Follow standing up with a skill movement done on command.
- Follow standing up with a tennis ball catch.
- Vary the commands given both audibly and visually.

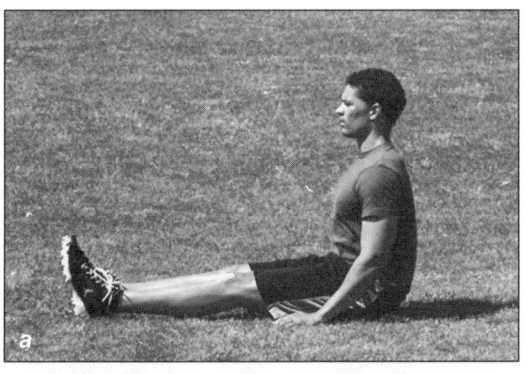
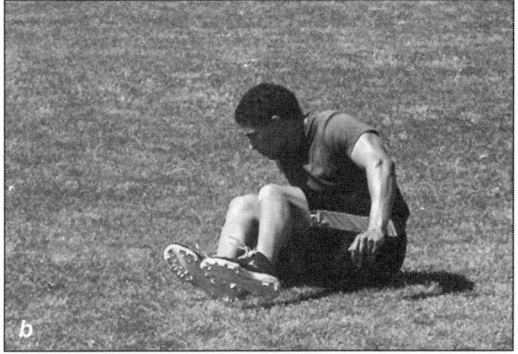
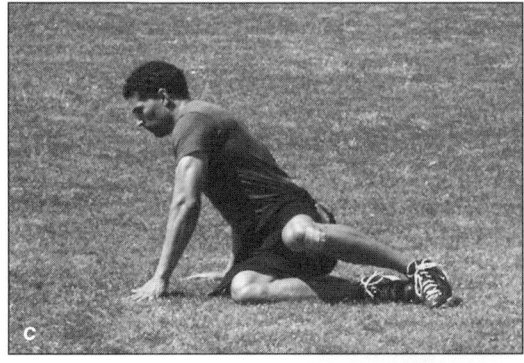
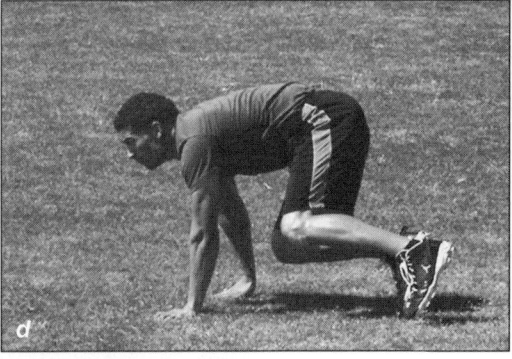
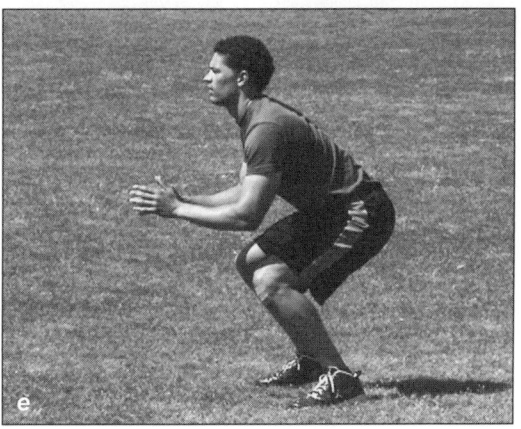

240
Lying-to-Stand Pop-Up

Purpose
To improve mental processing speed, total body agility, kinesthetic awareness, and quickness.

Procedure
- Start by lying in a supine position on the ground and wait for a signal (see figure *a*).
- Explode as fast as possible as you stand up (see figure *b-e*).

Variations
- Follow standing up with a skill movement done on command.
- Follow standing up with a tennis ball catch.
- Vary the commands given both audibly and visually.

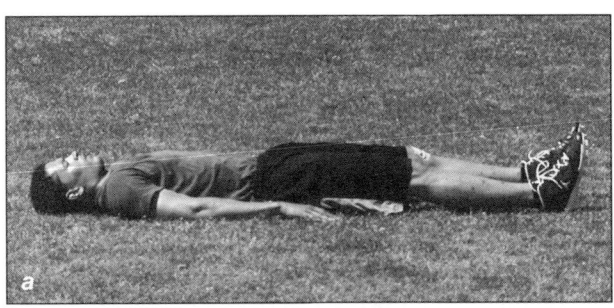
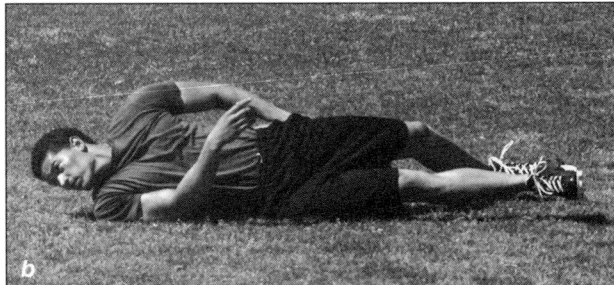
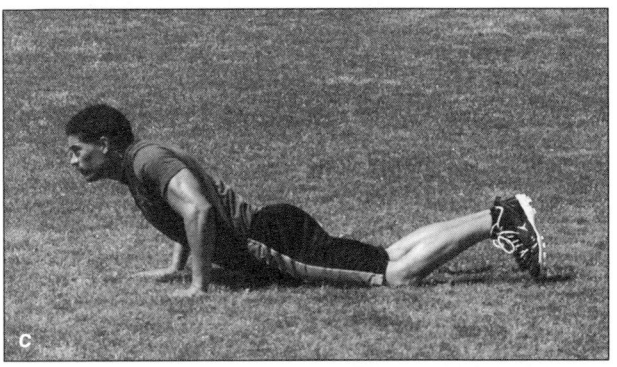
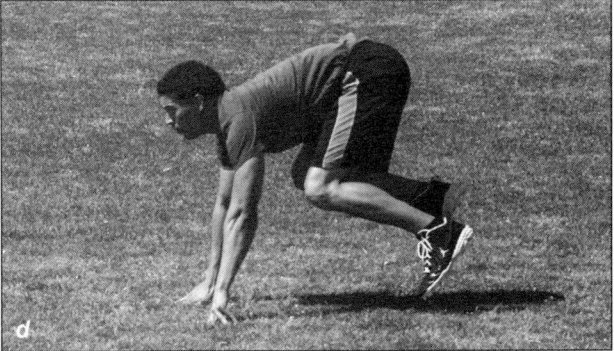
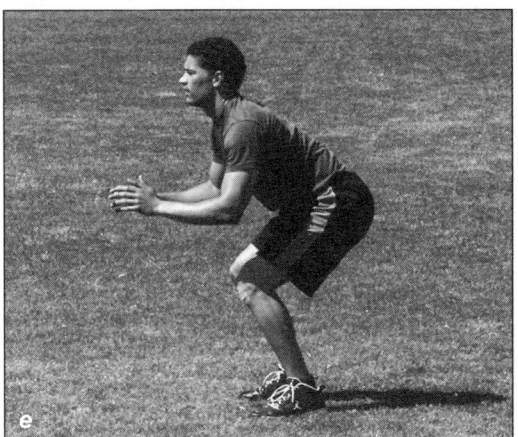

241
Sprawl-to-Stand Pop-Up

Purpose
To improve mental processing speed, total body agility, kinesthetic awareness, and quickness.

Procedure
- Start in an athletic stance and wait for a signal (see figure *a*).
- Perform a sprawl and get up as quickly as possible (see figure *b-e*).

Variations
- Follow standing up with a skill movement done on command.
- Follow standing up with a tennis ball catch.
- Vary the commands given both audibly and visually.

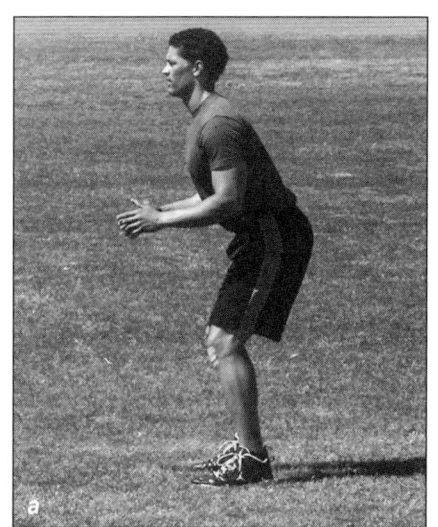
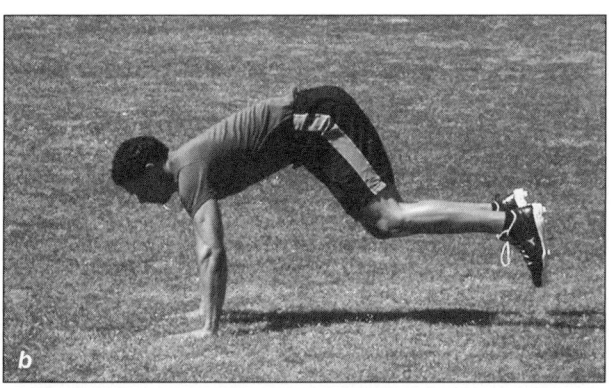
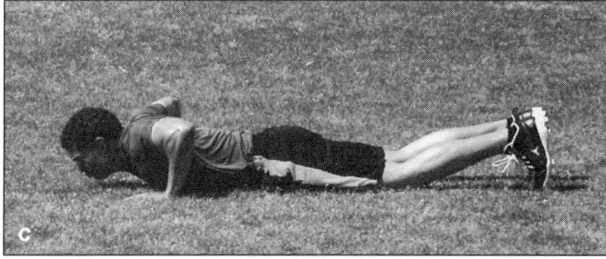
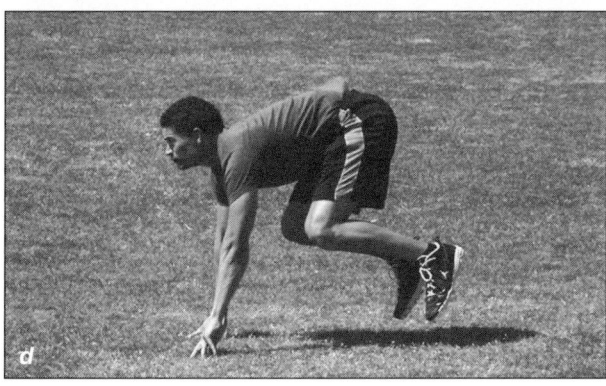
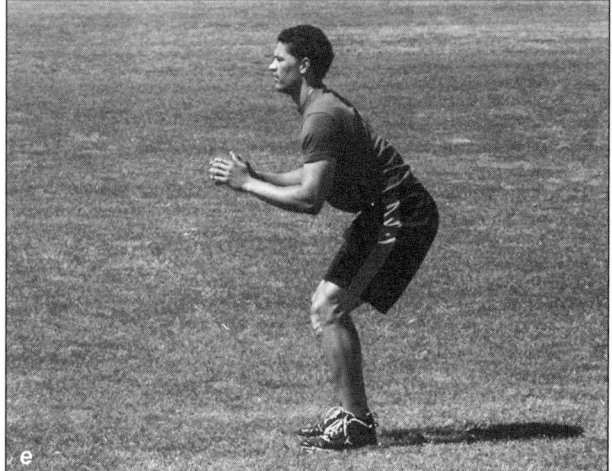

242

Crazy Ball Drill

Purpose

To improve mental processing speed, total body agility, kinesthetic awareness, and quickness.

Procedure

- Throw a ball in the air (see figure *a*).
- Perform a sprawl and get up as quickly as possible (see figure *b* and *c*).
- Catch the ball before it bounces twice.

Variations

- Attempt to touch the floor and catch the ball before it bounces twice.
- Use a reaction ball to enhance your multidirectional reaction time.
- Have a partner throw the ball during your sprawl.

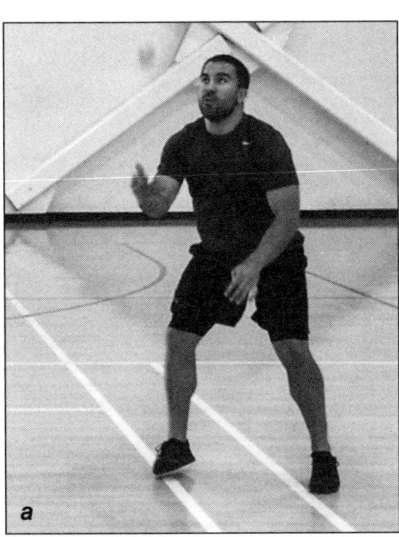
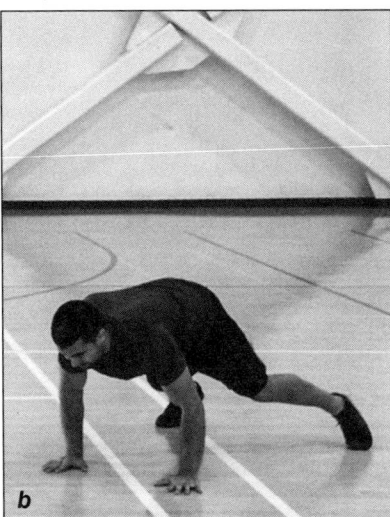
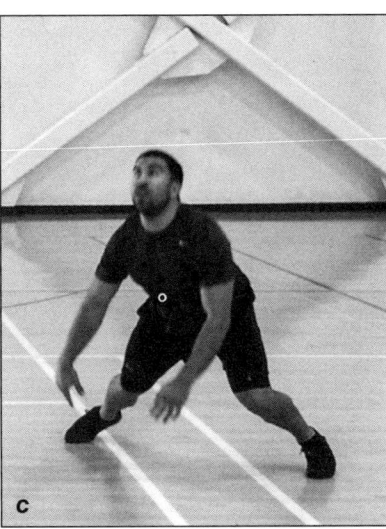

HAND-SPEED DRILLS

243
Hot Hands

Purpose
To improve mental processing speed, upper body reaction time to visual stimuli, and quickness.

Procedure
- Put your hands together (palm to palm) in front of you.
- A partner stands in front of you with her hands at her side (see figure).
- Your partner tries to quickly touch (i.e., to lightly slap) your hands while you try to react and avoid being touched.

Variations
- Both you and your partner assume a ready position.
- Follow the same procedure but use two separate contact targets instead of one.

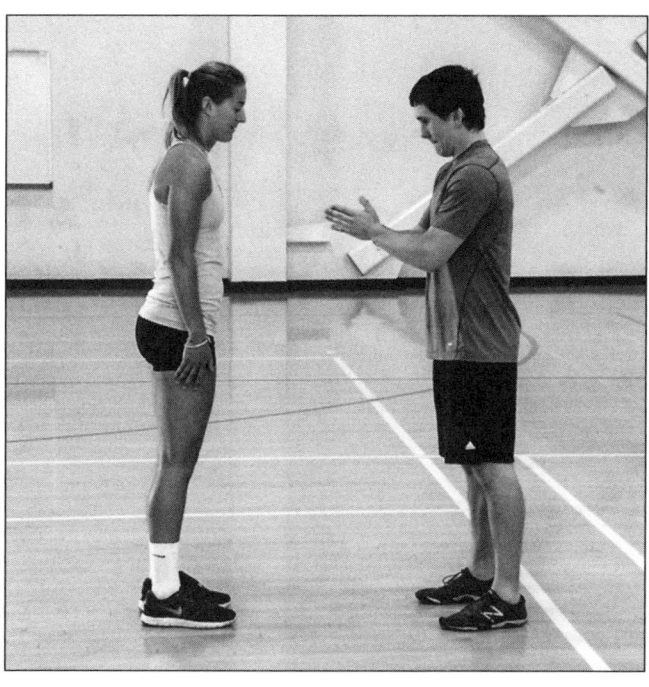

244
Ball Release

Purpose
To improve mental processing speed, upper body reaction time to visual stimuli, and quickness.

Procedure
- You assume a ready position and your partner holds two tennis balls out in front of you at shoulder height (see figure *a*).
- Your partner releases one of the two tennis balls without advance notice; you react and attempt to catch it in midair (see figure *b*).

Variations
- Have your partner use the contralateral hand to catch the tennis ball.
- Release both tennis balls simultaneously.

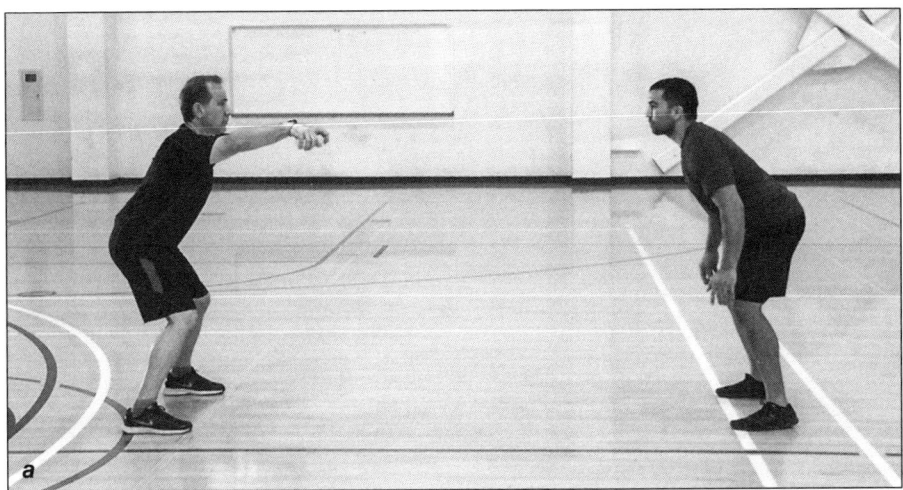

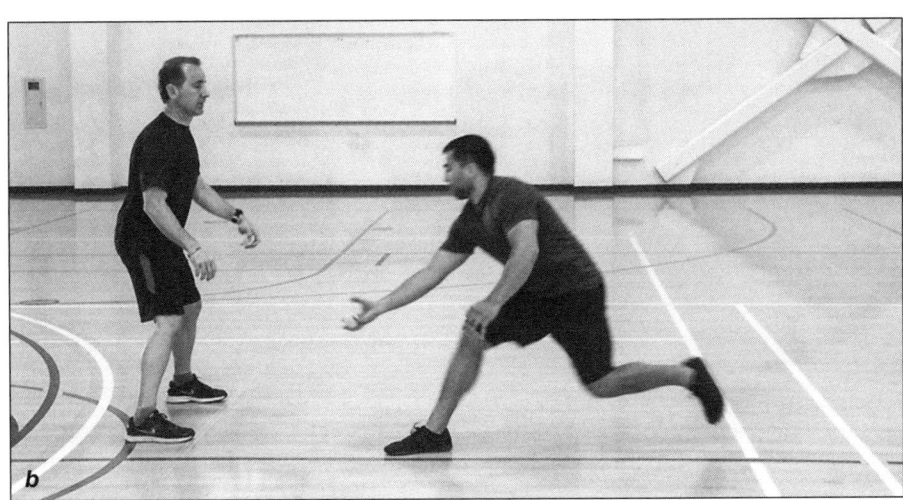

245

Card Snatching

Purpose
To improve upper body quickness and reaction ability to visual stimuli.

Procedure
- You stand in a ready position and a partner holds a playing card at shoulder height (see figure).
- You initiate the drill by attempting to snatch the card out of your partner's hand.
- Your partner reacts by attempting to move the card so as to prevent you from snatching it.

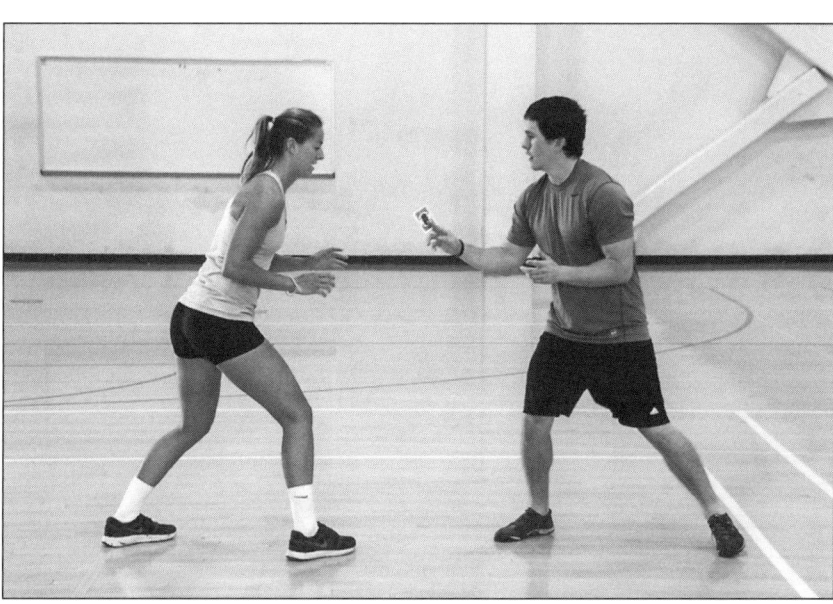

246

Ruler Drop

Purpose

To improve upper body quickness and reaction to a stimulus while providing feedback.

Procedure

- You hold your hand open with the arm extended and your partner holds a ruler at shoulder height (see figure).
- Your partner's thumb and index finger should be even with the 0 measurement at the end of the ruler.
- Your partner releases the ruler and you attempt to catch it as quickly as possible.
- The goal is to catch the ruler without letting it fall on the ground.

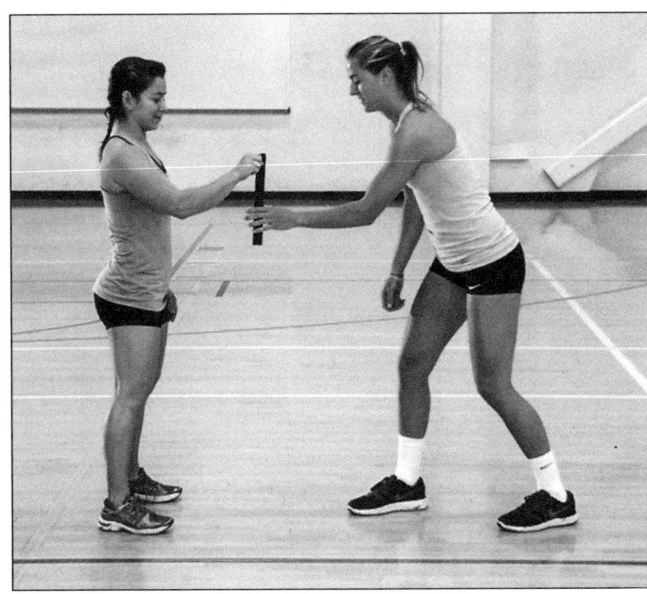

Focus Mitt

Purpose

To improve mental processing speed, upper body reaction time to visual stimuli, eye–hand coordination, and total body quickness.

Procedure

- Stand in the ready position or in a position particular to your sport and a partner stands in front of you (see figure *a*).
- Using a focus mitt, your partner initiates the drill by presenting the mitt as a target to which you are to deliver a predetermined punch or slap (see figure *b*).
- Your attack may mimic sport-specific movements, such as a tennis forehand or football lineman's hand technique.

Variations

- Add an additional mitt for complex response decisions.
- Throw multiple punches or combinations to specific targets.

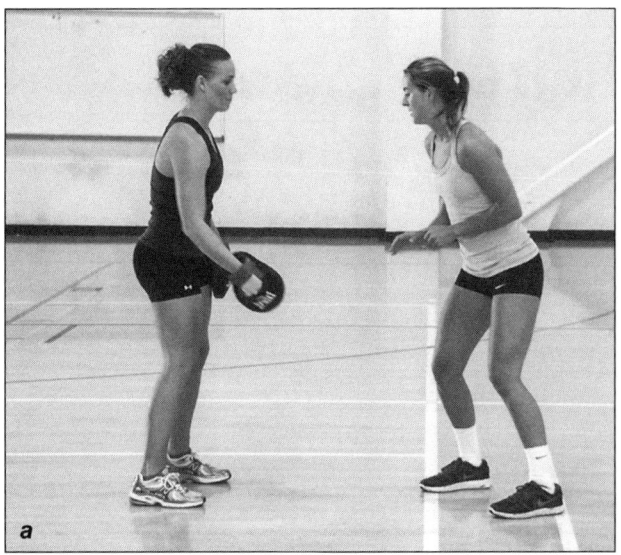 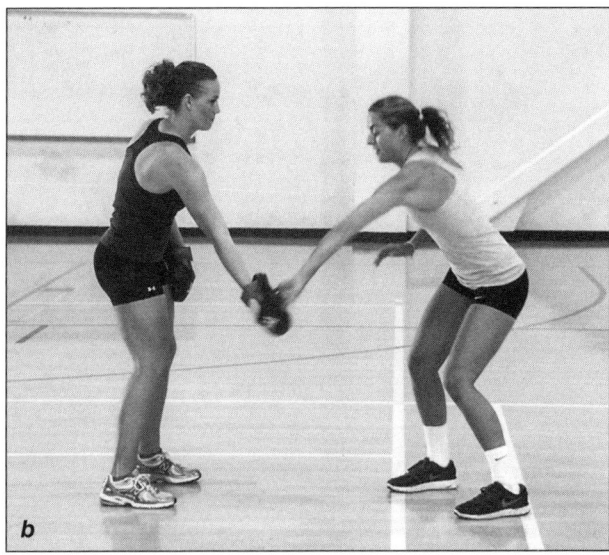

WHOLE-BODY REACTION DRILLS

248

Dodge Ball

Purpose

To improve mental processing speed and total body reaction time to visual stimuli.

Procedure

- This game can be played against a wall with two to four players or in a circle with five or more players.
- Using soft balls, multiple players throw while other players evade ball contact.

249

Rapid Fire

Purpose

To improve mental processing speed, total body reaction time to visual or audible stimuli, and total body quickness.

Procedure

- Assume a ready position and wait for a start signal.
- On the signal (either a visual or audible cue), begin to tap your feet alternately as fast as possible until the next command.
- React to each command (e.g., to do a lateral shuffle, forward or backward sprint, jump, sprawl) as quickly as possible.

250
Barrel Roll to Reaction

Purpose
To improve mental processing speed, total body reaction time to visual or audible stimuli, and total body agility.

Procedure
- Start in a two-point stance with the left foot forward.
- Bend over and start to fall forward.
- Roll over on the left shoulder just before making contact with the floor, and return to a ready position.
- React to your coach's audible or visual cue.

Variation
Add a sport-specific skill after the roll (such as a volleyball dig, right or left sprawl, cover tip, or lateral shuffle).

251
Backward Roll to Reaction

Purpose
To improve mental processing speed, total body reaction time to visual or audible stimuli, and total body agility.

Procedure
- Start in a ready position.
- Squat, bend over, and start to fall backward.
- Roll over on the left or right shoulder, and return to the ready position.
- React to your coach's audible or visual cue.

Variation
Add a sport-specific skill after the roll (such as a volleyball dig, right or left sprawl cover tip, or lateral shuffle).

252
Slalom With Reaction

QUICKNESS

Purpose
To improve mental processing speed, court sense, total body reaction time to visual or audible stimuli, total body agility, and general athleticism.

Procedure
- Start in a two-point stance with the right foot inside the first square of the ladder and the left foot outside the first square.
- Jump forward and diagonally to the right, and land the left foot inside the second square of the ladder and the right foot on the outside of the second square.
- Immediately upon landing, jump forward and diagonally to the left, landing the right foot inside the third square of the ladder and the left foot on the outside of the third square.
- Repeat this sequence throughout the ladder while reacting to your coach's visual commands (e.g., call out the number of fingers she holds up) continuously throughout the drill.

Variations
- Add a sport-specific skill at the end of the ladder.
- Call out only odd or even numbers as your coach shows both.
- Your coach can work a semicircle around the end of the ladder to enhance your peripheral vision. Two or three coaches can compose the semicircle, flashing numbers to further enhance your court vision and reaction times to stimuli on the periphery of your vision. Practicing reacting to stimuli on the periphery of your vision enhances reaction time to stimuli picked up in your central vision. Likewise, practicing reacting to stimuli picked up in your central vision enhances peripheral vision reaction time.
- Add a two- or three-step run-in to increase linear speed and quickness requirements through the ladder.

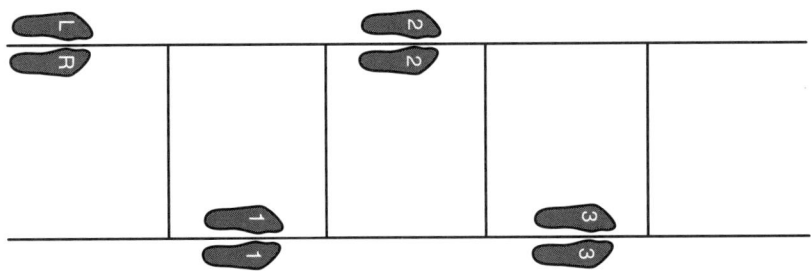

253
Hopscotch With Reaction

Purpose
To improve mental processing speed, court sense, total body reaction time to visual or audible stimuli, total body agility, general athleticism, and elastic strength in the ankle complex.

Procedure
- Start with both feet inside the first square of the ladder.
- Jump with both feet, landing each foot outside the ladder.
- Immediately upon landing, jump and land both feet inside the next square of the ladder.
- Repeat this sequence throughout the ladder while reacting to your coach's visual commands (e.g., call out the number of fingers he holds up) continuously throughout the drill.

Variations
- Add a sport-specific skill at the end of the ladder.
- Call out only odd or even numbers as your coach shows both.
- Your coach can work a semicircle around the end of the ladder to enhance your peripheral vision. Two or three coaches can compose the semicircle, flashing numbers to further enhance your court vision and reaction times to stimuli on the periphery of your vision. Practicing reacting to stimuli on the periphery of your vision enhances reaction time to stimuli picked up in your central vision. Likewise, practicing reacting to stimuli picked up in your central vision enhances peripheral vision reaction time.
- Add a two- or three-step run-in to increase linear speed and quickness requirements through the ladder.

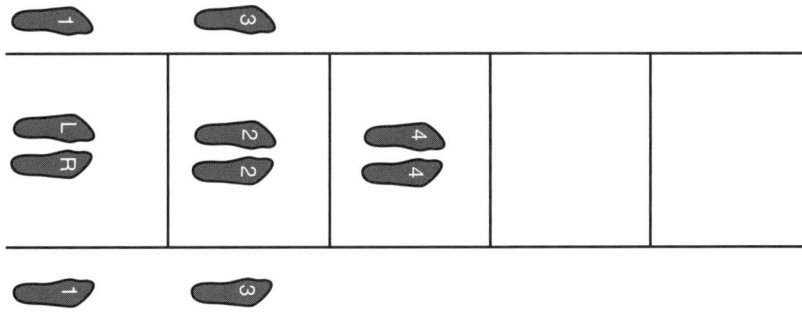

254
T Drill With Ball Toss

Purpose
To enhance change of direction skills and reactive agility.

Procedure
- Start at cone A.
- On the command of the coach, sprint to cone B.
- Side shuffle sideways to cone C.
- Carioca to the right to cone D.
- Shuffle back to cone B, touch it, and run backward to cone A.

Variation
The coach stands at the top of the T with a ball. Perform the drill pattern continuously, and when you receive the ball toss, reverse the direction of the drill pattern.

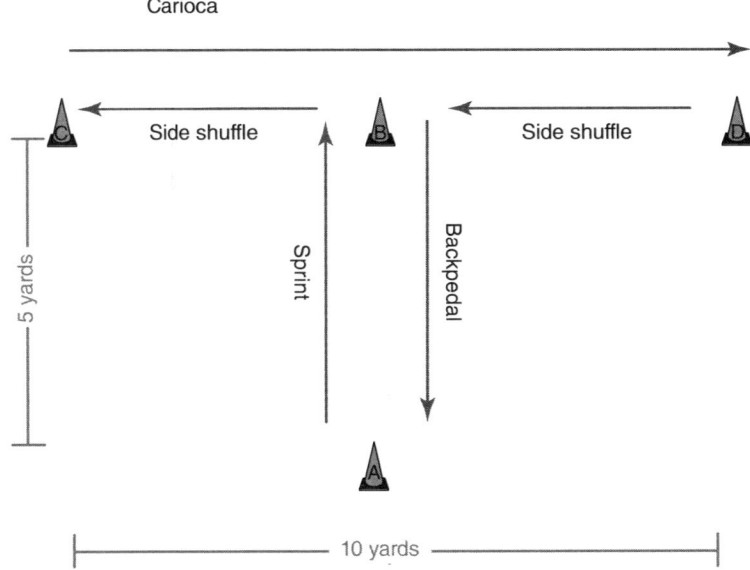

QUICK FEET DRILLS

255

Icky Shuffle With Reaction

Purpose
To improve mental processing speed, court sense, total body reaction time to visual or audible stimuli, total body agility, and general athleticism.

Procedure
- Start on the left side of an agility ladder.
- Step laterally with the right foot and place it in the first square of the ladder.
- Advance the left foot to inside the same box.
- Step laterally with the right foot to the right side of the ladder and the left foot to its next square.
- Bring the right foot to the same square in which you have your left foot.
- Step laterally to the left of the ladder, and advance the right foot to the next square. Repeat this pattern to the end of the ladder.
- React to your coach's visual commands (e.g., call out the number of fingers she holds up) continuously throughout the drill.

Variations
- Add a sport-specific skill at the end of the ladder.
- Call out only odd or even numbers as your coach shows both.
- Your coach can work a semicircle around the end of the ladder to enhance your peripheral vision.
- Two or three coaches can compose the semicircle, flashing numbers to further enhance your court vision and reaction times to stimuli on the periphery of your vision. Note that seeing objects with different sections of the eyes produces different reaction times. Stimuli picked up by the cones (or the nerves at the center of the eyes) register information faster than objects picked up by the rods (or nerves along the outside portion of the eyes). Practicing reacting to stimuli on the periphery of your vision enhances reaction time to stimuli picked up in your central vision. Likewise, practicing reacting to stimuli picked up in your central vision enhances peripheral vision reaction time.
- Add a two- or three-step run-in to increase linear speed and quickness requirements through the ladder.

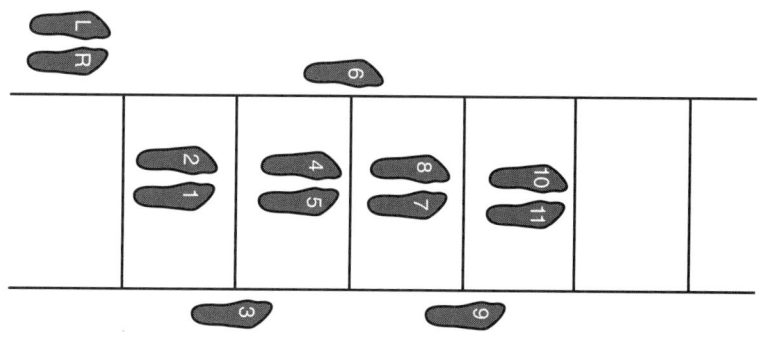

256

Backward Icky Shuffle With Reaction

Purpose
To improve mental processing speed, court sense, total body reaction time to visual or audible stimuli, total body agility, and general athleticism.

Procedure
- Start on the left side of an agility ladder, facing backward.
- Step laterally with the right foot, and place it in the first square of the ladder.
- Step with the left foot to inside the same box.
- Step laterally and drop-step with the right foot to the right side of the ladder, and step back with the left foot to its next square.
- Bring the right foot to the square in which you have your left foot.
- Step laterally and drop-step to the left side of the ladder, and step back with the right foot to its next square. Repeat this pattern to the end of the ladder.
- React to your coach's visual commands (e.g., call out the number of fingers he holds up) continuously throughout the drill.

Variations
- Add a sport-specific skill at the end of the ladder.
- Call out only odd or even numbers as your coach shows both.
- Your coach can work a semicircle around the end of the ladder to enhance your peripheral vision.
- Two or three coaches can compose the semicircle, flashing numbers to further enhance your court vision and reaction times to stimuli on the periphery of your vision. Note that seeing objects with different sections of the eyes produces different reaction times. Stimuli picked up by the cones (or the nerves at the center of the eyes) register information faster than objects picked up by the rods (or nerves along the outside portion of the eyes). Practicing reacting to stimuli on the periphery of your vision enhances reaction time to stimuli picked up in your central vision. Likewise, practicing reacting to stimuli picked up in your central vision enhances peripheral vision reaction time.

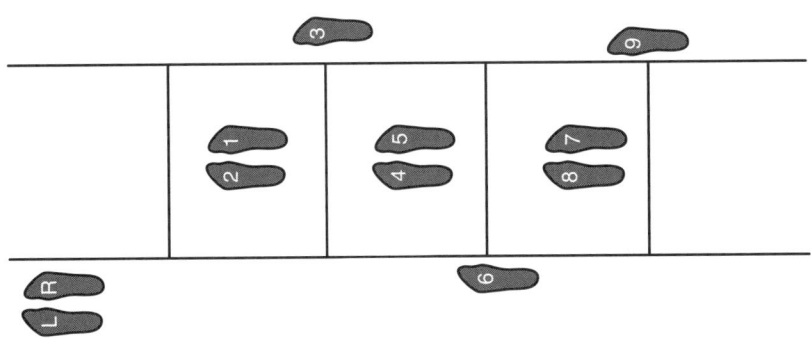

257

In–Out Shuffle With Reaction

Purpose
To improve mental processing speed, court sense, total body reaction time to visual or audible stimuli, total body agility, and general athleticism.

Procedure
- Start in a two-point stance, facing one side of the ladder.
- Step with the right foot straight ahead into the first square.
- Follow with the left foot into the first square.
- Step back and diagonally with the right foot until it is in front of the second square.
- Follow with the left foot until it is in front of the second square.
- Repeat this sequence throughout the ladder, making sure each foot hits each box.
- React to your coach's visual commands (e.g., call out the number of fingers she holds up) continuously throughout the drill.

Variations
- Add a sport-specific skill at the end of the ladder.
- Call out only odd or even numbers as your coach shows both.
- Your coach can work a semicircle around the end of the ladder to enhance your peripheral vision.
- Two or three coaches can compose the semicircle, flashing numbers to further enhance your court vision and reaction times to stimuli on the periphery of your vision. Note that seeing objects with different sections of the eyes produces different reaction times. Stimuli picked up by the cones (or the nerves at the center of the eyes) register information faster than objects picked up by the rods (or nerves along the outside portion of the eyes). Practicing reacting to stimuli on the periphery of your vision enhances reaction time to stimuli picked up in your central vision. Likewise, practicing reacting to stimuli picked up in your central vision enhances peripheral vision reaction time.

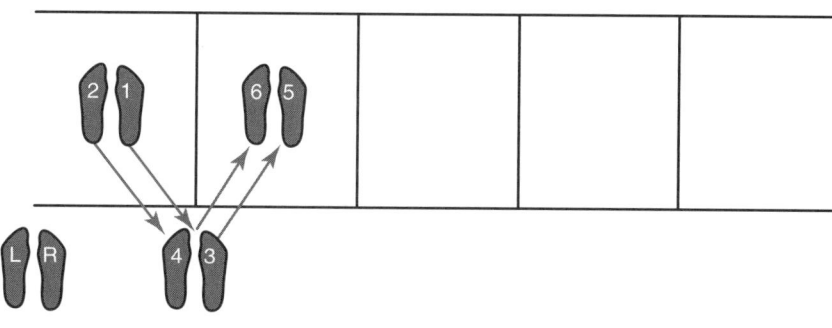

QUICKNESS

258

Snake With Reaction

Purpose
To improve mental processing speed, court sense, total body reaction time to visual or audible stimuli, total body agility, general athleticism, and elastic strength in the ankle complex.

Procedure
- Start in a two-point stance, straddling one side of the ladder.
- Keeping both feet together, perform a series of quarter-turn jumps.
- The direction the feet should point for each jump is as follows: straight ahead, left, straight ahead, right, straight ahead, and so on.
- Keep the shoulders relatively square while rotating the hips.
- Repeat this sequence throughout the ladder while reacting to your coach's visual commands (e.g., call out the number of fingers he holds up) continuously throughout the drill.

Variations
- Add a sport-specific skill at the end of the ladder.
- Call out only odd or even numbers as your coach shows both.
- Your coach can work a semicircle around the end of the ladder to enhance your peripheral vision.
- Two or three coaches can compose the semicircle, flashing numbers to further enhance your court vision and reaction times to stimuli on the periphery of your vision. Note that seeing objects with different sections of the eyes produces different reaction times. Stimuli picked up by the cones (or the nerves at the center of the eyes) register information faster than objects picked up by the rods (or nerves along the outside portion of the eyes). Practicing reacting to stimuli on the periphery of your vision enhances reaction time to stimuli picked up in your central vision. Likewise, practicing reacting to stimuli picked up in your central vision enhances peripheral vision reaction time.
- Add a two- or three-step run-in to increase linear speed and quickness requirements through the ladder.

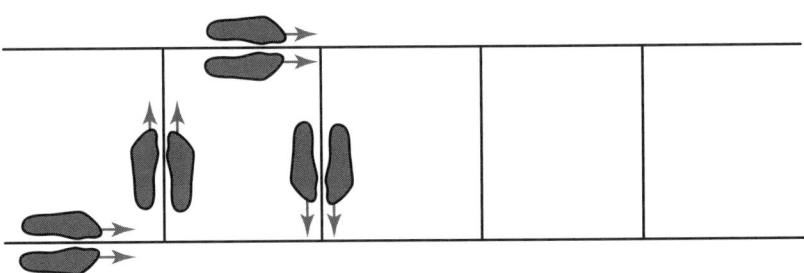

259
Chubby Checker With Reaction

Purpose
To improve mental processing speed, court sense, total body reaction time to visual or audible stimuli, first-step quickness, and general athleticism.

Procedure
- Start in a two-point stance, facing the ladder on its far left side.
- Jump laterally to the right with both feet, landing the left foot inside the first square of the ladder and the right foot outside the first square.
- Immediately upon landing, jump laterally to the right, with both feet landing outside the ladder.
- The hips should rotate so that the feet are diagonal to the ladder when the left foot is in the square and perpendicular to it when both feet are outside the ladder.
- Repeat this sequence while advancing the length of the ladder and reacting to your coach's visual commands (e.g., call out the number of fingers she holds up) continuously throughout the drill.

Variations
- Add a sport-specific skill at the end of the ladder.
- Call out only odd or even numbers as your coach shows both.
- Your coach can work a semicircle around the end of the ladder to enhance your peripheral vision.
- Two or three coaches can compose the semicircle, flashing numbers to further enhance your court vision and reaction times to stimuli on the periphery of your vision. Note that seeing objects with different sections of the eyes produces different reaction times. Stimuli picked up by the cones (or the nerves at the center of the eyes) register information faster than objects picked up by the rods (or nerves along the outside portion of the eyes). Practicing reacting to stimuli on the periphery of your vision enhances reaction time to stimuli picked up in your central vision. Likewise, practicing reacting to stimuli picked up in your central vision enhances peripheral vision reaction time.

QUICKNESS

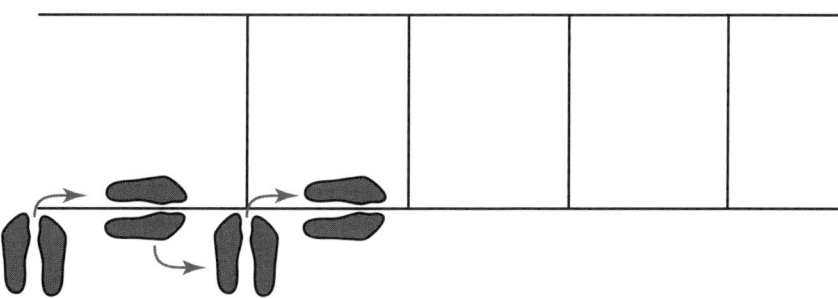

BIOMOTOR REACTIVE DRILL

260

Backpedal

Purpose

To improve quickness and flexibility in the hip flexors.

Procedure

- In an athletic stance, maintain your center of gravity over your base of support and run backward.
- Increase your stride length with good form.

Variation

On command, use an open step and sprint to a designated cone.

Here we have presented a variety of both simple and complex drills that train the variables that influence quickness. Reaction and quickness drills should always be executed with proper technique and form. Reinforcing good mechanics will allow better transfer to sport and activity skills while also reducing the risk of injury. The drills also provide advanced variations for long-term gains that make movements faster, more fluid, and more unconscious to provide athletes with greater opportunities for fun and success in their athletic development. By understanding and training the different levels of responses in the appropriate drills, the athlete may yield significant improvements in quickness that can inspire the next level of performance no matter the performance level or sport.

PART II

Training Programs

Chapter 7

Developing a Customized Program

Vance A. Ferrigno, Andrea M. Du Bois, Lee E. Brown

The following chapters are sport-specific programs that show you how to arrange an assortment of exercises into an 8-week program. These are not meant to be templates for specific exercises for the specific sports, however; they are meant to show you how to progress the exercises from easy to hard and simple to complex over the 8 weeks. Progression is a very individual thing because no two athletes will progress exactly the same. We show complex progressions in some of the 8-week programs that certain athletes may not see until 10 or 12 weeks or even longer. In other cases, athletes who already have a strong foundation of movement skills may see some of those complex progressions in the first 4 weeks. Every athlete has distinctive needs and goals that should be addressed, but all athletes want to improve the efficiency of their ability to move.

Choosing Your Drills

Mixing drills randomly will build the global movement skills of young athletes but may not be the most effective way to train athletes of higher movement development (Bompa 1995). In the early stages of athletic development, more is often better, providing a varied mix of skill development and keeping the young athlete engaged. As the athlete develops, however, the drills must be refined to address the very specific movement qualities you are trying to improve. The data collected in the chapter 2 assessment will help determine the specific exercises the coach would choose for the athlete to start with.

Once the athlete begins working on the drills, the next drills are chosen from the success or lack of success the athlete has had with the previous drills. Build on success! If the athlete is performing a task that is too difficult, it may discourage him. Conversely, if the drills are too easy, the athlete may lose interest. Coaches should change any drill that is not working or getting the desired results. This doesn't mean the drill was bad; it just wasn't the right drill for that moment. The coach can return to that drill when the athlete's progression is better prepared.

Another consideration in choosing drills is to mix up the various planes of body locomotion. Because all human motion is three-dimensional, the drills should also be three-dimensional (Gray 2004). What we mean by that is the drills shouldn't be all linear. For example, in a skipping drill, the athlete should skip forward, backward, laterally in both directions, and rotationally in both directions.

Each sport has different biomotor and metabolic demands, and even within a sport, the various positions can have different requirements. For example, when designing a program for baseball in chapter 8, there are nine player positions, with each position requiring somewhat different biomotor skills. Every player would have various speed, agility, and quickness drills in his program, but the emphasis of each would vary according to position and test results. For example, an outfielder might have more emphasis on acceleration abilities, whereas an infielder may have more emphasis on lateral agility. To take it one step further, a third baseman would have to work more on reactive skills than would a shortstop, who needs a little bit more range where the lateral agility becomes more important.

Determining Training Volume and Intensity

When deciding on how many repetitions of each drill to perform, over what distance to perform them, and what the rest intervals should be, you need to consider both the biomotor qualities you are trying to improve and the metabolic demand of the sport, and in some cases the position within that sport as well (Gambetta 1998). For example, in training a baseball player versus a basketball player, the star drill can be used for both sports. However, the repetitions and recovery intervals would look very different because the metabolic demands of each sport are very different. Also, in the following programs we give you two drills for each of the biomotor skills (speed, agility, and quickness). This is just a general guide for simplicity's sake. You may choose to use three speed drills, four for agility, and one for quickness. It is very individual to the goals you are trying to achieve in-season versus off-season (Murphy and Forney 1997).

There are several ways to set the duration, intensity, and recovery intervals. In many of the drills, such as the line drills, the distance is set but the recovery intervals can vary. In the purest essence of improving speed, agility, or quickness, adequate recovery between sets is needed to allow the energy systems and nervous system a chance to recover before performing the next drill. Work-to-rest ratios of 1:3 or 1:4 are often used as guides, but even longer intervals can be used to ensure the athlete can put as much power and intensity into the last drill as into the first.

When using speed, agility, and quickness training for conditioning, match the work-to-rest ratio of the target sport to make the training metabolically specific. With continued development of the athlete, being able to explode late in a game requires that at some point in training the volume must increase or the recovery interval decrease, or a combination of the two, to prepare the athlete to perform at a high intensity late into a game. Because of individual differences, specific recommendations on the volume and intensity of exercises are impossible to make. The sample programs show a variety of ways to set the recovery intervals, but these are just examples; the athlete's response to today's drill parameters will have an impact on what ratios of work to rest are used in the next workout.

Designing a Workout

In designing daily workouts, coaches and athletes need to put some thought into the various aspects of the workout, not just improvise. Start with the goal of that particular workout. Don't train just to train, train with a purpose. What should the warm-up be? How is today's warm-up different from yesterday's, and how long should it last? Where do the rest periods fit in, and how long they should they be? What you are looking for is a smooth flow, where the warm-up transitions to the main body of the workout, which transitions to the cool-down and restoration phases. Writing out the workout on paper will help you create this flow and provide for a smooth workout. With that said, the written plan isn't written in stone. Once the workout begins, the coach should watch for and listen to the athlete's response and make adjustments if needed.

Warm-Up

The warm-up is a critical part of each workout. Many athletes and even some coaches think the warm-up is something you do before the workout and don't see it as part of the workout itself. That is a mistake in thinking because the warm-up drills are the very same drills used in the main body of the program, only performed at a lower amplitude. If an athlete performs a 10-minute comprehensive warm-up at the outset of each workout, over the course of a year, the cumulative warm-up time adds exponentially to the training volume, which has an impact on the athlete's fitness. The other obvious benefit of the warm-up is reducing the risk of injuring soft tissue by gently bringing the body from a resting state to a heightened state of performance (Knudson 2008). Remember, the warm-up drills should also be three-dimensional. Most of the basic locomotor drills (skipping, shuffling, carioca, and running) can be performed forward, backward, laterally in both directions, and rotationally in both directions.

The following list of exercises makes up a sample 10- to 15-minute warm-up using the drills in the book. Each locomotion drill is performed over 15 to 20 yards or meters. Start off with easy flowing motions, and slowly increase the amplitude of the movements as the warm-up progresses. The athlete should perform each drill two to four times depending on her needs.

- Multidirectional Skipping (p. 133)
- Acceleration Heel Kicks (p. 44)
- Lateral Shuffles with 180- and 360-degree turns (p. 103)
- Carioca with 180- and 360-degree turns (p. 140)
- Figure-Eight Cone Drill (p. 134)
- Backward Run (p. 166)
- Crossover Run (p. 101)
- Lying-to-Stand Pop-Up (p.234) with 10-yard burst (p. 53)

Breaks and Cool-Down

Water breaks are a great way to provide rest and well-needed hydration to the body, especially in hot climates. Keep water close by, and take a water break immediately after the warm-up, in the middle of the main body of the session, and at the end of the main body of the session (i.e., right before flexibility work). Athletes are not always very conscientious about hydrating properly before a training session, so it's better for the coach to make sure they stay hydrated.

The cool-down, or flexibility session, is a time for gearing down, working on range of motion (ROM) issues using static flexibility exercises, and positively reflecting on the session. The cool-down should not turn into a flexibility contest. Rather, it should focus on improving individual ROM deficits. Most stretching should be performed from a standing position so that gravity and ground reaction can load the muscles, joints, and connective tissues in a triplane environment consistent with what happens while competing and training (Gray 2007).

Finish every session with positive affirmations. Focus on the successes of the session, not the failures. Speak of needed improvements in a positive manner, and communicate an eagerness to accomplish all goals. No athlete likes to be reminded of or constantly badgered about her shortcomings. Athletes will respond better to a positive and respectful coaching style. Developing a good work ethic and desire to perform at the highest level possible begins with mutual respect and admiration between the coach and athlete.

Tweaking Drills for Progression

Coaches should not feel compelled to switch drills too quickly. An athlete should be able to perform a drill smoothly and consistently before moving on. This may happen in a single session, or it may take several sessions. Once the athlete performs the drill with symmetry and efficiency, he can move to a complex variation that some of the drills provide before the coach needs to choose a completely new or more complex drill. Feel free to change a drill or to combine it with a sport-specific skill or another drill. All these drills were developed through experimentation. This is where a coach or athlete can get creative with program design. As the athlete continues to develop, drills can be combined to add biomotor complexity and metabolic demand. Again, it is important to make sure the athlete masters the basic movement patterns before taking on more complex drills or combining them with another skill. If a complex drill is done sloppily, it will do more harm than good by reinforcing poor movement patterns and potentially putting the athlete in a position where he can get injured.

Every athlete is an individual with individual needs to improve in her given sport. A comprehensive training plan for any athlete must take numerous variables into account. Using the information gained through the chapter 2 assessment and the demands of the sport and position of that sport, coaches and athletes can customize a plan accordingly. Be creative and use smart progressions. If you are to err, do so on the conservative side. It is easier to dial up a program than to scale back after coming out too aggressively and risking injury. Most of all, coaches should listen to their athletes' feedback and test frequently so the program can be adjusted to ensure improvement is occurring.

Chapter 8

Baseball and Softball

Andrea M. Du Bois, Lee E. Brown, Vance A. Ferrigno

Baseball and softball are sports that combine skill, speed, agility, and quickness. Although the games are very similar to one another, different field dimensions and game lengths require slightly different training programs. Some aspects of the sport of softball are slower than baseball; however, players are still required to execute the same skills of hitting, throwing, and catching quickly and efficiently in order to be successful.

Defensively, baseball and softball players are required to respond quickly, powerfully, and accurately to catch a hit ball and then immediately react by accurately throwing the ball to a respective player. For example, Major League Baseball players can reach first base in 4.56 seconds (Barret and Burton 2002). This means the defensive athlete must be able to catch the ball, change direction, and throw the ball with accuracy to first base within this time frame to complete a successful defensive play. Offensively, the athlete must be able to respond to a thrown ball, swing the bat at a high velocity, and then accelerate quickly to first base.

Previous research demonstrates the time to reach first base in Major League Baseball is highly related to the sprint time in the first 13.7 meters (45 feet) of the run (from home plate to the foul line). Therefore, training speed and acceleration in the first 13.7 meters will help improve the player's chances of success (Barret and Burton 2002). Typically this sprinting is linear, but if a player is running past first base, he must be able to change direction (in a more rounded fashion) to head toward second. Sprinting is also important defensively because players must sprint to catch a hit ball. However, unlike sprinting the bases, players may require specialized footwork including forward sprinting, side shuffling (at any angle), backpedaling, or any combination thereof to catch the ball. Depending on the direction the athlete is facing when he catches the ball, he might then have to immediately change direction to throw the ball. This action must be done both quickly and accurately for a successful completion of the play. Not all balls are caught from sprinting, and there are times an athlete must jump to catch the ball. Jumping can occur vertically or to either side. Like changes in direction in sprinting, the player must be agile enough to catch the ball and throw if needed to complete the play.

Research has demonstrated that baseball infielders are required to throw at a variety of angles and often while off balance (McFarland and Wasik 1998). However, these requirements are not unique to infielders and apply to other baseball and softball positions, with the differences lying in the throwing distance. From Little League to Major League Baseball, the throwing distance for a baseball infielder can range from 5 to 180 feet (1.5 to 55 m) depending on the play requirement and position within the infield (Axe, Windley, and Snyder-Mackler 2001). Because of their placement on the field, the shortstop and second baseman must be able to respond quickly to a hit ball and often must immediately throw that ball (to first or third) with one smooth and continuous motion. The first baseman often throws in the same direction with each play (toward second or third), if required to throw at all, and does not need as much quickness. Outfielders might have to sprint over a greater distance because of their position on the field and often require some degree of deceleration before subsequently throwing the ball. Catching, like throwing, can also require coordinated movements of the upper and lower body at a variety of angles. Baseball and softball athletes are often required to respond to the caught ball with an immediate throw, and therefore they must maintain some degree of balance and remain agile to complete successive tasks.

BASEBALL AND SOFTBALL PROGRAM

When designing a program for an athlete, the coach needs to consider the demands in a particular game as well as the demands of the sport. Baseball has a very long in-season with numerous games per week. It is therefore very important that speed, agility, and quickness programming works in conjunction with and takes into consideration weekly games, skill-based practice, and strength and conditioning training.

The following program has been designed for a baseball infielder. However, this program can be adapted to other players on the team by manipulating the drill type, volume, intensity, or duration. The thought process in the speed drills is to start the player with some fundamental acceleration drills before moving on to resisted and assisted drills in week 5. Each week the previous week's drill is carried over and a new drill added. With the agility drills, we used a quick, short explosive Lateral Shuffle to address the initial explosive reaction to a hit ball. In week 2, a hand reach to the ground was added to the quick shuffle to help the athlete get down more efficiently to field a ball. In week 3, athletes field a ball that the coach rolls to the side they are moving to. In week 5's T drill, as the athlete accelerates toward the first cone, the coach rolls a ball to one of the lateral cones, forcing the athlete to react and get to the ball. Once the ball is fielded, he completes the drill. The quickness drills focus on lower and total body explosiveness. The medicine ball drills focus on rotational explosiveness.

	SPEED		AGILITY		QUICKNESS	
	1	2	3	4	5	6
Week 1	A skip (p. 50) 5 × 20 yd; jog to start and repeat	Falling starts (p. 70) 5 × 30 yd; walk to start and repeat	Quick 3-5 step lateral shuffle (p. 103) Walk to start and repeat in opposite direction. That equals 1 rep.; 10 reps; 10 sec RI between reps Pro Agility 5 × 45 sec between sets	Backpedal (p. 252) 10 × 10 yd; walk to start and repeat	Push-off box shuffle (p. 209) 5 × 10; 30 sec RI	Medicine ball wall side toss (p. 194) 3 × 10 each side; 60 sec RI between sets
Week 2	Falling starts (p. 70) 5 × 30 yd; walk to start and repeat	Resist from behind (p. 64) 5 × 30 yd; walk to start and repeat	Quick 3-5 step lateral shuffle (p. 103) and touch ground between legs on the last shuffle. Walk to start and quickly shuffle opposite direction and repeat (=1 rep). 5 Reps = 1 Set; 10 sec RI between reps; Perform 2 sets; 90 sec RI	Sprint and backpedal on command (p. 228) 10 × 5 yd backpedal and 10 yd sprint	Scissor jumps (p. 202) 5 × 10; 50 sec RI	Medicine ball wall side toss with perpendicular stance (p. 194) 3 × 10 each side; 60 sec RI between sets
Week 3	Resist from front (p. 63) 5 × 30 yd; walk to start and repeat	Partner-assisted tubing acceleration (p. 68) 5 × 30 yd; walk to start and repeat	Add a lateral shuffle to ball pickup and throw (p. 103) 5 × 15; 45 sec RI	20-yard square (p. 108) 5×; 30 sec RI	Scissor jumps with forward movement (p. 202) 5 × 10 yd; 50 sec RI	Medicine ball wall overhead throw (p. 195) 5 × 10; 30 sec RI
Week 4	Partner-assisted tubing acceleration (p. 68) 5 × 30 yd; walk to start and repeat	Quick feet and high knees (p. 43) 10 × 10 yd; 20 sec RI	30-yard T drill (p. 91) 5×; 30 sec RI	20-yard square (p. 108) with catch and throw 5×; 30 sec RI	Lateral skaters (p. 203) 5 × 10; 50 sec RI	Single-leg medicine ball wall overhead throw (p. 195) 5 × 10 each leg; 30 sec RI
Week 5	Quick feet to acceleration (p. 55) 10 × 15 yd: (quick feet 5 yd and accelerate 10 yd); 40 sec RI	Light sled pull (p. 60) 5 × 20 yd; 60 sec RI	T drill with ball toss (p. 246) 5×; 30 sec RI	X-pattern multiskill (p. 109) 5×; 30 sec RI	Lateral skaters with forward movement (p. 203) 5 × 10 yd; 50 sec RI	Single-leg medicine ball wall overhead throw (p. 195) 5 × 10 each leg; 30 sec RI
Week 6	Light sled pull (p. 60) 5 × 20 yd; 60 sec RI	Stadium stairs (p. 62) 6 × 5 steps; 30 sec RI	V drill (p. 128) 5×; 30 sec RI	X-pattern multiskill with catch and throw (p. 109) 5×; 30 sec RI	Lateral skaters (p. 203) 5 × 5 yd each direction; 50 sec RI	Medicine ball wall chest pass (p. 193) 5 × 10; 30 sec RI
Week 7	Stadium stairs (p. 62) 6 × 5 steps; 30 sec RI	Uphill acceleration runs (p. 62) 6 × 5; 30 sec RI	Icky shuffle (p. 135) 4 × ladder's length; walk to start and repeat	Sprawl-to-stand pop-up (p. 235); 5 sets × 5 reps; 60 sec RI between sets	Single-leg hop (p. 215) 5 × ½ ladder's length each leg	Single-arm medicine ball wall chest pass (p. 193) 5 × 10 each leg; 30 sec RI
Week 8	Uphill acceleration runs (p. 62) 6 × 5 sec; 30 sec RI	Medicine ball scoop toss to uphill acceleration runs (p. 73 and p. 62) 10 × 5 sec; 60 sec RI	Icky shuffle while fielding ball (p. 135) ½ ladder's length	Sprawl-to-stand pop-up (p. 235) 5 sets × 3 reps with 15-20 sec between reps; 60 sec between sets	Single-leg hop (lateral) (p. 215) 5 × ½ ladder's length each leg	Single-leg and single-arm medicine ball wall chest pass (p. 193) 5 × 10 each leg; 30 sec RI

RI = rest interval.

Chapter 9

Football and Rugby

Andrea M. Du Bois, Lee E. Brown, Vance A. Ferrigno

Football is characterized by bursts of high-intensity activity separated by short periods of either passive or active rest. The level of demand varies by position, but most players are required to possess speed, quickness, and agility in order to be successful. Over the course of the game, there will be periods of repeated sprints in multiple directions. Over the course of a sprint, a player might be required to accelerate, change direction with cuts or spins, avoid or withstand contact, and decelerate. Any of the skills may be executed repeatedly within a single play. These movements often require coordination with hand-offs, short passes, throwing, or catching. The specific positional requirements are discussed later in the chapter.

Rugby, like football, is a high-contact and high-intensity sport. There are two forms of rugby, sevens and the traditional 15-player rugby. This section focuses on the increasingly popular sevens rugby; however, the demands of each version are very similar, with only slight differences in the rules. The game is played in two 7-minute halves separated by a 2-minute halftime (as compared with 10-minute halves in 15-player). These shorter games allow multiple games to be played per day, increasing the physical demands and injury risk for the players. Rugby is a very high-intensity sport, with the demands increasing on players in the sevens format as compared with the 15-player format. Depending on position, specific demands vary slightly, but overall all players must possess speed, agility, quickness, strength, and power. Play is often divided into periods of high-intensity work separated by brief periods of active or passive rest. A rugby player is required to avoid or withstand contact while sprinting down the field in a variety of directions. This movement requires periods of acceleration, linear sprinting, change of direction in the form of cuts and spins, and deceleration. These skills are executed repeatedly over the course of the 14-minute game.

Often a player is required to accurately throw and catch the ball while running, therefore requiring coordination of the upper and lower body. Because of the high frequency of contacts, a player is often placed in vulnerable positions, and injury risk is high. speed, agility, and quickness training can assist in the development of strength, agility, quickness, and speed to excel in each of the aforementioned skills and to help reduce injuries (Meir 2012).

Although positional demands vary in the sport of football, there are some common speed, agility, and quickness requirements. GPS tracking studies demonstrate that across positions (offensive, defensive, nomadic), players cover 11.7 to 12.3 km (7.3 to 7.6 mi) at a mean velocity of 6.8 to 7.5 km/h (4.2 to 4.7 mph) over the course of a single game in their 105 minutes of playing time. Upon further examination, players execute 237 to 248 accelerations greater than 4 km/h (2.5 mph) in 1 second and 77 to 89 surges over 18 km/h (11.2 mph). Furthermore, players sustain 20 km/h (12.4 mph) for 10 to 11 seconds and spend 20 to 25 minutes above 8 km/h (5 mph) and 4.5 to 5.5 minutes above 18 km/h (11.2 mph) (Wisbey et al. 2010). This study shows that players perform multiple high-velocity sprints over the course of the game. These sprints require acceleration, change of direction, deceleration, and at times reacceleration. It is also important to remember that this occurs while players attempt to avoid or withstand contact from opposing players, thus requiring cuts, spins, and agility to maintain balance after a contact. Players need to develop explosiveness to react to the start of a play as well as acceleration and deceleration to complete the play. Changes of direction are also essential for success and should be developed in a variety of directions and movement styles. Sprint length can vary from a couple yards to a maximum of 109 yards depending on the length of the play, and therefore sprint speed should be developed across these distances and according to positional demands. Furthermore, players are required to sprint multiple times over the course of a single game; therefore, repeated sprint ability is essential for success. The faster, more agile player avoids contact and successfully completes the plays. speed, agility, and quickness training is therefore of the utmost importance for an athlete's success.

Similar to football, positional demands vary in rugby, but there is also the common theme of speed, agility, and quickness. GPS tracking studies of elite women's sevens rugby players demonstrate that players cover 4.9 to 6.5 km (3 to 4 mi) in a single game, with backs covering more distance than forwards. When this distance was broken down, 9.5 percent of the distance was medium intensity, 1.8 percent high intensity, and 1.2 percent sprinting. Average speed over the course of the game was 4.0 km/h (2.5 mph), with average maximum speeds of 22.9 km/h (14.2 mph). Over the course of a game, an athlete performs around five sprints, ranging from 6 to 12 yards or meters in length (Suarez-Arrones et al. 2014). Like football, these sprints require explosiveness, acceleration, and deceleration while avoiding or withstanding contact. Players withstood 705 impacts per game, and of these 65 were heavy, 43 very heavy, and 6 severe (Suarez-Arrones et al. 2014). As a result, similar to football, speed, agility, and quickness training should focus on developing explosiveness, acceleration, speed, change of direction, agility, and deceleration.

FOOTBALL AND RUGBY PROGRAM

The following program has been designed for a football running back. However, this program can be adapted to other players on the team by manipulating the drill type, volume, intensity, or duration. Because of the high-contact nature of American football and rugby, special care should be taken to reduce non-contact injuries. A player must be healthy before beginning any speed, agility, and quickness training. Furthermore, speed, agility, and quickness training can help develop the physiological characteristics needed to reduce these injuries. As with any sport, skill-based practice should be balanced with strength and conditioning and speed, agility, and quickness training. Appropriate tapering before games is required as the won–lost record over the course of a season determines eligibility for championship games.

	SPEED		AGILITY		QUICKNESS	
	1	2	3	4	5	6
Week 1	Prancing (p. 46) 5 × 15 yd; jog to start and repeat	A skip (p. 50) 5 × 30 yd; walk to start and repeat	Multidirectional skipping (p. 133) 5 × 15 yd; 30 sec RI; add speed as drill is mastered	Cone zigzag (p. 115) 5×; 30 sec RI	Push-off box shuffle (p. 209) 5 × 10 sec; 30 sec RI	Quick feet (p. 212) 5 × ladder's length; 30 sec RI
Week 2	Single-leg A skip (p. 51) 5 × 20 yd; walk to start and repeat	Run-through (p. 78) 5 × 15 yd; walk to start and repeat	20-yard square (p. 108) 5×; 30 sec RI	Snake drill 2 (p. 127) 5×; 30 sec RI	Scissor jumps (p. 202) 5 × 10 sec; 50 sec RI	Quick feet (lateral) (p. 212) 5 × ladder's length each side; 30 sec RI
Week 3	Run-through (p. 78) 5 × 15 yd; walk to start and repeat	Ins and outs (p. 52) 5 × 75 yd; walk to start and repeat	20-yard square with catch (p. 108) 5×; 30 sec RI	Lateral weave (p. 158) 5×; 30 sec RI	Scissor jumps with forward movement (p. 202) 5 × 10 yd; 50 sec RI	Quick feet with 5-yard approach (p. 212) and type of ladder drill called out as athlete finishes 5×; 30 sec RI
Week 4	Ins and outs (p. 52) 5 × 90 yd; walk to start and repeat	Harness pull (p. 66) 10 × 30 yd; 20 sec RI	H movement (p. 132) 5×; 30 sec RI	Lateral weave with catch (p. 158) 5×; 30 sec RI	Lateral skaters (p. 203) 5 × 10 yd; 50 sec RI	Lunge with power-up jump (p. 208) 5 × 5 each leg; 30 sec RI
Week 5	Harness pull (p. 66) 10 × 30 yd; 20 sec RI	Gears (p. 52) 5 × 100 yd; 60 sec RI	H movement with catch (p. 132) 5×; 30 sec RI	Star drill (sprint-carioca-backpedal) (p. 133) 5×; 30 sec RI	Lateral skaters with forward movement (p. 203) 5 × 10 yd; 50 sec RI	Lunge with power-up jump (p. p. 208) 5 × 10 sec each leg; 30 sec RI
Week 6	Gears (p. 52) 5 × 100 yd; 60 sec RI	Partner-assisted tubing acceleration (p. 68) 6 × 20 yd; 30 sec RI	Z-pattern cuts (p. 115) 5×; 30 sec RI	Star drill (sprint-backpedal-shuffle) (p. 133) 5×; 30 sec RI	Lateral skaters with lateral movement (p. 203) 5 × 10 yd each direction; 50 sec RI	Mirror two-box drill (p. 225) 5 × 30 sec; 30 sec RI
Week 7	Partner-assisted tubing acceleration drill (p. 68) 6 × 20 yd; 30 sec RI	Heavy sled pull (p. 61) 6 × 20 yd; 30 sec RI	Squirm (p. 89) 5×; walk to start and repeat	X-pattern multiskill (p. 109) 5×; 60 sec RI	Containing opponent drill (p. 220) 5 × 30 sec; 30 sec RI	Triangle drills with commands (p. 222) 5 × 10 sec each leg; 30 sec RI
Week 8	Heavy sled pull (p. 61) 6 × 20 yd; 30 sec RI	Uphill acceleration runs (p. 62) 10 × 5 sec; 60 sec RI	Squirm while catching ball at 2nd turn (p. 89) 5×; walk to start and repeat	X-pattern multiskill with ball catch at various points (p. 109) 5×; 60 sec RI	Partner-resisted lateral shuffle and chase (p. 219) 5 × 30 sec; 30 sec RI	Triangle drills with commands and partner chase (p. 222) 5 × 10 sec each leg; 30 sec RI

RI = rest interval.

Chapter 10

Basketball and Netball

Andrea M. Du Bois, Lee E. Brown, Vance A. Ferrigno

Basketball requires a combination of skill, speed, agility, and quickness. Players must run (multiple directions), dribble, pass, catch, jump, and shoot in order to be successful. During a men's NCAA Division II game, players engage in a variety of multidirectional movements that consist of running, dribbling, and shuffling at a variety of velocities. During a 40-minute game, players cover 4,500 to 5,000 meters (2.8 to 3.1 miles). When broken down for time, 57 percent of the game time is spent walking, 33 percent running, 9 percent standing, and 1.5 percent jumping (Narazaki et al. 2009). Taylor (2003) studied the movements of one individual player in the Australian National Basketball League over the course of two years. In the four games evaluated, the player played an average of 35 total minutes per game. In terms of intensity ratios (high intensity:submaximal intensity), a 1:1.12 ratio resulted. Of all the high-intensity efforts, 52 percent lasted 1 to 5 seconds, and 97 percent lasted 1 to 15 seconds. With regard to submaximal efforts, 38 percent lasted 5 to 10 seconds, 25 percent lasted 10 to 20 seconds, and 94 percent lasted 1 to 20 seconds. Overall, there were a total of 19 efforts per series (period of time between time-outs). Players also participated in intermittent stops throughout play for a total of 25 stops per playing time. This resulted in a 1:11 ratio (stop:effort), with ranges of 1:10 to 1:20 (Taylor 2003). These efforts were not broken down by movement type, but it can be assumed they consisted of running, jumping, dribbling, and shuffling.

Similar to other sports, the position played influences the specific requirements of the player and helps guide manipulation of the critical variables (chapter 1). Basketball positions can be generally divided into forwards, centers, and guards. With regard to speed, agility, and quickness needs, the forwards and centers must be able to explode off the ground, rebound a ball, and then either shoot the ball (offensively) or pass the ball to another player. They must be able to do this even if they are off balance. Sprints on the court will be relatively short in duration. Athletes may be required to pivot, shuffle, and backpedal while under the pressure of opposing players in order to successfully execute an offensive or defensive play. Forwards and centers tend to be some of the larger players on the team, so developing jump and rejump ability is essential. Guards also need to be able to explode off the ground to either rebound or shoot. This movement may be followed by a jump, pivot, shuffle, or sprint. Guards tend to be the players that bring the ball down the court. This requires guards to sprint over a moderate distance while avoiding opposing players through rapid changes of direction and spins. speed, agility, and quickness training for the guards should be focused on moderate-distance sprints, rapid cuts and changes of direction, jump and rejump ability, and multidirectional movement.

Netball is an international sport that is very similar to basketball in structure but does exhibit significant differences. A netball court is 100 feet (30 m) in length and 50 feet (15 m) wide. The court is divided lengthwise into three equal parts. On either end, the thirds are referred to as the goal third, while the middle third is referred to as the center third. Within each goal third, there is a semicircle (goal circle) with a 16-foot (5 m) diameter, located at the end of the court (International Federation of Netball Associates 1999). Over the course of the game, players are restricted to specific portions of the court. Similar to basketball, there is a ring located within the goal circle, and players are required to throw the ball into the 10-foot (3 m) ring. However, unlike basketball, there is no backboard behind the ring. Furthermore, all goals must be scored within the goal circle, and therefore only two players on the seven-person team can score a goal. The game of netball consists of four quarters of 15 minutes in duration. Players receive a 3-minute break after quarters one and three and a 5-minute break after the second quarter.

Netball requires players to catch and throw the ball rapidly in multiple directions while maintaining balance. Defensively, players must try to block the thrown balls without making contact with the player. This sounds very similar to the sport of basketball. However, unlike basketball, a player cannot dribble and run with the ball. Players are required to catch and then release the ball within 3 seconds while being allowed only to pivot or step once to throw the ball. As a result, netball requires a variety of quick and explosive movements to pass and catch the ball. Players must also have the speed to run down the court (33 to 66 feet [10 to 20 m] maximum depending on player position) to either catch or defend the ball (International Federation of Netball Associates 1999). On average, a total of 173 forward jumps, 134 vertical jumps, and 109 lateral jumps are recorded in a single game (Lavipour 2009). Of the 173 forward jumps, there are an equal number of jumps landed unilaterally and bilaterally as well as an equal number of jumps that include a turn versus no turn. However, in both the lateral and forward jumps, a unilateral landing position with no turn in the air is completed more frequently. Overall, 65 percent of the total jumps are landed on a single leg, and 28 percent of the total jumps require an immediate jump or quick change of direction to complete the pass (Lavipour 2009). As a result, jumping speed, agility, and quickness are essential for success in netball. Although players cannot run with the ball, they must develop multidirectional speed in order to appropriately position themselves for a play. Therefore, speed, agility, and quickness training programs should focus on developing both agility and quickness during repeated jumps in a variety of directions and landing styles and speed in various directions.

BASKETBALL AND NETBALL PROGRAM

The following program has been designed for a power forward. However, this program can be adapted to other players on the team by manipulating the drill type, volume, intensity, or duration. As with all sports, it is essential to balance skill-based training with strength and conditioning and speed, agility, and quickness training. The speed, agility, and quickness sample program given here helps improve agility, speed, and quickness to allow the athlete to better move on the court. However, skill-based practice should not be replaced by these drills (even when very sport specific) because the player is still required to accurately throw the ball to opposing players as well as shoot the ball into the ring or hoop.

Because basketball and netball are defined by explosive starts and stops that strongly rely on agility and quickness, those two biomotor qualities are emphasized over speed.

	SPEED		QUICKNESS	AGILITY		QUICKNESS	
	1	2	3	4	5	6
Week 1	Skip for max height and distance (p. 47) 10 × 10 yd; 20 sec RI	Stadium stairs (p. 62) 15 × 10 steps; 45 sec RI	Zigzag crossover shuffle (p. 155) 5-7×; walk to start and repeat	40-yard line shuffle (p. 92) 3-4×; 40 sec RI	In-place ankle jumps (p. 201) 10 × 20 sec; 10 sec RI	Medicine ball upper-body shuffle (p. 197) 5 × 10; 30 sec RI
Week 2	Split-squat jumps (p. 79) 5 × 5 each leg; 30 sec RI	Resist from front (p. 63) 5 × 10 yd; walk to start and repeat	Snake drill 2 (p. 127) 5-7×; walk to start and repeat	55-yard line sprint to backpedal (p. 94) 5×; 30 sec RI	Medicine ball upper-body shuffle (p. 197) 5 × 10; 30 sec RI	Speed skips (p. 208) 7 × 10 yd; use easy backward skip to recover, and return to start and immediately begin again
Week 3	Heavy sled pull (p. 61) 5 × 10 yd; 30 sec RI	Skip for max height and distance (p. 47) 10 × 10 yd; 20 sec RI	Star drill (sprint–backpedal–shuffle) (p. 133) 5 × 40 sec; 20 sec RI	40-yard square multiskill (p. 125) 5 × 20 sec; 10 sec RI	In-place tuck jumps (p. 204) 10 × 5; 30 sec RI	Medicine ball wall scoop toss (p. 194) 10 × 5 tosses; 30 sec RI
Week 4	Bounding (p. 53) 7 × 15 yd; 30 sec RI	Stadium stairs (p. 62) 20 × 10 steps; 60 sec RI	40-yard square multiskill (p. 125) 5 × 20 sec; 10 sec RI	Star drill (sprint-carioca-backpedal) (p. 133) 5 × 40 sec; 20 sec RI; perform passing drills	Tuck jumps (p. 204) with linear motion 10 × 5 yd; 30 sec RI	Single- or double-arm medicine ball wall overhead throw (p. 195) 5 × 10; 10 sec RI
Week 5	Harness pull (p. 66) 10 × 15 yd; 20 sec RI	Heavy sled pull (p. 61) 7 × 15 yd; 45 sec RI	15-yard turn drill (p. 107) 5-7×; 20 sec RI	Cone zigzag (p. 115) 10×; 20 sec RI	Single-leg medicine ball wall overhead throw (p. 195) 7-8 × 10; 20 sec RI	Repeated vertical jumps (p. 205) 10 × 20 sec; 40 sec RI
Week 6	Single-arm medicine ball wall chest pass (p. 193) to ins and outs (p. 52) 5 × 4 cones 10 yd apart; 60 sec RI	Resist from front (p. 63) 10×; 30 sec RI	Backward zigzag (p. 116) 10×; 20 sec RI	X-pattern multiskill (p. 109) 5-7×; 20 sec RI	Plyo push-ups (p. 192) with a clap 10 × 10 sec; 30 sec RI	Repeated vertical jumps (p. 205) with lateral shuffle (p. 103) (3 jumps, 3-step shuffle left, 3 jumps, 3-step shuffle, right 3 jumps) 4×; 60 sec RI
Week 7	Stadium stairs (p. 62) 15 × 10 steps; 20 sec RI	Partner-assisted tubing acceleration (p. 68) 10 × 15 yd; 45 sec RI	X-pattern multiskill (p. 109) while dribbling ball 5-7×; 20 sec RI	E movement (p. 130) while passing ball 5×; 20 sec RI	Lunge with power-up jump (p. 208) 10 × 5; 40 sec RI	Barrier jump with cut and sprint (p. 207) 10 × 5 yds; 40 sec RI
Week 8	Uphill acceleration runs (p. 62) 10×; 30 sec RI	Medicine ball overhead throw (p. 195) to uphill acceleration runs (p. 62) 10 × 5 yd; 60 sec RI	E movement (p. 130) while dribbling or passing ball 5×; 20 sec RI	H movement (p. 132) while dribbling ball 5×; 60 sec RI	Single-leg hop (p. 215) with linear motion forward, backward, and lateral while passing ball 10 × 20 sec each leg; 50 sec RI	Sprint and backpedal on command (p. 228) using various court lines 5 × 40 sec; 20 sec RI

RI = rest interval

Chapter 11

Combat Sports

Andrea M. Du Bois, Lee E. Brown, Vance A. Ferrigno

Combat sports encompass a variety of martial arts including, but not limited to, kickboxing, muay Thai, judo, wrestling, grappling, and mixed martial arts (MMA). Regardless of the type, speed, agility, and quickness are not only essential for success but also important for preventing injury. Combat sports are explosive in nature. These fast movements require speed, accuracy, and coordination of multiple body parts including legs, arms, and trunk in order to successfully execute strikes (Lenetsky, Harris, and Brughelli 2013). Furthermore, the legs are the underlying drive for most upper body movements. Therefore, athletes must be able to both act and react quickly to a variety of opponent strikes and in different directions, often moving from upright to the ground and back in a matter of seconds. Slowness can result in a landed strike from the opponent as well as placing the body in a position that compromises joint structure (especially the knee).

Given the numerous forms of martial arts, the following sections will discuss speed, agility and quickness requirements for popular forms of martial arts.

Kickboxing and Muay Thai

Both kickboxing and muay Thai require athletes to execute a variety of skills including punching, kicking, kneeing, elbowing, clinching, takedowns, and grappling (Buse and Santana 2008; Turner 2009). Punches require triple extension (ankle, knee, and hip) and synchronization of multiple joints and muscle groups. This same synchronization is also required for kicking, kneeing, and elbowing (Turner 2009). Athletes are required to execute all the aforementioned skills not only quickly and forcefully but also repeatedly, and therefore development of the stretch–shortening cycle through plyometric training is essential (Buse and Santana 2008; Turner 2009).

Judo

Judo is a very dynamic sport consisting of high-intensity bouts intermixed with periods of lower intensity. Judo requires athletes to execute complex skills quickly and efficiently. These skills require throwing, pinning, and submission, which result from the coordinated movements of multiple joints. Execution of these skills is required in several directions and often from standing to the ground and back to standing (Henry 2011).

Wrestling

Wrestling takes on a variety of forms, each with specific rules, but overall all forms are similar in nature. Wrestlers are required to use either their upper body or lower body to attack and control the opponent's body. Speed, power, agility, balance, quickness, and coordination are essential for success in the sport (Ratamess 2011). These characteristics allow athletes to act both offensively and defensively to control their opponent through close holds, takedowns, and submissions.

Mixed Martial Arts

Mixed martial arts (MMA), a sport that has gained popularity recently, combines Brazilian jiu-jitsu, muay Thai, kickboxing, and wrestling into one. MMA requires athletes to quickly change direction, pivot, and execute a series of rapid punches, kicks, and takedowns, essentially the skills of all the aforementioned combat sports. To be successful, athletes must be able to execute a variety of movements including standing strikes, clinching, and grappling. Strikes may be long range or close range and include punches, kicks, knees, and elbows. Clinching is a standing form of grappling and can include close-range elbows and knees as well as trips, throws, and takedowns. Grappling requires athletes to perform movements similar to wrestling including holds, pins, and submissions. A high-intensity burst may often require a combination of the three aforementioned movements in several directions (Lenetsky and Harris 2012). Therefore, athletes need to develop speed, agility, and quickness in multiple directions including from standing to the ground and back again. Plyometric training can not only improve athletic performance but also help prevent injuries, especially in the knee in female athletes (Schick, Brown, and Schick 2012).

COMBAT SPORTS PROGRAM

The development of speed, agility, and quickness plays an important role not only in the success of the combat sport athlete but also in the prevention of injury. Slow movements result in landed punches and kicks as well as successful takedowns and submissions by the opponent. Because of the twisting nature of the sport, speed, agility, and quickness training can also help protect the integrity of the joints, especially the knee. Even though punches are considered an upper body movement, they originate from the lower body. Therefore lower body training should be emphasized. Because of the aggressive nature of the sport, athletes engage in few matches or tournaments throughout the year relative to other sports. In short, MMA requires comprehensive training of skill, strength, and speed, agility, and quickness but must also include appropriate periodization and rest so as to avoid overtraining.

It is suggested that athletes perform speed, agility, and quickness training two times per week in the off-season and only one time per week during the season.

	SPEED		AGILITY		QUICKNESS	
	1	2	3	4	5	6
Week 1	Skip for max height and distance (p. 47) 10 × 15 yd; 20 sec RI	Stadium stairs (p. 62) 15 × 10 steps; 45 sec RI	Backward roll over shoulder (p. 172) 10-12×	40-yard square multiskill (p. 125), bear crawl 4 sets: 75 sec btwn sets	Rope skipping (p. 201) 5 × 3 min; 60 sec RI	Four-point pop-up (p. 232) 10× with no RI or 3-5 sets with 40 sec RI between sets
Week 2	Skip for max height and distance (p. 47) 10 × 15 yd; 20 sec RI	Heavy sled pull (p. 61) 5 × 15 yd; 30 sec RI	Backward roll over shoulder (p. 172) 10-12×	40-yard square multiskill (p. 125): at each cone, drop and go, get up 4 sets: 75 sec btwn sets	Bob, weave, and parry (pp. 216, 218, 217) 5-7 × 45 sec; 15 sec RI; mix combinations of each drill	Tuck jump with forward, backward, lateral, or rotational motion (p. 204) 10 × 10 jumps; 30 sec RI
Week 3	Split-squat jumps (p. 79) 5 × 5 each leg; 30 sec RI	Uphill to flat contrast speed runs (p. 80) 10 × 20 yd; 60 sec RI	Forward roll over shoulder (p. 171) 10-12×	10 plyo push-ups (p. 193) to star drill (sprint–bear crawl–shuffle) (p. 133) 5×; 60-90 sec RI	Mirror partner sprints (p. 220) 5×; 30 sec RI	Rope skipping (p. 201) 10 × 45 sec; 15 sec RI; jump at highest speed possible; mix in single leg
Week 4	Resist from front (p. 63) 10 × 10 yd; walk to start and repeat	Stadium stairs (p. 62) 15 × 10 steps; 30 sec RI	Forward roll–backward roll combination (p. 173) 10-12×	Z-pattern cuts (p. 115) performed as a bear crawl with push-ups at every cone 5 cones × 5 push-ups; 60 sec RI	Tuck jumps (p. 204) to bob (p. 216) 5 × 10 jumps to 45 sec of bobs; 60 sec RI	Four-point pop-up (p. 232) to tuck jumps (p. 204) 10× with no RI; 3-5 sets; 40 sec RI between sets
Week 5	Mirror partner sprints (p. 220) 5-7×; 30 sec RI	Heavy sled pull (p. 61) 5 × 20 yd; 30 sec RI	Medicine ball forward scoop toss, bounce and catch to any roll (p. 185) 5-7 × 10; 60 sec RI	Icky shuffle (p. 135) performed on hands in push-up position with pop-up at end of ladder and shuffle back to start 5×; 60 sec RI	Mirror partner sprints (p. 220) to focus mitts (p. 241) 45 sec sprints and 5 × focus mitts; 40 sec RI	Medicine ball scoop toss (p. 73) 5 × 30 sec; 15 sec RI
Week 6	Harness pull (p. 66) 10 × 20 yd; 20 sec RI	Sit-to-stand pop-up (p. 233) to bounding (p. 53) 8 × 10 yd; 30 sec RI	50 mountain climbers (p. 59) to 3 forward roll over shoulder (p. 171) from kneeling position 3×; 60-90 sec RI	Slalom jumps (p. 143) performed on hands in push-up position; perform forward and backward. 5× 60-90 sec RI	Medicine ball scoop toss (p. 73) 5× to medicine ball wall single arm chest pass 5×. Repeat with opposite arm. Perform combo 5×; 45 sec RI	Single-arm medicine ball wall chest pass (p. 193) 10 × 10 each side; 30 sec RI

	SPEED		AGILITY		QUICKNESS	
	1	2	3	4	5	6
Week 7	Split-squat jumps (p. 79) 8 × 5 each leg; 30 sec RI	Lying-to-stand pop-up (p. 234) to downhill speed runs (p. 80) 10 × 15 yd; 30 sec RI	Slalom jumps (p. 143) performed on hands ½ ladder in push-up position; perform pop up and perform weave drill (p. 218) for 45 sec; Repeat 3x for one set. 3-5 sets; 90 sec RI	Icky shuffle (p. 135) performed on hands in push-up position; complete ladder up and back; pop up and perform shuffle on feet up and back 5×; 60 sec RI	Sprawl-to-stand pop-up (p. 235) to medicine ball lateral shuffle with pass (p. 103) 10 × 20 sec; 20 sec RI	Upper body box shuffles (p. 199) 10 × 10 each side; 30 sec RI
Week 8	Sprawl-to-stand pop-up (p. 235) to uphill acceleration runs (p. 62) 10 × 10 yd; 60 sec RI	Heavy sled pull (p. 61) 8 × 15 yd; 30 sec RI	Single leg bound (p. 54) to cone zig zag (p. 115). (This is a speed drill for power tied into an agility drill for foot work.) 3-5 bounds to ten cones; 3-5 sets per leg	40-yard line sprint (p. 90) to 10 explosive reclined pulls (p. 200) 4-5×; RI as short as athlete can handle	Barrel roll to reaction (p. 243) to parry (p. 217), bob (p. 216), or weave (p. 218); athlete starts with a roll, pops up, and reacts to parry, bob, or weave; when coach calls roll the athlete rolls again, pops up, and finishes drill 5 × 45 sec; 60 sec RI	Medicine ball wall chest passes (one-arm and one-leg) (p. 193) 10 × 10 each side; 30 sec RI

RI = rest interval.

Chapter 12

Track and Field

Andrea M. Du Bois, Lee E. Brown, Vance A. Ferrigno

Track and field is a sport of many disciplines including sprinting, endurance running, jumping, and throwing. The athlete who can run the fastest, jump the highest, and throw the farthest is the winner; therefore, the development of speed and quickness is essential for success regardless of the specific event. Agility does not play a major role in this sport. Sprinting requires coordination of the lower body musculature to effectively generate speed (Kyröläinen, Komi, and Belli 1999; Kyröläinen, Avela, and Komi 2005; Miller, Umberger, and Caldwell 2012). Research demonstrates increased sensitivity of the stretch–shortening cycle can lead to improvements in sprint time (Kyröläinen, Komi, and Belli 1999; Miller, Umberger, and Caldwell 2012; Komi 2000). Therefore, including plyometrics in a training program can lead to improved performance (Brown and Vescovi 2012; Behrens and Simonson 2011). Jumping and throwing sports require athletes to quickly generate both lower body and upper body power, often in a coordinated fashion. Generally, track and field can be divided into four groups of athletes: sprinters, distance runners, jumpers and throwers. An understanding of the requirements for each of these categories of athletes can assist in guiding the drill choice and manipulation of the critical variables to address the specific needs of the athlete.

Sprinters

Sprinting events range from 100 meters to 400 meters in length. Sprinting success is dependent on a rapid reaction to the race start, acceleration out of the starting blocks, and linear speed over the course of the race. Hurdlers are a unique subset of sprinters who not only have to develop linear speed similar to sprinters but also effectively coordinate their muscles to maintain this speed while jumping over the hurdles. This jump appears as an exaggerated stride in elite-level hurdlers, requiring athletes to develop specific skills that propel them vertically to clear the hurdle as well as horizontally to maintain speed. speed, agility, and quickness training will help develop these skills as well as the dynamic balance required.

Distance Runners

Distance events in track and field can range from 800 meters to 10,000 meters in length. Although top linear speed isn't the main training focus of these athletes, linear speed does influence performance. There are many times within the course of a race when an athlete is required to surge past a competitor on the track. This surge requires acceleration, speed, and a smooth deceleration to settle back into the athlete's pace. Linear speed and acceleration are also very important at the end of the race because even long-distance events can end in a photo finish. Therefore, linear speed and acceleration can play a significant role in the athlete's success. Steeplechasers, like hurdlers, are a special subset of distance runners who must maintain their running speed while jumping over large hurdles, one of which has a water pit. These athletes must develop skills that allow them to propel themselves vertically and horizontally in order to safely navigate these obstacles.

Jumpers

Jumping events include the long jump, triple jump, high jump, and pole vault. Each event has slightly different requirements, but all are highly dependent on the athlete's ability to coordinate sprinting and then jumping off a single leg. In the long and triple jump, the athlete must rapidly accelerate down the track in a consistent fashion so he is able to begin his jump as accurately as possible from the designated position. The athlete must then successfully transfer the energy developed in the sprint into a horizontal jump off a single leg. In the triple jump, the athlete must perform two leaps, or bounds, before performing the final long jump. During these leaps, it is important that the athlete preserve the speed developed during the sprint. In the high jump, the athlete must also accelerate toward the jump location, but this is done in a curved manner so the athlete can begin her jump with her back to the bar. Unlike in the long and triple jump, the goal of this athlete is to jump as high as possible, and therefore success is dependent on her ability to transfer the horizontal energy from the run into vertical energy. Pole-vaulters are required to rapidly accelerate and sprint down the track while holding a pole that could be 15 feet (4.5 m) or more in length. At the end of the sprint, the athlete is required to place the tip of the pole in a pit while jumping off one foot and swinging his legs into the air. This requires that the athlete successfully coordinate his upper and lower body movements. Regardless of the jumping events, speed and quickness are important training components that will assist athletes in their performance.

Throwers

Throwing events include the hammer, shot put, discus, and javelin throw. Throwing technique and throwing object weight vary between the different events, but success in all events is dependent on the ability to develop rotational power through the coordination of the lower and upper body. Discus and hammer throwers rapidly spin before object release, requiring quick, coordinated movements of the feet. A javelin thrower runs before object release and therefore needs to develop lower body speed and acceleration in coordination with throwing. Although shot-putters have limited movement before throwing, success is dependent on rapid rotational acceleration.

TRACK AND FIELD PROGRAM

Speed, agility, and quickness training is important for every event within the sport of track and field and should be incorporated into the regular training program. However, speed is the predominate factor leading to track success. Unlike the more traditional sports, track and field athletes may have only a few meets a year, with qualification for championships often requiring only that the athlete meet the required mark once in a given season. Therefore, more time can be dedicated to training, while periodization should reflect appropriate tapering before significant events. Although the following program has been designed for 100- and 110-meter hurdlers, this program can be adapted to other track and field events by manipulating the drill type, volume, intensity, or duration.

	SPEED		QUICKNESS	
	1	2	3	4
Week 1	A skip (p. 50) 10 × 10 yd; walk to start and repeat	Falling starts (p. 71) 10 × 10 yd; walk to start and repeat	In-place ankle jumps (p. 201) 10 × 15; 20 sec RI	Quick feet (p. 212) 5×; walk to start and repeat
Week 2	Punch wall drill (p. 37) 7×; walk to start and repeat	Hurdle fast legs (p. 79) 7×; walk to start	Scissor jumps (p. 202) 5 × 5 each leg; 30 sec RI	Medicine ball forward scoop toss, bounce, and catch (p. 185) 7 × 15 yd; 30 sec RI
Week 3	Drive wall drill (p. 38) to ladder quick run with sprint (p. 156) 5×; 30 sec RI	Acceleration heel kicks (p. 44) 10×; 30 sec RI	Icky shuffle (p. 135) 7×; walk to start and repeat	Lateral skaters (p. 203) 7 × 10 sec; 20 sec RI
Week 4	Split-squat jumps (p. 79) 5 × 5 each leg; 30 sec RI	Uphill acceleration run (p. 62) 10 × 15 yd; 60 sec RI	Single-leg hop (p. 215) 7×; walk to start and repeat	Barrier jumps (p. 206) 6 × 3 jumps; 30 sec RI
Week 5	Skip for max height and distance (p. 47) 7 × 20 yd; 30 sec RI	Stadium stairs (p. 62) 10 × 10 steps; 30 sec RI	Push-off box shuffle (p. 209) 5 × 10 each leg; 45 sec RI	Scissor jumps (p. 202) 7-8 × 5 each leg; 30 sec RI
Week 6	Contrast parachute running (p. 82) 7 × 20 yd; 45 sec RI	Bounding (p. 53) 7 × 15 yd; 30 sec RI	Barrier jump with cut and sprint (p. 207) 5 × (with 20 yd sprint); 45 sec RI	Chubby checker with reaction (p. 251) 8×; walk to start and repeat
Week 7	Downhill speed runs (p. 80) 10 × 15 yd; 45 sec RI	Partner-assisted tubing acceleration drill (p. 68) 10 × 20 yd; 45 sec RI	Lunge with power-up jump (p. 208) 10 × 5 each leg; 60 sec RI	Quick feet (p. 212) 10×; walk to start and repeat
Week 8	Single-leg bounds (p. 54) 5× each leg × 4 sets; 30 sec RI	Bullet belt (p. 67) 10 × 20 yd; 60 sec RI	Medicine ball forward scoop toss, bounce, and catch (p. 185) 8 × 20 yd; 60 sec RI	Lateral skaters (p. 203) 5-7 × 10 sec; 20 sec RI

RI = rest interval.

Chapter 13

Soccer

Andrea M. Du Bois, Lee E. Brown, Vance A. Ferrigno

Soccer is an explosive sport that is also very aerobic in nature. When evaluating the movement patterns of female soccer players, it has been found that they can cover anywhere from 9.1 to 11.9 km (5.7 to 7.4 mi) per game. These movements include not only submaximal aerobic work but also sprinting and jumping. When further examining these movements, on average a female soccer player will engage in 250 intense anaerobic actions per game. This includes 39 repeated sprints, with the athlete being required to sprint every 90 seconds for 2 to 4 seconds' duration. During these sprints, speed is essential for success because it determines whether the player can gain ball possession, score goals, or defend goals. A female soccer player will sprint for a total of 1,025 meters (.6 mi) per game (Turner et al, 2013).

Sprinting is not the only requirement of soccer players. Further analysis demonstrates that a female player engages in 111 on-ball activities and changes direction 90 to 100 times in a single game. During these activities, athletes are required to strike the ball, turn, jump, accelerate, decelerate, and cut (Turner, Munro, and Comfort 2013). Both acceleration and deceleration occur in multiple directions and from different starting points. For example, a player might receive the ball and then immediately turn 90 to 180 degrees and sprint in a new direction. When playing offensively or defensively without the ball, players are required to backpedal and side shuffle during game play (Jeffreys 2008). Therefore, it should be obvious why speed, agility, and quickness training is essential for success in soccer. The faster and more powerful player will be able to gain ball possession through either foot control or heading, maintain ball possession, take the ball down the field, and successfully score. From a defensive position, the quicker and more powerful athlete can better defend opposing players, thus preventing breakaways and shots on goal.

Generally speaking, soccer athletes are required to execute both offensive and defensive responsibilities over the course of the game. Depending on the specific assignment of the player, relative distribution of the responsibilities may vary. Overall, there are fundamental skills that a soccer athlete must possess, including acceleration, speed, change of direction, and deceleration. Players are also required to coordinate various body segments to dribble, pass, kick, and head the ball as well as jump and tackle in order to gain ball possession. Generally speaking, soccer sprints can cover 5 to 30 yards or meters and often include running without the ball, but ball contact may occur at the beginning or end of the run (Hedrick 1999).

The offensive and defensive requirements of a soccer athlete rely on the same basic skills. Upon reception of a ball from a fellow player, a soccer athlete is required to carry the ball down the field via dribbling, kicking, or passing. The basic act of receiving a ball can require rapid acceleration to the ball, change of direction along the path to the ball, and jumping. As the athlete advances the ball downfield, she must avoid opposing players and may be required to cut, spin, and weave. These movements often involve quick execution followed by rapid acceleration. Defensively, a player must be able to quickly accelerate to the position of the play in an attempt to steal the ball from an opposing player. A contest for a ball could include jumping in order to head the ball, a sprint in order to intercept a ball, or a tackle in order to steal the ball. In any of these instances (offensively and defensively), the faster and more agile player gains and maintains ball possession. Therefore, the quicker, faster, and more agile player is the more successful player.

SOCCER PROGRAM

Soccer players, particularly females, have a high risk of ACL injury. Speed, agility, and quickness training may ameliorate this risk. Furthermore, soccer players have the unique responsibility (with the exception of the keeper) of maintaining both aerobic fitness and anaerobic power. As a result of these conflicting demands, a coach will not be able to fully develop either of these characteristics to their fullest potential. Regardless, speed, agility, and quickness training should be executed in conjunction with aerobic training, skill-based practice, and resistance training. Soccer (when played internationally) is a year-round sport. Often you cannot pick a main event (e.g., the World Cup) or when you want an athlete to peak, as soccer depends on numerous qualification rounds and games to reach the championship round. Therefore, a more undulating periodization program should be adopted.

It is suggested that athletes perform speed, agility, and quickness training two times per week in the off-season and only one time per week during the season.

	SPEED		AGILITY		QUICKNESS	
	1	2	3	4	5	6
Week 1	Ankling (p. 45) 10 × 10 yd; walk to start and repeat	Falling starts (p. 71) 10 × 10 yd; walk to start and repeat	40-yard line backpedal to sprint (p. 93) 5×; 20 sec RI	Icky shuffle (p. 135) 4×; 15 sec RI	Four-point pop-up (p. 232) to 10-yard sprint 5×; 15 sec RI	Medicine ball wall overhead throw (p. 195) 5 × 10; 20 sec RI
Week 2	Ladder quick run with sprint (p. 156) 7×; walk to start and repeat	Gears (p. 52) 4×; walk to start and repeat	40-yard line shuffle (p. 92) 5×; 20 sec RI	In-out shuffle (p. 136) 7×; 15 sec RI	Four-point pop-up (p. 232) to half-ladder icky shuffle (p. 135) 5×; 15 sec RI	Medicine ball wall overhead throw with single-leg hops (p. 195) 5 × 5 each leg; 20 sec RI
Week 3	Falling starts (p. 71) to ladder quick run with sprint (p. 156) 5×; 30 sec RI	Gears (p. 52); space cones at 10 yd to Z-pattern runs (p. 110) next block 4×; 90 sec RI	Z-pattern cuts (p. 115) 6×; 4 cones; 20 sec RI	Bag weave (p. 158) 8×; 20 sec RI	Mirror two-box drill (p. 225) 8-10 × 15 sec; 45 sec RI	Backpedal and cut on command (p. 278) 10 × 10 sec; 50 sec RI; vary biomotor skills
Week 4	Uphill acceleration run (p. 62) 10×; 30 sec RI	Ins and outs (p. 52); space cones 15 yd apart 5×; 40 sec RI	Squirm (p. 89) 5×; 40 sec RI	Combo zigzag (p. 116) 5×; 30 sec RI	Mirror two-box drill (p. 225) 8-10 × 15 sec; 45 sec RI	Barrier jumps (p. 206) 6 × 3 jumps; 30 sec RI
Week 5	Uphill acceleration run (p. 62) 10 × 15 yd; 60 sec RI	Falling starts (p. 71) to cone zigzag (p. 115) 5×; 40 sec RI	Cone zigzag (p. 115) 6×; 20 sec RI	60-yard line sprint (p. 91) 8-10×; 60 sec RI	Partner-resisted lateral shuffle and chase (p. 219) 5-7×; 20 sec RI	Barrier jumps with cut and sprint (p. 207) 8-10×; 40 sec RI
Week 6	Uphill acceleration run (p. 62) perform in gears (p. 52) format 10×; 60 sec RI	Bounding (p. 53) 7 × 15 yd; 30 sec RI	Cone zigzag (p. 115) using 5 cones with ball dribble to squirm (p. 89) 6×; 40 sec RI	55-yard line sprint to backpedal (p. 94) 8-10×; 60 sec RI	Triangle drill with commands (p. 222) 5×; 40 sec RI	Lateral barrier jumps with cut and sprint (p. 207) 8-10×; 40 sec RI
Week 7	Bounding (p. 53) with backpedal to start and repeat 5 × 15 yd; 90 sec RI	Harness pull (p. 66) 5 × 15 yd; 40 sec RI	Wheel drill (p. 159) 8-10×; 40 sec RI	H movement (p. 132) 5×; 40 sec RI	Sprint and backpedal on command (p. 228) 10 × 15 yd; 40 sec RI	Triangle drill with commands and partner variation (p. 222) 5×; 40 sec RI
Week 8	Single-leg bounds (p. 54) 5 × each leg × 4 sets; tie into one of the cone drills	Bullet belt (p. 67) 10 yd; after release tie into cone drill with ball skill	Wheel drill (p. 159) to any cone drill 8-10×; 40 sec RI	H movement (p. 132) to ball skill 5×; 40 sec RI	Backward icky shuffle with reaction (p. 248) 5-7×; 20 sec RI	Lateral skaters (p. 203) to any cone drill 5-7×; 20 sec RI

RI = rest interval.

Chapter 14

Lacrosse

Andrea M. Du Bois, Lee E. Brown,
Vance A. Ferrigno

Lacrosse combines the physiological demands of football, soccer, basketball, and hockey. Like soccer, lacrosse requires both aerobic fitness and anaerobic power. Activity is intermittent over the course of play as players alternate between periods of explosive, high-intensity movements and active and passive rest. Over the course of the game, there is a balanced ratio between sprinting, jogging, and walking. Players are required to perform frequent explosive movements in a variety of directions as well as engage in quick change of direction. Some of these skills are similar to basketball in that players must cut and spin while continuing to maintain explosive power and speed. Rapid changes from offensive movements to defensive movements are also essential for success (Gutowski and Rosene 2011). Players must possess speed and agility in the lower body, and these movements must be coordinated with throwing and catching skills. Throwing and catching require quick yet accurate movements under the pressure of contact with an opposing player. As a result, speed, agility, and quickness training can help develop the lower body explosiveness required to move on the field as well as the agility required to maintain balance and accuracy to throw and catch the ball in dynamic and full-contact situations.

Although positional responsibilities vary among players, athletic success in all positions is dependent on the athlete's speed, agility, and quickness. Offensively, the athlete's main responsibility is to score goals. In order to accomplish this, the athlete must possess speed, agility, and superb stick skills. Success depends on the ability to outrun and avoid contact with opposing players, thus requiring rapid changes of direction along with periods of acceleration and deceleration (Gutowski and Rosene 2011). These movements need to be coordinated with accurate passes and catches as well as shots on goal. When contacted during play, the player must maintain balance and be able to reaccelerate or quickly react and pass the ball to a fellow player. As in baseball, upper body and lower body speed, agility, and quickness need to be developed and synchronized to execute the aforementioned skills. A slow player will be hit and risk losing control of the ball; therefore, a fast and agile player will be successful. Defensively, a player must also possess the ability to rapidly accelerate, change direction, and decelerate to prevent an opposing player from scoring a goal or completing a successful pass to a teammate. As in soccer, it is not uncommon for a player to need to rapidly switch between offensive and defensive responsibilities.

LACROSSE PROGRAM

Lacrosse is a high-contact sport, with players engaging in contact 88 percent of the game. As a result, contact injuries are extremely common. It is important that athletes participate in speed, agility, and quickness training. Even though speed, agility, and quickness training is limited in its ability to prevent contact injuries, it can help reduce risk for some noncontact injuries and thus limit total injuries over the course of a season. It should also be emphasized that speed, agility, and quickness training is not used instead of specific ball-handling drills. Accurate passing and catching require skill-specific agility and accuracy and hours of repetitive practice to develop. As with all sports, there must be an equal balance between skill-based practice, strength and conditioning, and speed, agility, and quickness training.

	SPEED		AGILITY		QUICKNESS	
	1	2	3	4	5	6
Week 1	Single-leg fast leg (p. 77) 5× each leg; 45 sec RI	Gears (p. 52) 5×; 60 sec RI	Multidirectional skipping (p. 133) 5-7 × 25 yd; 60 sec RI	30-yard T drill (p. 91) 4-6×; 30 sec RI	Triangle drill with commands (p. 222) 8 × 20 sec; 20 sec RI	Single-arm medicine ball wall chest pass (p. 193) 3-4 × 10 each arm; 30 sec RI between arms
Week 2	Alternating fast leg (p. 77) 5×; 45 sec RI	Uphill acceleration run (p. 62) 5-7 × 15 yd; 60 sec RI	Snake drill 1 (p. 126) 6-8×; 30 sec RI	60-yard line sprint (p. 91) 4×; 40 sec RI	Dodgeball (p. 281) 4 × 45 sec; 15 sec RI	Four-point pop-up (p. 232) to sprint 5 × 15-20 yd; 30 sec RI
Week 3	Alternating fast leg (p. 77) 5×; 45 sec RI	Uphill acceleration run (p. 62) 5-7 × 15 yd; 60 sec RI	Snake drill 2 (p. 127) 5-7×; 40 sec RI	55-yard line sprint to backpedal (p. 94) 4×; 40 sec RI	Medicine ball bull in a ring (p. 182) 5-7 × 20 sec; 40 sec RI	Triangle chase drill (p. 222) 8 × 15 sec; 45 sec RI
Week 4	Parachute running (p. 81) 5 × 20 yd; 60 sec RI	Uphill to flat contrast speed runs (p. 80) 5-7 × 15 yd; 60 sec RI	In-out shuffle (p. 136) forward and backward with ball pass 6-8×; 30 sec RI	100-yard line shuttle (p. 95) 4×; 60 sec RI	Mirror two-box drill (p. 225) 5-7 × 20 sec; 40 sec RI	Backpedal and cut on command (p. 278) 5 × 15-20 yd
Week 5	Contrast parachute running (p. 82) 5 × 20; 45 sec RI	Uphill acceleration run (p. 62) 5-7 × 15 yd; 60 sec RI	Crossover shuffle (p. 154) to basic 40-yard model (p. 51) 5-7×; 45 sec RI	Z-pattern cuts (p. 115) to squirm (p. 89) 5×; 40 sec RI	Medicine ball lateral shuffle with pass (p. 183) with reaction change of direction 6-8 × 20 sec; 60 sec RI	Mirror partner sprints (p. 220) 5-7 × 20 yd; 40 sec RI
Week 6	Downhill speed runs (p. 80) 4-6 × 15-20 yd; walk to start and repeat	Harness pull (p. 66) 5-7 × 15 yd; 60 sec RI	Icky shuffle (p. 135) to 40-yard square carioca (p. 111) 5-7×; 90 sec RI	Cone zigzag (p. 115) to 15-yard turn drill (p. 107) performed with stick and ball; finish with shot on goal 5-7×; 90 sec RI	Containing opponent drill (p. 220) 6-8 × 20 sec; 60 sec RI	Four-point pop-up (p. 232) to mirror partner sprints (p. 220) 5-7×; 20 yd; 40 sec RI
Week 7	Downhill to flat contrast speed runs (p. 81) 4-6 × 15-20 yd; walk to start and repeat	Bullet belt (p. 67) 5-7 × 15 yd; 60 sec RI	Squirm (p. 89) 5-7×; 60 sec RI	Star drill (sprint-backpedal-shuffle) (p. 133) 5-7×; 75-90 sec RI	Mirror two-box drill (p. 225) with ball pass 5-7×; 20s; 40 sec RI	Partner-resisted lateral shuffle and chase (p. 219) 5-7×; 40 sec RI
Week 8	Partner-assisted tubing acceleration (p. 68) 5-7 × 15 yd; 60 sec RI	Heavy sled pull (p. 61) 6-8 × 20 yd; 90 sec RI	Z-pattern run (p. 110) and jog 10 yd downfield while performing a skill 5-7×; 60 sec RI	Four-point pop-up (p. 232) to V drill (p. 128) 6-8×; 45 sec RI	Medicine ball scoop toss (p. 73) to figure-eight cone drill (p. 134); 3 explosive tosses to figure eights 5×; 10 sec RI	Backward roll over shoulder (p. 172) with a pop up to 20-yard shuttle (p. 88) 5-7×; 60 sec RI

RI = rest interval.

Chapter 15

Tennis and Badminton

Andrea M. Du Bois, Lee E. Brown, Vance A. Ferrigno

Tennis is a sport in which speed, agility, and explosiveness correlate with enhanced performance. Breaking down the time spent in each activity shows that a player spends 4 to 10 seconds engaging in high-intensity activity during a point (Fernandez-Fernandez et al 2009). The International Tennis Federation requires 20 seconds of rest (active recovery) between points, 90 seconds of rest (seated) between games, and 120 seconds of recovery (seated) between sets (ITF 2013). These time frames result in an average match time of 1.5 hours (range of 1 to 5 hours or more) (Fernandez-Fernandez 2009). The surface of the court greatly affects the activity duration and requirements. Clay surfaces typically result in slower movements, giving the players more time to hit the ball, whereas hard surfaces are faster and require more explosive activity (Fernandez-Fernandez 2009). As a result, on a clay surface 20 to 30 percent of the total match time is spent playing, whereas on hard surfaces, only 10 to 15 percent of the total match time is spent playing.

During the action of a point, players must quickly change direction, accelerate for short periods of time, and execute powerful strokes. A ball can be served at speeds up to 130 miles per hour (210 km/h), requiring the player to quickly react to return a ball. On average, a player is required to run 3 yards or meters per shot and 8 to 15 yards or meters per point, which consists of approximately four changes of direction. During a match, a player may cover 1,300 to 3,600 yards or meters depending on the surface. When examining the distance required for a player to move for a shot, 80 percent of the shots (typically 2.5 to 3 per rally) occur within 2.5 yards or meters of the player and are completed standing. Ten percent of the shots occur within 2.5 to 4.5 yards or meters of the player and require a sliding movement. Less than 5 percent of the shots occur outside the range of 4.5 yards or meters and require a running pattern (Fernandez-Fernandez et al 2009). With regard to direction, 47 percent of shots require forward movement, 48 percent require lateral movement, and 5 percent require backward movement. Overall, quick reaction and lateral movement are essential for success in tennis, and the athlete must be able to rapidly change direction (Parsons and Jones 1998).

Badminton also requires explosive and highly reactive movements because the shuttlecock can travel at speeds up to 206 miles per hour (332 km/h). Success in badminton requires athletes to quickly react to a served shuttlecock, allowing them to reach the shot but also effectively and efficiently return the shot to the opposing player. The movement, although not very large, is very quick and explosive and can occur in multiple directions. During this explosive movement, the player must also be able to maintain an effective body posture while quickly changing directions forward and backward and side to side. Therefore, agility training is very important (Sturgess and Newton 2008).

TENNIS AND BADMINTON PROGRAM

Because tennis is more about agility and quickness, with very little true speed, the speed drills are kept to a minimum, with their primary focus being on leg strength and endurance. We are also making the assumption that this tennis player plays on both hard courts and clay courts. Therefore, the agility drills will need to be performed on the various court surfaces in tennis shoes. Finally, the average tennis point lasts 10 to 25 seconds, but the match can, at the highest levels, last 4 to 5 hours. So although it is an anaerobic power sport in nature, tennis requires extreme fitness in the later sets of a match. Therefore, the higher the level of play, the greater the volume of work needed to prepare athletes for longer matches. An RI of 20-90 seconds is used between most drills.

	SPEED		AGILITY		QUICKNESS	
	1	2	3	4	5	6
Week 1	Ins and outs (p. 52) 5×; 30 sec RI	Skip for max height and distance (p. 47) 5 × 10 yd; 20 sec RI	30-yard T drill (p. 91) performed on court baseline to service line 5×; 20 sec RI	20-yard shuttle (p. 88) 5×; 20 sec RI	Multidirectional skipping (p. 133) 10 × 10 sec on visual command	Jumping jacks (p. 211) sequence change on command 10 × 20 sec
Week 2	Skip for max height and distance (p. 47) to T drill (p. 91) 5×; 20 sec RI	Light sled pull (p. 60) 5 × 10 yd; 20 sec RI	20-yard shuttle (p. 88) with ball pick-up 7×; 20 sec RI	40-yard line shuffle (p. 92) 5×; 60 sec RI	Jumping jacks (p. 211) with locomotion; sequence change on command 10 × 20 sec	Jump rope with multi-directional jumps (p. 210), sequence change on command 10 × 20 sec
Week 3	Light sled pull (p. 60) 5 × 10 yd; 20 sec RI	Skip for max height and distance (p. 47) to backpedal (p. 252) 5 × 10 yd; 20 sec RI	40-yard line backpedal to sprint (p. 93) 5×; 60 sec RI	40-yard line shuffle (p. 92) 5×; 60 sec RI	Jump rope with multi-directional jumps (p. 210) with locomotion; sequence change on command 10 × 20 sec	Rapid fire (p. 242) 10×; 20 sec RI
Week 4	Light sled pull (p. 60) 8 × 10 yd; 20 sec RI	Uphill acceleration run (p. 62) 5 × 20 yd; walk to start and repeat	40-yard line shuffle (p. 92) with opposite-hand touch on line 5×; 60 sec RI	40-yard line backpedal to sprint (p. 93) 5×; 60 sec RI	Rapid fire (p. 242) with volley 10×; 20 sec RI	Side shuffle reactive (p. 230) sideline to sideline with cone touch 10 × 20 sec; 20 sec RI
Week 5	Uphill acceleration run (p. 62) with weight vest 10 × 10 yd	Heavy sled pull (p. 61) 10 × 20 yd; 60 sec RI	40-yard square carioca (p. 111) 5×; 60 sec RI	40-yard square carioca (p. 111) 5×; 60 sec RI	Side shuffle reactive (p. 230) sideline to sideline with visual cue 20 sec × 20 sec RI	Medicine ball wall side toss (p. 194) 10 × 5 each side; no RI side to side; 20 sec RI between sets
Week 6	Heavy sled pull (p. 61) 10 × 20 yd; 60 sec RI	Stadium stairs (p. 62) 10 × 10 steps; 60 sec RI	Star drill (sprint–carioca–backpedal) (p. 133) 5×; 60 sec RI	Star drill (sprint–carioca–backpedal) (p. 133) 5×; 60 sec RI	Lateral shuffle (p. 103) with medicine ball wall side toss (p. 194) 10 × 15 sec; 30 sec RI	Carioca (p. 140) with visual cue sideline to sideline 5×; 20 sec RI
Week 7	Stadium stairs (p. 62) with weighted vest 10 × 10 steps; 60 sec RI	Medicine ball scoop toss (p. 73) to uphill acceleration run (p. 62); 4 toss and sprints; 90 sec RI between sets	55-yard line sprint to backpedal (p. 94) 5×; 60 sec RI	55-yard line sprint to backpedal (p. 94) 5×; 60 sec RI	Carioca (p. 140) with volley sideline to sideline 5×; 20 sec RI	Lateral skaters (p. 203) 10 × 10 sec; 20 sec RI
Week 8	Medicine ball wall side toss (p. 194) to uphill acceleration run (p. 62) 4 toss and sprints; no RI between; 90 sec RI between sets	Downhill speed runs (p. 80) 5 × 20 yd; walk to start and repeat	55-yard line sprint to backpedal (p. 94) 5×; 60 sec RI	V drill (p. 128) 5×; 60 sec RI	Lateral skaters (p. 203) to T drill with ball pick-up (p. 91) 5×; 20 sec RI	Half ladder (p. 215) with reaction to volley 10×; 20 sec RI

RI = rest interval.

Chapter 16

Racquetball and Squash

Andrea M. Du Bois, Lee E. Brown, Vance A. Ferrigno

Racquetball and squash are fast-paced sports that require short explosive movements and quick reactions. In order to be successful, players must possess speed and agility in a variety of directions including forward, side to side, and backward. Because of the small size of the court, sprints are very short, and bounds, leaps, jumps, and dives are often used to reach the ball. The player must not only react quickly to a hit ball but also be able to powerfully return that ball. This often requires a change of direction and shot accuracy. These requirements are very similar to those of tennis. Therefore, from an offensive perspective, a successful player can hit the ball to a precise location on the court. From a defensive perspective, a player possesses speed, agility, and quickness in multiple directions in order to reach shots anywhere on the court (USA Racquetball 2008; World Squash Federation 2010).

RACQUETBALL AND SQUASH PROGRAM

Both racquetball and squash are played within confined areas (World Squash Federation 2013); therefore, speed, agility, and quickness training should be designed around short, explosive bursts. Players need lower body movements coordinated with those of the upper body to increase shot accuracy. Like other sports, this training should not replace skill-based training for accuracy but should be used to assist players in executing the skills with greater power.

	SPEED		AGILITY		QUICKNESS	
	1	2	3	4	5	6
Week 1	Skip for max height and distance (p. 47) 10 × 10 yd; walk to start and repeat	Falling starts (p. 71) 10 × 15 yd; walk to start and repeat	Carioca (p. 140) 10 × 10 yd each leg; walk to start and repeat	Crossover shuffle (p. 154) 5×; walk to start and repeat	Quick feet (p. 212) 5×; 30 sec RI	Medicine ball wall side toss (p. 194) 3 × 10 each side; 60 sec RI between sets
Week 2	Falling starts (p. 71) 10 × 15 yd; walk to start and repeat	Resist from front (p. 63) 10 × 15 yd; walk to start and repeat	20-yard square (p. 108) 5×; 30 sec RI	Zigzag crossover shuffle (p. 155) 5×; walk to start and repeat	Quick feet (p. 212) forward to backward 5×; 30 sec RI	Medicine ball wall side toss (p. 194); perpendicular stance 3 × 10 each side; 60 sec RI between sets
Week 3	Resist from front (p. 63) 10 × 15 yd; walk to start and repeat	Resist from behind (p. 64) 10 × 15 yd; walk to start and repeat	20-yard square (p. 108) with racket swing at the end 5×; 30 sec RI	V drill (p. 128) 5×; 30 sec RI	Quick feet (p. 212) reaction in all directions 5×; 30 sec RI	Medicine ball wall chest pass (p. 193) 5 × 10; 30 sec RI
Week 4	Resist from behind (p. 64) 10 × 15 yd; walk to start and repeat	Stadium stairs (p. 62) 5 × 10 steps, 40 sec RI	Multidirectional skipping (p. 133) 10 × 10 yd each leg; walk to start and repeat	V drill (p. 128) with racket and swing at ball 5×; 30 sec RI	Push-off box shuffle (p. 209) 5 × 10; 30 sec RI	Single-arm medicine ball wall chest pass (p. 193) 5 × 10 each arm; 30 sec RI
Week 5	Stadium stairs (p. 62) 8 × 10 steps, 40 sec RI	Skip for max height and distance (p. 47) 10 × 10 yd; walk to start and repeat	Cone zigzag (p. 115) 5×; 30 sec RI	X-pattern multiskill (p. 109) 5×; 30 sec RI	Scissor jumps (p. 202) 5 × 10; 50 sec RI	Medicine ball lateral shuffle with pass (p. 183) and change of direction 5 × 10; 30 sec RI
Week 6	Skip for max height and distance (p. 47) 10 × 10 yd; walk to start and repeat	Split-squat jumps (p. 79) 5 × 5 each leg; 30 sec RI	Cone zigzag (p. 115) with racket swing 5 ×; 30 sec RI	X-pattern multiskill (p. 109) with racket swing 5×; 30 sec RI	Scissor jumps (p. 202) with forward movement 5 × 10 yd; 50 sec RI	Upper body shuffles (p. 198) 5 × 10; 30 sec RI
Week 7	Split-squat jumps (p. 79) 5 × 5 each leg; 30 sec RI	Ins and outs (p. 52) 6 × 15 yd; walk to start and repeat	Icky shuffle (p. 135) 4 × ladder's length; walk to start and repeat	Star drill: sprint–backpedal–shuffle (p. 133) 5 × 30 sec; 30 sec RI	Lateral skaters (p. 203) with forward movement 5 × 10 yd; 50 sec RI	Medicine ball one-arm push-off (p. 196) 5 × 10; 30 sec RI
Week 8	Ins and outs (p. 52) 6 × 15 yd; walk to start and repeat	Partner-assisted tubing acceleration (p. 68) 10 × 15 yd; walk to start and repeat	Icky shuffle (p. 135) while hitting ball 4 × ladder's length; walk to start and repeat	Star drill: sprint–backpedal–shuffle (p. 133) on command 5 × 30 sec; 30 sec RI	Lateral skaters (p. 203) 5 × 5 yd each direction; 50 sec RI	Medicine ball upper body shuffles (p. 197) 5 × 10; 30 sec RI

RI = rest interval.

References

Chapter 1

Abad, C., Prado, M., Ugrinowitsch, C., Tricoli, V., and Barroso, R. 2011. Combination of general and specific warm-ups improves leg-press one repetition maximum compared with specific warm-up in trained individuals. *J Strength Cond Res* 25 (8): 2242-45.

Bradley-Popovich, G.E. 2001. Nonlinear versus linear periodization models. *Strength Cond J* 23 (1): 42.

Dierking, J., and Bemben, M. 1998. Delayed onset muscle soreness. *Strength Cond J* 20 (4): 44-48.

Graham, J. 2002. Periodization research and an example application. *Strength Cond J* 24 (6): 62-70.

Nazem, T., and Ackerman, K. 2012. The female athlete triad. *Sports Health: A Multidisciplinary Approach* 4 (4): 302-11.

Parsons, L., and Jones, M. 1998. Development of speed, agility, and quickness for tennis athletes. *Strength Cond* 20:14-19.

Plisk, S. 2000. Speed, agility, and speed-endurance development. In *Essentials of Strength Training and Conditioning*, ed. T.R. Baechle and R.W. Earle, 457-85. Champaign, IL: Human Kinetics.

Plisk, S. 2004. Periodization: Fancy name for a basic concept. *Olympic Coach* 16 (2): 14-18.

Chapter 2

Brown, L.E., Khamoui, A.V. & Jo, E. 2013. Test administration and interpretation. In *Conditioning for Strength and Human Performance*. 2nd ed. Ed T.J. Chandler and L.E. Brown pp. 165-193. Philadelphia: Lippincott, Williams & Wilkins.

Gambetta, V. 1998. *The Gambetta Method*. Sarasota, FL: Gambetta Sports Training Systems.

Gray, G. 2004. *Knee 1.1*. Functional Video Digest. Adrian, MI: Gray Institute.

Gray, G. 2006a. *Coordination/Agility*. Fast Function Series. Adrian, MI: Gray Institute.

Gray, G. 2006b. *Fundamentals/Skills*. Fast Function Series. Adrian, MI: Gray Institute.

Harman, E. 2008. Principles of test selection and administration. In *Essentials of Strength and Conditioning*, 3rd ed., ed. T.R. Baechle and R.W. Earle. pp. 237-247. Champaign, IL: Human Kinetics.

Chapter 3

Butler, R.J., and Hardy, L. 1992. The performance profile: Theory and application. *Sport Psychol* 6:253-64.

Gould, D., and Eklund, R.C. 2007. The application of sport psychology for performance optimization. In *Essential Readings in Sport and Exercise Psychology*, ed. D. Smith and M. Bar-Eli, 231-40. Champaign, IL: Human Kinetics.

Jones, G., Hanton, S., and Connaughton, D. 2002. What is this thing called mental toughness: An investigation of elite sport performers. *J Appl Sport Psychol* 14:205-18.

Loehr, J. 1986. *Mental Toughness Training for Sports: Achieving Athletic Excellence*. Lexington, MA: Stephen Greene Press.

Moran, A. 2011. Concentration/attention. In *Routledge Handbook of Applied Sport Psychology*, ed. S. Hanrahan and M. Andersen, 500-509. New York: Routledge.

USOC. 2002. *U.S. Olympic Committee Coaches Guide: Sport Psychology Training Manual*. Colorado Springs, CO: USOC Coaching and Sport Sciences.

Vernacchia, R., McGuire, R., and Cook, D. 1996. *Coaching Mental Excellence*. Portola Valley, CA: Warde.

Chapter 4

Cronin, JB, Green, JP, Levin, GT, Brughelli, ME, and Frost, DM. Effect of starting stance on initial sprint performance. J Strength Cond Res 21:990-992, 2007.

Cusick J, Lund R, and Ficklin T. A comparison of three different start techniques on sprint speed in collegiate linebackers. *J Strength Cond Res.* 2014. DOI: 10.1519/JSC.0000000000000453. Post Acceptance March 11, 2014.

Duthie, G.M., Pyne, D.B., Marsh, D.J., & Hooper, S.L. Sprint patterns in rugby union players during competition. J Strength Cond Res. 20(1) 208-214, 2006.

Gambetta, V. Getting Gait Right *Training & Conditioning,* 11.4, May/June 2001, www.momentummedia.com/articles/tc/tc1104/gait.htm

Harland.MJ and Steele,JR Biomechanics of the sprint start. *Sports Med.* 1997 Jan; (23)11-20.

Jeffreys I (2009) Gamespeed: Movement Training for Superior Sports Performance. Monterey CA. Coaches Choice

Chapter 5

Arthur, M., and Bailey, B. 1998. Agility drills. In *Complete Conditioning for Football,* 191-237. Champaign, IL: Human Kinetics.

Barnes, M., and Attaway, J. 1996. Agility and conditioning of the San Francisco 49ers. *Strength Cond* 18 (4): 10-16.

Brittenham, G. 1996. Athleticism for basketball. In *Complete Conditioning for Basketball,* 69-87. Champaign, IL: Human Kinetics.

Brown, L., and Khamoui, A.V. 2012. Agility training. In *NSCA's Guide to Program Design,* ed. J.R. Hoffman, 143-164. Champaign IL: Human Kinetics.

Cissik, J., and Barnes M. 2011. *Sport Speed and Agility,* 2nd ed, Monterey, CA: Coaches Choice.

Costello, F., and Kreis, E.J. 1993. Introduction to agility. In *Sports Agility,* 2-3. Nashville, TN: Taylor Sports.

Halberg, G.V. 2001. Relationships among power, acceleration, maximum speed, programmed agility, and reactive agility: The neural fundamentals of agility. Master's thesis, Central Michigan University.

Harman, E. 2008. The biomechanics of resistance exercise. In *Essentials of Strength Training and Conditioning,* 3rd ed., ed. T.R. Baechle and R.W. Earle, 65-91. Champaign IL: Human Kinetics.

Hoffman, J.R. 2012. Anaerobic conditioning. In *NSCA's Guide to Program Design,* ed. J.R. Hoffman, 119-129. Champaign IL: Human Kinetics.

Murphy, P., and Forney, J. 1997. Agility training. In *Complete Conditioning for Baseball,* 126-36. Champaign, IL: Human Kinetics.

Plisk, S. 2008. Speed, agility, and speed-endurance development. In *Essentials of Strength Training and Conditioning,* 3rd ed., ed. T.R. Baechle and R.W. Earle. Champaign IL: Human Kinetics.

Chapter 6

Clark, M. 2001. *Integrated Training for the New Millennium.* Thousand Oaks, CA: National Academy of Sports Medicine.

Guyton, A.C. 1991. *Textbook of Medical Physiology,* 6th ed. Philadelphia: Saunders.

Jeeves, M.A. 1961. Changes in performance at a serial reaction task under conditions of advance and delay of information. *Ergonomics* 4:329-38.

Leonard, J.A. 1953. Advance information in sensori-motor skills. *Q J Exp Psychol* 5:141-9.

Prentice, W.E., and Voight, M.I. 1999. *Techniques in Musculoskeletal Rehabilitation.* Chicago: McGraw-Hill.

Schmidt, R.A., and Lee, T.D. 1998. *Motor Control and Learning: A Behavioral Emphasis,* 3rd ed. Champaign, IL: Human Kinetics.

Schmidt, R.A., and Wrisberg, C.A. 2000. *Motor Learning and Performance,* 2nd ed. Champaign, IL: Human Kinetics.

Young, W. and Farrow, D. 2013. The Importance of a Sport-Specific Stimulus for Training Agility. *Strength & Conditioning Journal* 35:39-43.).

Chapter 7

Bompa, T. 1995. *From Childhood to Champion Athlete*. Toronto: Veritas.
Gambetta, V. 1998. *The Gambetta Method*. Sarasota, FL: Gambetta Sports Training Systems.
Gray, G. 2004. *Running 2.7*. Functional Video Digest. Adrian, MI: Gray Institute.
Gray, G. 2007. *Flexibility/Mobility*. Fast Function Series. Adrian, MI: Gray Institute.
Knudson, D. 2013. Warm-up and flexibility. In *Conditioning for Strength and Human Performance*, 2nd ed. ed. J. Chandler and L. Brown, 194-209. Philadelphia: Lippincott, Williams & Wilkins.
Murphy, P., and Forney, J. 1997. *Complete Conditioning for Baseball*. Champaign, IL: Human Kinetics.

Chapter 8

Axe, M.J., Windley, T.C., and Snyder-Mackler, L. 2001. Data-based interval throwing programs for baseball position players from age 13 to college level. *J Sport Rehabil* 10:267-86.
Barrett, D.D., and Burton, A.W. 2002. Throwing patterns used by collegiate baseball players in actual games. *Res Q Exer Sport* 73 (1): 19-27.
McFarland, E.G., and Wasik, M. 1998. Epidemiology of collegiate baseball injuries. *Clin J Sport Med* 8 (1): 10-13.

Chapter 9

Meir, R. Training for and competing in sevens rugby: Practical considerations from experience in the International Rugby Board world series. *Strength Cond J* 34(4): 76-86, 2012.
Suarez-Arrones, L., Portillo, J., Pareja-Blanco, F., Sáez de Villareal, E., Sánchez-Medina, L., and Munguía-Izquierdo, D. 2014. Match play activity profile in elite women's rugby union players. *J Strength Cond Res* 28:452-8.
Wisbey, B., Montgomery, P.G., Pyne, D.B., and Rattray, B. 2010. Quantifying movement demands of AFL football using GPS tracking. *J Sci Med Sport* 13:531-6.

Chapter 10

International Federation of Netball Associates. 1999. Official Rules of the International Federation of Netball Associations. Available: http://simnetball.tripod.com/netball_rules.pdf
Lavipour, D. 2009. *Development of a Netball Specific Dynamic Balance Assessment*. Auckland, NZ: Auckland University of Technology.
Narazaki, K., Berg, K., Stergiou, N., and Chen, B. 2009. Physiological demands of competitive basketball. *Scand J Med Sci Sports* 19:425-32.
Taylor, J. 2003. Basketball: Applying time motion data to conditioning. *Strength Cond J* 25:57-64.

Chapter 11

Buse, G.J, and Santana, J.C. 2008. Conditioning strategies for competitive kickboxing. *Strength Cond J* 30 (4) : 42-8.
Henry, T. 2011. Resistance training for judo: Functional strength training concepts and principles. *Strength Cond J* 33 (6): 40-9.
Lenetsky, S., and Harris, N. 2012. The mixed martial arts athlete: A physiological profile. *Strength Cond J* 34 (1): 32-47.
Lenetsky, S., Harris, N., and Brughelli, M. 2013. Assessment and contributors of punching forces in combat sports athletes: Implications for strength and conditioning. *Strength Cond J* 35 (2): 1-7.
Ratamess, N.A. 2011. Strength and conditioning for grappling sports. *Strength Cond J* 33 (60): 18-24.
Schick, M.G, Brown, L.E., and Schick, E.E. 2012. Strength and conditioning considerations for female mixed martial artists. *Strength Cond J* 43 (1): 66-75.

Turner, A.N. 2009. Strength and conditioning for muay Thai athletes. *Strength Cond J* 31 (6): 78-92.

Chapter 12

Behrens, M.J., and Simonson, S.R. 2011. A Comparison of the various methods used to enhance sprint speed. *Strength Cond J* 33:64-71.

Brown, T.D., and Vescovi, J.D. 2012. Maximum speed: Misconceptions of sprinting. *Strength Cond J* 34:37-41.

Komi, P.V. 2000. Stretch–shortening cycle: A powerful model to study normal and fatigued muscle. *J Biomech* 33:1197-1206.

Kyröläinen, H., Avela, J., and Komi, P.V. 2005. Changes in muscle activity with increasing running speed. *J Sports Sci* 23:1101-9.

Kyröläinen, H., Komi, P.V., and Belli, A. 1999. Changes in muscle activity patterns and kinetics with increasing running speed. *J Strength Cond Res* 13:400-406.

Miller, R.H., Umberger, B.R., and Caldwell, G.E. 2012. Sensitivity of maximum sprinting speed to characteristic parameters of the muscle force–velocity relationship. *J Biomech* 45:1406-13.

Chapter 13

Hedrick, A. 1999. Soccer-specific conditioning. *Strength Cond J* 21 (2): 17-21.

Jeffreys, I. 2008. Movement training for field sports: Soccer. *Strength Cond J* 30 (40): 19-27.

Turner, E., Munro, A.G., and Comfort, P. 2013. Female soccer: Part 1—a needs analysis. *Strength Cond J* 35 (1): 51-7.

Chapter 14

Gutowski, A.E., and Rosene, J.M. 2011. Preseason performance testing battery for men's lacrosse. *Strength Cond J* 33 (2): 16-22.

Chapter 15

Fernandez-Fernandez, J., Sanz-Rivas, D., and Mendez-Villanueva, A. 2009. A review of the activity profile and physiological demands of tennis and match play. *Strength Cond J* 31 (4): 15-26.

International Tennis Federation. 2013. *ITF Rules of Tennis*. London: ITF.

Parsons, M.S., and Jones, M.T. 1998. Development of speed, agility, quickness for tennis athletes. *Strength Cond J* 20 (3): 14-19.

Sturgess, S., and Newton, R.U. 2008. Design and implementation of a specific strength program for badminton. *Strength Cond J* 30 (3): 33-41.

Chapter 16

USA Racquetball. 2008. Intro to Racquetball Rules and Play. Available: www.usaracquetballevents.com/how_to_play_racquetball.pdf.

World Squash Federation. 2010. World Squash Singles Rules 2010. Available: www.ussquash.com/wp-content/uploads/2012/08/WSF-Singles-Rules.pdf.

World Squash Federation. 2013. Court Specifications. Available: www.worldsquash.org/ws/resources/court-construction.

About the Editors

Lee E. Brown, EdD, CSCS*D, FNSCA, FACSM, is a previous President of the National Strength and Conditioning Association (NSCA) Board of Directors. In 2014 Brown received the NSCA's Lifetime Achievement award for his work with the Association.

Brown holds both a master's degree in exercise science and a doctorate in educational leadership from Florida Atlantic University. Formerly a high school physical education teacher and coach of many sports, Brown is now a professor of strength and conditioning in the department of kinesiology at California State University, Fullerton. He and his wife, Theresa, reside in Buena Park, California.

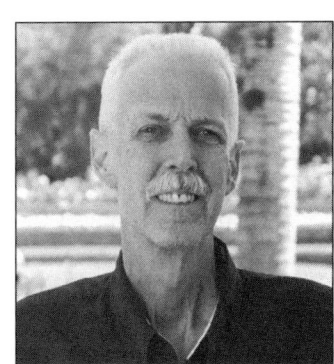

Vance Ferrigno, B.S. FAFS is President of F3 Training Systems, LLC and is also a Nike NG 360 Golf Performance Specialist for the Cliffs Clubs overseeing the golf performance program. Ferrigno earned his bachelor's degree in exercise science from Florida State University and a Fellow of Applied Functional Science from the Gray Institute. His certifications include American College of Sports Medicine's Health Fitness Specialist and Health Fitness Director, National Strength and Conditioning Association's Certified Strength and Conditioning Specialist, USA Weight Lifting Club Coach, USA Cycling Level 2 Coach and Nike NG 360 Golf Performance Specialist. He resides in Travelers Rest, SC.

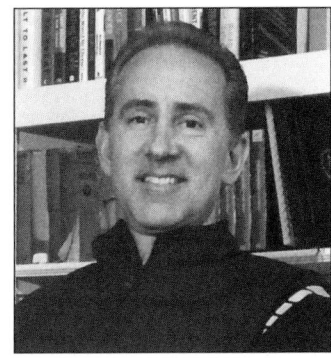

About the Contributors

Tori Beaudette, MS, earned her master's degree in kinesiology from California State University at Fullerton where she studied the effects of overspeed vertical jumping and was director of the Human Performance Laboratory. Beaudette was a performance specialist for EXOS at Google Mountain View and is now an adjunct faculty member of the kinesiology department at California State University at San Bernardino.

Jay Dawes, PhD, is an assistant professor of strength and conditioning at the University of Colorado at Colorado Springs. Jay has worked as a strength and performance coach, personal trainer, educator, and postrehabilitation specialist for more than 15 years and continues to act as a performance consultant for a variety of athletes, law enforcement officers, and those in physically demanding occupations. He is a certified strength and conditioning specialist (CSCS) and a certified personal trainer (CPT) by the National Strength and Conditioning Association (NSCA) and is certified by the American College of Sports Medicine as a health fitness specialist (ACSM-HFS), USA Weightlifting as a club coach, and the Australian Strength and Conditioning Association as a level 2 strength and conditioning coach. Additionally, Jay was recognized as a fellow of the NSCA (FNSCA) in 2009.

Andrea Du Bois, MS, HFS, is a certified health fitness specialist (HFS) with the American College of Sports Medicine (ACSM). Andrea earned a master of science degree in kinesiology from California State University at Fullerton with a research emphasis in strength and conditioning and sport performance. During her time at Fullerton, Andrea was a teaching and research assistant in the department of kinesiology and lab director for the Human Performance Laboratory. Before earning her MS, Andrea worked as a fitness and aquatics coordinator for California State University at San Bernardino (CSUSB) recreational sports. She also served as the assistant coach for the CSUSB women's cross country team. Andrea is pursuing a PhD in biokinesiology at the University of Southern California. As part of her studies, Andrea is a teaching assistant in the doctorate of physical therapy program and a research assistant in the Jacquelin Perry Musculoskeletal Biomechanics Research Laboratory.

John Graham, MS, HFS, CSCS*D, RSCC*D, FNSCA, is the senior director of sports and human performance at St. Luke's University Health Network in Allentown and Bethlehem, Pennsylvania. He is an adjunct professor at the College of New Jersey in the department of health and exercise science and at DeSales University in the department of sport and exercise science. John is on the industry advisory panel for the American Council on Exercise (ACE) and an associate editor for the *Strength and Conditioning Journal*. He chairs the NSCA certification committee, of which he is also a fellow. John is a certified strength and conditioning specialist, registered strength and conditioning coach, and ACSM-certified health fitness specialist.

John was on the NSCA board of directors from 2001 to 2003 and was vice president in 2002 and secretary–treasurer in 2003. He was awarded the NSCA *Strength and Conditioning Journal* Editorial Excellence Award in 2000. He has been recognized by the Medical Fitness Association, National Multiple Sclerosis Society, *Eastern Pennsylvania Business Journal*, Pennsylvania State Senate and House of Representatives, and Hamot Health Systems for his contributions to fitness and sport performance.

Doug Lentz, MS, CSCS*D, RSCC*E, is the director of fitness and wellness at Results Therapy and Fitness in Chambersburg, Pennsylvania. Doug is also a national coach with USA Weightlifting. Since his graduation from Penn State University in 1981, Doug has coached professional, Olympic, collegiate, high school, and adolescent athletes on strength and speed in 16 sports. Lentz was the strength coach for 1992 Olympic marathoner Steve Spence throughout most of his professional racing career. Doug now works with Neely Spence Gracey, who runs professionally with the Hansons-Brooks Distance Project. Doug's focus with his sprinters and distance runners is power development and acceleration mechanics. Doug was the Pennsylvania state director for the National Strength and Conditioning Association (NSCA) from 1992 to 1998 and was the chairperson for the NSCA Conference Committee from 1994 to 2004. Lentz was a clinic advisor for the American Running Association from 1991 to 2005.

Logan Schwartz, MEd, CSCS, FAFS, is the assistant strength and conditioning and performance coach for the University of Texas men's basketball program. Before joining the UT staff, Schwartz spent four years at Austin-based Train 4 The Game as a performance specialist and strength coach and director of the intern program. He holds a bachelor's degree in kinesiology as well as a master's degree in exercise physiology from the University of Texas at Austin. Schwartz is a certified strength and conditioning specialist (CSCS) by the National Strength and Conditioning Association and is a fellow of Applied Functional Science (FAFS) and certified in functional manual reaction (FMR) by the Gray Institute for Functional Transformation (GIFT). Logan also holds a certification in applied functional science (CAFS) and is a Nike Golf NG360 performance specialist. Schwartz is also a practitioner for the prescription and fabrication of biomechanical foot orthoses as well as a practitioner of functional soft tissue transformation.

Traci Statler, PhD, CC-AASP, CSCS, is an associate professor of sport and performance psychology at California State University at Fullerton and a certified consultant (CC-AASP) through the Association of Applied Sport Psychology. She is a strength and conditioning specialist (CSCS) through the National Strength and Conditioning Association (NSCA) and has worked as a sport psychology consultant and cognitive performance coach for the U.S. track and field team for 15 years. As a college professor, Statler teaches classes in applied, theoretical, and consulting issues in sport psychology as well as legal and ethical issues in kinesiology. She has been working in applied sport psychology for two decades and has consulted with collegiate, professional, and Olympic athletes in numerous sports as well as with doctors, medical practitioners, and police officers throughout Southern California.

Diane Vives is president and performance training director of Vives Training Systems and Fit4Austin in Austin, Texas. Coach Vives is passionate about guiding her team of performance coaches in innovative training methods that are driven by evidence-based systems. Her performance training reaches both athletes and the general population with a focus on small-group and team training. Vives is also the education director and a lead instructor for Functional Movement Systems. She was the only female on the Under Armour Performance Training Council from 2008 to 2013. She served on the National Strength and Conditioning Association board of directors from 2006 to 2009. Vives coauthored *Speed, Agility, and Quickness, Second Edition*, as well as *Developing Speed*, both published by Human Kinetics. She has produced video courses for Training the Female Athlete, SMARTsets Training Volumes 1 to 4, and H2O Innovative Training With Active Resistance. Vives is a mentor to trainers and strength coaches worldwide as well as a contributing presenter to many of the leading international organizations to create a positive impact on the sport performance and fitness industries.

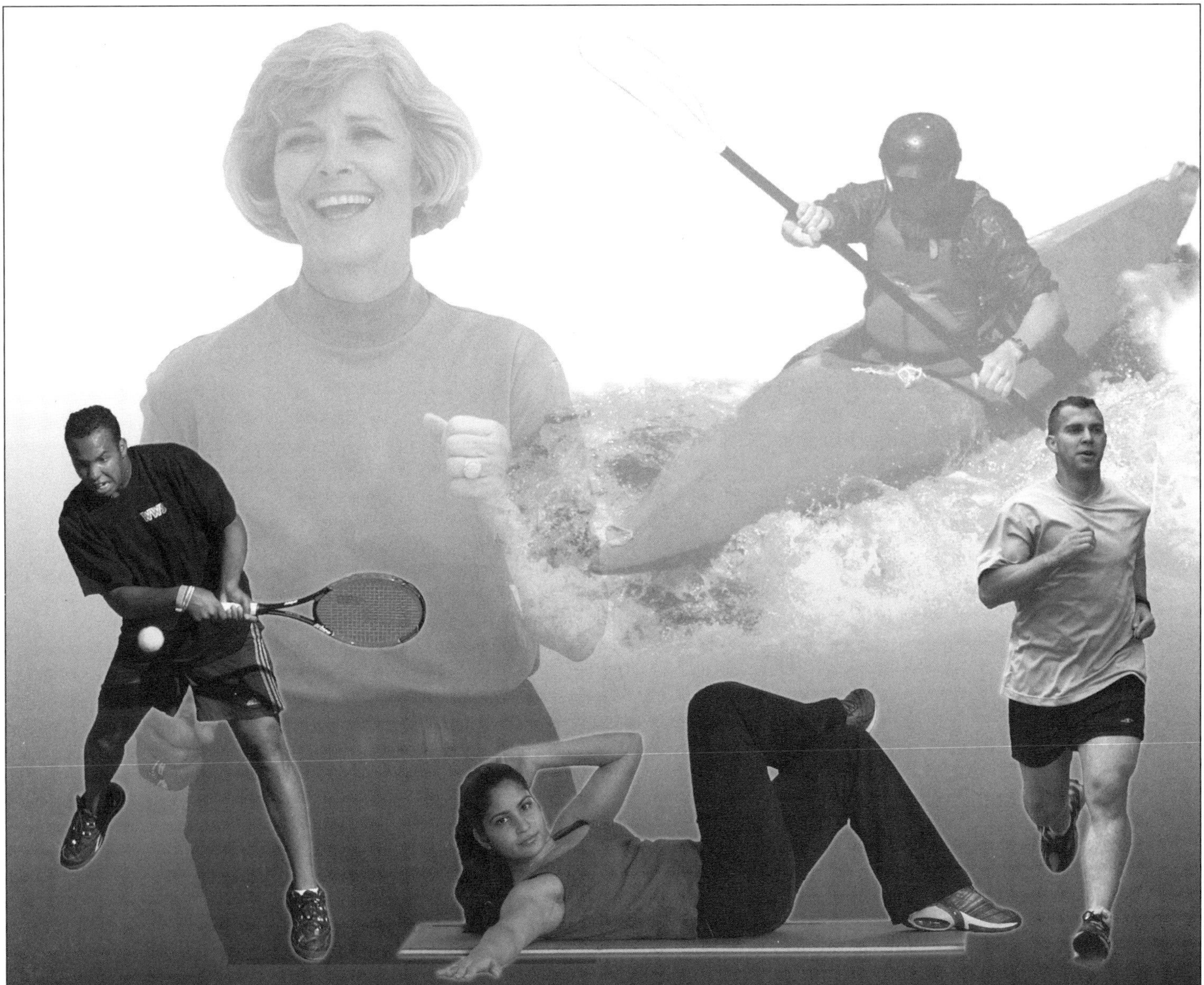

You'll find other outstanding sports and fitness resources at

www.HumanKinetics.com

In the U.S. call 1-800-747-4457

Australia 08 8372 0999 • Canada 1-800-465-7301
Europe +44 (0) 113 255 5665 • New Zealand 0800 222 062

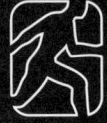
HUMAN KINETICS
The Premier Publisher for Sports & Fitness
P.O. Box 5076 • Champaign, IL 61825-5076 USA

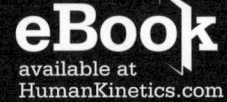
eBook available at HumanKinetics.com